Essentials of
Pharmaceutical Technology
Second Edition

Essentials of Pharmaceutical Technology
Second Edition

Ajay Semalty
M. Pharm., MBA, Ph. D., PDF (Japan)
Assistant Professor
Department of Pharmaceutical Sciences, School of Sciences,
H.N.B. Garhwal University (A Central University)
Srinagar (Garhwal), Uttarakhand
Visiting Scientist
Faculty of Pharmacy, Meijo University Nagoya, Japan

Mona Semalty
M. Pharm., MBA, Ph. D.
Assistant Professor
Department of Pharmaceutical Sciences, School of Sciences,
H.N.B. Garhwal University (A Central University)
Srinagar (Garhwal), Uttarakhand

M.S.M. Rawat
M. Sc., Ph. D. (IIT Delhi)
Former Vice Chancellor
& Founder Head Department of Pharmaceutical Sciences
H.N.B. Garhwal University (A Central University)
Srinagar (Garhwal), Uttarakhand

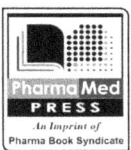

PharmaMed Press
An imprint of Pharma Book Syndicate

A unit of BSP Books Pvt. Ltd.
4-4-309/316, Giriraj Lane,
Sultan Bazar, Hyderabad - 500 095.

Essentials of Pharmaceutical Technology, *Second Edition*
by *Ajay Semalty, Mona Semalty,* and *M.S.M. Rawat*
Copyright © 2019 *by Publisher,* All rights reserved.

No part of this book or parts thereof may be reproduced, stored in a retrieval system or transmitted in any language or by any means, electronic, mechanical, photocopying, recording or otherwise without the prior written permission of the publishers.

Published by

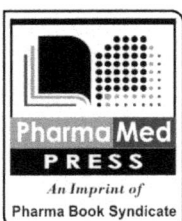

PharmaMed Press
An imprint of Pharma Book Syndicate
A unit of BSP Books Pvt. Ltd.
4-4-309/316, Giriraj Lane, Sultan Bazar, Hyderabad - 500 095.
Phone: 040-23445688, 23445600; Fax: 91+40-23445611
E-mail: info@pharmamedpress.com
www.pharmamedpress.com/pharmamedpress.net

ISBN: 978-93-85433-17-7 (Hardback)

Preface to Second Edition

After the huge success and demand of the first edition of the book we are pleased and honored to extend the second edition of the book for the Pharmacy students, researchers and academicians. For the flawless reading and understanding of readers we have made many modifications in many chapters. In revising the book we have kept the book's main features (easy language, to-the-point coverage of topics, pictorial/graphical and tabular presentation) intact and moreover made it more effective. Many new figures and tables have been incorporated. The efforts have been made to provide the contents in the form of self-explanatory figures and tables. Apart from the previous chapters, a glossary of verbatim official definitions has been added at the end. This will serve as ready reference for the students for preparing for their exams including GPAT.

As we have got the huge response from readers for the first edition we again hope that this book shall be very useful to students as well as teachers as ready source of basics of each and every covered topic. We welcome the opinion about the book and the suggestions to further improve the work, from students and teachers.

Authors

Preface to First Edition

Delivering the active medicament to the body system for a certain therapeutic action is the central idea of Pharmaceutical technology. A Pharmaceutical drug is delivered through various routes of administration with the help of various kinds of dosage forms. Moreover a drug product should be effective, safe and stable. All the aspects of pharmaceutical texts, dealing with drug delivery, basically target these three issues.

Each profession is built by good professional texts. State of the art texts are strengthening the pharmacy profession. More and more texts are coming with the latest trends and developments in pharmaceutical technology. But the good quality basic texts are always in demand. The students of pharmaceutical science have always felt a need of student friendly text. There are very few good books which really cater the needs of students studying pharmaceutics. Many state of the art textbooks are either unavailable/unaffordable or too wide in covering the topics that the students don't find it easy to understand and decide what to read and learn on exam point of view. This work is an effort to fulfill this ever felt need of pharmacy students.

The book covers basics of dissolution study, bioavailability and stability studies (and ICH guidelines) in detail with recent guidelines. The most common and popular dosage forms viz. tablet, capsule, parenterals, suspension and emulsion have been discussed. Other topics discussed include controlled release products, oral protein delivery etc. The USPs of the book are easy language, to-the-point coverage of topics, pictorial/graphical and tabular presentation which make this work unique. We hope that this book shall be very useful to students as well as teachers as ready source of basics of each and every covered topic. We welcome the opinion about the book and the suggestions to further improve the work, from students and teachers.

Authors

Acknowledgements

We would like to thank all the persons who helped in designing, planning and finishing this book. Firstly we would like to thank our family members for their continued encouragement, support and assistance. Without them, it would not have been possible to complete the book.

As Benjamin Franklin said *"There are no slow learners, there are only slow teachers"* this is the teacher who is solely responsible for quality of teaching and learning process. In the process of teaching and learning, we also learned lot of many things about the likes and dislikes of the students regarding the choice of books and reading habits. We have tried to focus our efforts on those points, to make the book student friendly. We are thankful to our students whose input again helped in designing and planning this book.

"Who dares to teach, must never cease to learn"- This statement by John Cotton Dana is absolutely true because the learning is a never ending process that will positively enhance our awareness and knowledge and will positively contribute to our abilities as teachers. So we are also thankful to all the respected teachers who read, refer and recommend this book to their students.

We warmly acknowledge Mr. Lokesh Adhikari, Project Fellow, UGC-DAE CSR project, Department of Pharmaceutical Sciences, H.N.B. Garhwal (Central) University Srinagar (Garhwal) for his vital help and support in revising the book.

We also thank Prof. S.H. Ansari, Faculty of Pharmacy, Hamdard University, New Delhi; Prof. Pawan Kumar Dubey, Director, Vivekananda College of Pharmacy, Indore; Prof. Rajesh Kumar, Head-Pharmacy, D.A.B. University, Indore; Prof. M.S. Ranawat, Dean Pharmacy, B.N. University Udaipur (Raj.); Prof. Y. S. Tanwar, B. N. College of Pharmacy, B.N. University Udaipur (Raj.); Prof. Vandan S. Panda, K.M. Kundanani College of Pharmacy, Mumbai; Prof. N.S. Hari Narayana Moorthy, Dean Pharmacy, Indira Gandhi National Tribal University, Amarkantak, Prof. S.H. Bodakhe, Guru Ghasidas University, Bilaspur, Chhatisgarh; Prof. Vijay Juyal, Head- Pharmacy, Kumaun University, Nainital, Dr. Abdul Faruk, Head Department of Pharmaceutical Sciences, H.N.B. Garhwal (Central) University Srinagar (Garhwal) and all the other well-wishers who always keep triggering us time to time for the work like this.

Acknowledgements

We are thankful to all the researchers, staff members of Department of Pharmaceutical Sciences and Department of Chemistry, H.N.B. Garhwal (Central) University Srinagar (Garhwal) for their moral support.

We humbly acknowledge the publisher (Pharma Book Syndicate Hyderabad, India), in particular Mr. Anil Shah, Mr. Avadesh Kumar, Mr. Tiwari, Mr. Naresh Davergave and all other members of his expert team for their efforts, guidance and timely support in preparation of this work.

Last but not the least, we thank God almighty for giving strength, patience and determination to complete this work on time in present form.

Authors

Contents

Preface to Second Edition ....(v)
Preface to First Edition.. (vii)
Acknowledgements ....(ix)

Chapter 1
Bioavailability.. 1

Chapter 2
Dissolution Study 37

Chapter 3
Tablets and Tablet Coating..................................... 65

Chapter 4
Capsules 102

Chapter 5
Suspensions 118

Chapter 6
Emulsions 141

Chapter 7
Oral Controlled Release Products....................... 170

Chapter 8
Oral Drug Delivery of Proteins and Peptides.... 196

Chapter 9
Aerosols 208

Chapter 10
Parenteral Products 243

Chapter 11
Sterile Processing: Quality Assurance and Validation 290

Chapter 12
Stability Studies 303

Chapter 13
ICH Guidelines on Stability 321

Appendix
Glossary 336

CHAPTER 1

Bioavailability

Introduction

Biopharmaceutics is the study of the interrelationship of the physicochemical properties of the active pharmaceutical ingredient (API), and its pharmacokinetic and pharmacodynamic behavior. Pharmacokinetics is "What the body does with the drug", while the pharmacodynamics is "what the drug does to the body". Biopharmaceutics also considers the formulation of the drug product including excipients, the method of manufacturing, and the route of drug administration. In terms of regulatory product quality attributes, results from bioequivalence (BE) studies and certain bioavailability (BA) studies may be viewed as "product quality performance specifications". A specific regulatory challenge is to validate the methods used to assess the results from these studies to assure that the BA and BE data generated relate in a well-defined and meaningful way to safety and efficacy of the drug product.

Bioavailability is defined in various ways. For drugs and other substances that act within the body (as contrasted to within the gut), it is generally considered to be the quantity or fraction of an administered dose of a substance that gets into the circulation and then is not metabolized, complexed or excreted before it can exert its intended biological effect.

Bioavailability is defined in § 320.1 of US FDA guidelines for industry as: *the rate and extent to which the active ingredient or active moiety is absorbed from a drug product and becomes available at the site of action. For drug products that are not intended to be absorbed into the bloodstream, bioavailability may be assessed by measurements intended to reflect the rate and extent to which the active ingredient or active moiety becomes available at the site of action.*

Usually, the "bioavailability" is the fraction of an extravascular dose that goes to the central blood compartment. But the exceptions exist e.g. Topical dosing (bioavailability is then drug delivered to site of action). Intravenous (IV) doses are 100% bioavailable and are the basis for absolute bioavailability calculations.

If the BA of two or more products are found almost similar (on comparison), they are called as Bioequivalent (BE). More precisely, Bioequivalence (BE) means the absence of a greater-than-allowable difference between the systemic bioavailability of a test product and that of a reference product.

Importance of Studying Bioavailability

Except the parenterals, the "true dose" is not the drug administered, but is the drug available to exert its effect. The drug becomes available to the systemic circulation for exerting the effect after dissolution (dissolving into the gastrointestinal fluid), absorption (permeation across the biological membranes) and surviving metabolism. The drug may show very low bioavailability due to one (or more) of the following reasons.

- Dosage form or drug may not dissolve readily
- Drug may not be readily pass across biological membranes (or be absorbed)
- Drug may be extensively metabolized during absorption process (first-pass, gut wall, liver)

So it can be understood that a variable bioavailability may produce variable exposures and thus variable effects.

Concept of Bioavailability

A schematic illustration of the steps involved in the release and absorption of a drug taken as an oral solid dosage form is presented in Fig. 1.1.

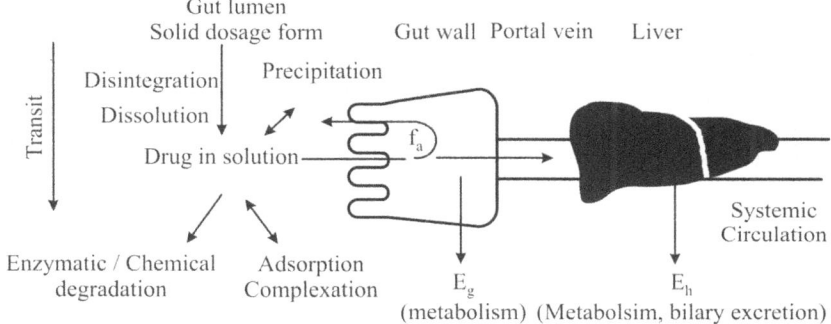

Fig. 1.1 Processes influencing the bioavailability of orally administered drugs.

The oral bioavailability can be divided into three major determinants, according to the following equation:

$$F = f_a \cdot (1 - E_g) \cdot (1 - E_h)$$

where f_a is the fraction of the dose that is absorbed across the apical cell membrane of the enterocyte and E_g and E_h are the extraction of the drug over the gut and liver, respectively.

The f_a may be limited by all the reactions that may happen in the lumen and at the apical membrane. This includes the dissolution of the drug in the gastrointestinal (GI) tract, since in order to be absorbed in the GI, a drug has to be dissolved. This can be a problem with poorly water-soluble substances, for which the dissolution often limits the absorption after oral administration. Most of the new substances in drug development today are highly lipophilic, and the solubility and dissolution rates in gastric and intestinal fluids (IF) are therefore often critical for the oral bioavailability.

Biopharmaceutical Classification System (BCS)

The Biopharmaceutical Classification System (BCS), which was proposed by Amidon et al. in 1995, classifies drugs into four different groups (Table 1.1), depending on their solubility and permeability. BCS is a drug development tool that allows estimation of the contribution of three fundamental factors including dissolution, solubility and intestinal permeability, which govern the rate and extent of drug absorption from solid oral dosage forms. Drug dissolution is the process by which the drug is released, dissolved and becomes ready for absorption. Permeability is referred to the ability of the drug molecule to permeate through a membrane into the systemic circulation. The intention of the system (BCS) was to set up a theoretical basis for correlating the *in vitro* dissolution profiles with *in vivo* bioavailability of drugs. BCS is also a fundamental guideline for determining the conditions under which *in vitro in vivo* correlations (IVIVCs) are expected. It is also used as a tool for developing the *in vitro* dissolution specification. The BCS can be employed as a tool to develop a strategy for improving the bioavailability of new chemical entities. Additionally, the system provides information about whether a compound's BA is solubility or permeability limited.

Table 1.1 The biopharmaceutical classification system

Class	Solubility	Permeability	General properties of drugs of the class	Examples of the Class
I	High	High	Water Soluble, (high C_S value resulting in a high C_{Aq} value); well absorbed from GIT (larger P values); lipophilic with a MW $\leq$ 500Da and aqueous solubility $\geq$ 1 mg/mL; D : S $\leq$ 250mL	Paracetamol, piroxicam*, propranolol, theophylline, rofecoxib
II	Low	High	relatively lipophilic and water insoluble drugs (C_S $\leq$ 0.1 mg/mL); well absorbed from GIT (large P values); D : S $\geq$ 250 mL	Carbamazepine, digoxin, cinnarizine, glibenclamide, miconazole, nimesulide, nifedipine, phenytoin, spironolactone, tolbutamide, Itraconazole
III	High	Low	Water Soluble (high C_S and high C_{Aq}); do not readily permeate biomembranes (low P); D : S $\leq$ 250mL	Acyclovir, atenolol, ranitidine, diphenhydramine

Table 1.1 contd...

Class	Solubility	Permeability	General properties of drugs of the class	Examples of the Class
IV	Low	Low	water-insoluble (Low C_S and low C_{Aq}). do not readily permeate biomembranes (low P); D : S ≥ 250mL	Furosemide, cyclosporine A

* *piroxicam is practically insoluble in water but is a potent drug with low enough D : S ratio to be classified as a class I drug.*
C_S is saturation solubility of the drug in the aqueous fluid; C_{Aq} is the drug concentration in the aqueous exterior immediately adjacent to the mucosal surface; P is permeability coefficient of the drug through the lipophilic mucosa; D:S is dose to solubility ratio.

When a drug shows a dose to solubility ratio (D:S) of 250 ml or lower at 37 °C over a **pH range of 1.2–6.8**, it can be classified as "**highly soluble**". The pH was decreased from 7.5 in the FDA guidance to 6.8 in WHO Expert Committee on Specifications for Pharmaceutical Preparations, 40th Report, 2006, this reflects the need to dissolve the drug before it reaches the mid-jejunum to ensure absorption from the gastrointestinal tract. A drug is classified as "**highly permeable**" if the fraction absorbed is **> 85 %** (from solution). In WHO revisions to the criteria for BCS classification, the permeability criterion was relaxed from 90% in the FDA guidance (40th Report, 2006) to 85%, which shifted some BCS class III drugs to class I drugs e.g. paracetamol, acetylsalicylic acid, allopurinol, lamivudine and promethazine.

Modeling of BCS and Key Parameters

The BCS is based on a simple absorption model, in which the intestine is a cylindrical tube where absorption occurs; particles are spheres of the same size; there are no reactions (i.e., there is no metabolism) in the intestine; solubility is independent of the particle size and the intestinal pH gradient; and no aggregation occurs. Amidon et al. have demonstrated that the key parameters controlling drug absorption are three dimensionless numbers: an Absorption Number, A_n; a Dissolution Number, D_n; and a Dose Number, D_o; representing the fundamental processes of membrane permeation, drug dissolution and dose, respectively:

Absorption Number (A_n)

The Absorption Number (A_n) is the ratio of the Mean Residence Time (T_{res}) to the Mean Absorption Time (T_{abs}) and is calculated by equation 1.

$$A_n = T_{res} / T_{abs} \quad \ldots(1)$$

or $\quad A_n = (P_{eff} / R) \, T_{res}$

where T_{res} is the mean residence time (~180 min), P_{eff} is the effective permeability, and R is the radius of the intestinal segment.

Dissolution Number (D_n)

The Dissolution Number (D_n) is the ratio of T_{res} to Mean Dissolution Time (T_{diss}) and could be estimated using equation 2.

$$D_n = T_{res} / T_{diss} \quad \ldots(2)$$

T_{diss} is the time required for a drug particle to dissolve

Dose Number (D_o)

The Dose Number (D_o) is calculated using equation 3.

$$D_o = (M_o/V_o) / C_s \quad \ldots(3)$$

where M_0 is the dose of drug administered, V_0 is the initial gastric volume (~250 ml), C_s is the saturation solubility,

Class I compounds such as metoprolol exhibit a high absorption (A_n) and a high Dissolution (D_n) number. The rate-limiting step to drug absorption is drug dissolution or gastric emptying rate if dissolution is very rapid.

Class II drugs such as phenytoin has a high absorption number, A_n, but a low dissolution number, D_n. *In vivo* drug dissolution for Class II drugs is, therefore, a rate limiting factor in drug absorption (except at very high dose number, D_o) and consequently absorption is usually slower than Class I and takes place over a longer period of time.

Class III drugs, such as cimetidine, are rapidly dissolving and permeability is the rate controlling step in drug absorption.

Class IV drugs are low solubility and low permeability drugs. This class of drugs exhibit significant problems for effective oral delivery. It is anticipated that inappropriate formulation of drugs fall in class IV, as in the case of class II drugs, could have an additional negative influence on both the rate and extent of drug absorption.

Types of Bioavailability

Bioavailability Dose: Dose available to the patient to give therapeutic effect is called as bioavailable dose, which is always less than the administered dose.

Systemic bioavailability: The amount of drug that reaches the systemic circulation is known as 'Systemic bioavailability'.

Bioavailable fraction: It refers to the fraction of administered dose.

F = Bioavailable dose / Administered dose

Absolute bioavailability: Comparison between systemic availability of orally administered drug with IV administered one. (Denoted by F).

or *"Absolute bioavailability"* compares an extravascular formulation to an IV formulation

Relative bioavailability: Comparison between systematic availability of orally administered drug with an oral standard of same drug. Denoted by F_r.

Or "Relative bioavailability" compares 2 extravascular formulations

Bioavailability Calculations	
Systemic clearance	CL(iv) = Dose(iv) / AUC(iv)
Apparent (oral) clearance	CL(oral) = CL(iv) / F = Dose(oral) / AUC(oral)
Set CL(iv) equivalent	CL(iv) = Dose(iv) / AUC(iv) = (Dose(oral) • F)/ AUC(oral)
Absolute bioavailability	F = [Dose(iv) •AUC(oral)] / [Dose(oral) •AUC(iv)]

Objectives of Bioavailability Studies

Bioavailability studies are done in clinical, academic, and regulatory interest. The latter includes agencies that approve the sale of products in their nation(s), as well as regulatory agencies. Applications from manufacturers seeking regulatory approval for a new drug (New Drug Application (NDA) must furnish exhaustive information about a drug's pharmacokinetics. Typically, such evidence involves studies wherein the drug has been orally administered. While such trials may broadly be viewed as bioavailability studies, many are apparently designed to assess the drug's safety and efficacy via strategies of dose escalation and chronic administration. The more pertinent interest in bioavailability relates to questions about absolute extent of absorption (absolute bioavailability), the importance of product formulation changes that are made during a new drug's development process, the comparability of different oral

dosage forms (e.g. modified-release versus conventional products), and whether the products can be administered with meals. Therefore, objective of BA studies can be summarized as followed.
1. Development of new drug entity.
2. Determination of influence of
   - Excipients.
   - Patient related factors.
   - Possible interaction with other drugs.
3. Development of new formulations.
4. To control the quality of drug.
5. To determine the
   - Processing factors.
   - Storage
   - Stability on drug absorption.

Factors Affecting Bioavailability

Bioavailability following oral doses may vary because of either patient-related or dosage-form-related factors. Patient factors can include the nature and timing of meals, age, disease, genetic traits and gastrointestinal physiology. The dosage form factors include:
1. the chemical form of the drug (salt vs. acid),
2. its physical properties (crystal structure, particle size), and
3. an array of formulation (non-active ingredients) and manufacturing (tablet hardness) variables. Some important factors affecting BA are described as followed.

- **Food effects**

  Co-administration of food with oral drug products may influence drug BA and/or BE. Food effect BA studies focus on the effects of food on the release of the drug substance from the drug product as well as the absorption of the drug substance. BE studies with food focus on demonstrating comparable BA between test and reference products when co-administered with meals. Usually, a single-dose, two-period, two-treatment, two-sequence crossover study is recommended for both food-effect BA and BE studies. -FDA

    (i) Food may increase, decrease, or have no effect on the rate and/or the extent of absorption.
       - May affect rate and extent independently

- Food affects GI motility and also can increase solubilization of drugs
- Change may depend on content of meal

(ii) Food may mitigate nausea. Vomiting tends to decrease bioavailability

(iii) Dose time and food: Timing of dose with respect to food also affects the bioavailability of administered drugs.

- **Physiology related factors**

   Bilayer structure of cell membranes

   A drug when administered to the body, first dissolves into the gastric fluid (hydrophilic environment) and then it permeates across the biological membranes (lipophilic environment), finally reaching into the blood. For good bioavailability, a drug must have an adequate hydrophilicity (for dissolution into gastrointestinal fluid) as well as an adequate lipophilicity (to permeate across the lipidic biomembrane). So, the drugs too lipophilic won't dissolve while the drugs too hydrophilic won't transverse lipid outer layer of cell. Thickness and blood supply of membranes also play the role in BA.

   GI transit time

   How much time a drug spends in transit through GIT is responsible factor in BA. Acetaminophen is a useful probe drug to assess GI transit

   pH environment

   GIT shows a variety of pH (pH 6.6 (buccal), pH 1.2 (stomach), pH 6.8 duodenum, pH 7-8 (small intestine)) throughout its length from oral cavity to colon. Depending on pKa, drug may be charged or uncharged in different regions and its absorption and hence the BA may vary (pH partition hypothesis: Un-ionized drug is absorbed through membranes; Charges species don't get through easily; Ionization of drug molecule depends on pH of the site e.g. weakly acidic drugs are unionized at acidic pH of stomach and hence absorbed from the gastric region). For acids, a pH below the pKa enhances absorption, while for bases; a pH above the pKa enhances absorption.

Metabolic activity (induction, inhibition or first pass metabolism)

Several drugs selectively increase or decrease the activity of cytochrome P450, these are called enzyme inducer and enzyme inhibitors, respectively (Table 1.2). Enzyme induction usually occurs within several days and increases liver weight, microsomal protein content and biliary secretion. Enzyme induction usually increases the activity of glucuronyl transferase, and thus enhances drug conjugation. In some instances, drugs may induce their own metabolism (auto-induction). On the other hand enzyme inhibition may increase plasma concentrations of other concurrently used drugs, resulting in drug interactions.

Table 1.2 Drugs inducing or inhibiting Cytochrome P450

Inducers	Inhibitors
Barbiturates	Imidazoles (cimetidine, etomidate, ketoconazole, omeprazole)
Phenytoin	
Carbamazepine	Macrolide antibiotics (erythromycin, clarithromycin)
Rifampicin	
Griseofulvin	Antidepressants
Alcohol (chronic consumption)	HIV protease inhibitors
Polycyclic hydrocarbons (tobacco Amiodarone smoke, grilled meat)	Cyclosporin Gestodene

Another most common metabolic factor governing the bioavailability of a large number of drugs is first pass or presystemic metabolism. After oral administration, some drugs are extensively metabolized by the gut wall (e.g. chlorpromazine, dopamine) or by the liver (e.g. lidocaine, pethidine) before they enter the systemic circulation. In these conditions, oral administration may not produce adequate plasma concentrations in the systemic circulation and may result in an impaired response to drugs. As hepatic, renal and cardiac diseases are important factors affecting the variable response to drugs, the pathological changes may also affect the metabolism and clearance of drugs in an unpredictable manner. In severe hepatic disease (e.g. cirrhosis or hepatitis), the elimination of drugs that are primarily metabolized may be impaired.

Surface area for absorption

Mucosal surface area is more extensive in the upper small intestine than the stomach, and hence most drugs, whether acids or bases, are predominantly absorbed from the duodenum.

- **Drug related factors**

    Particle size of drug

    In general reduction of particle size of a drug increases the effective surface area (surface area of drug available for dissolution) and hence the bioavailability. But particle size reduction in hydrophobic drugs (like aspirin) results in decrease in effective surface area and hence the (lowered) absorption.

    Crystal structure

    In general the amorphous drugs are more soluble than the crystalline one in aqueous (gastric) fluids. So the amorphous drugs are more absorbed.

    Polymorphic forms

    If a drug shows polymorphism (existence of more than one crystalline forms of a drug), some of its ploymorphs show more bioavailability than the others. Chloramphenicol palmitate is found in 3 polymorphic forms (A, B, C). Out of the three forms form B shows best bioavailability while the form A is virtually inactive biologically.

    Drug-Drug interactions

    Drug interactions which occur mainly due to enzyme induction or inhibition, change in gastric motility and gastric pH affect the bioavailability of concomitant drugs. Enzyme induction (in the gut or liver) lowers the bioavailability, while enzyme inhibition increases the bioavailability of a drug. On the other hand, drugs affecting gastric motility can modify drug dissolution, and influence the rate, but not the extent, of drug absorption. In particular, drugs that slow gastric emptying (e.g. atropine, morphine) decrease the rate of drug absorption. Other drug interactions, as between tetracyclines and iron, or colestyramine and digoxin, may affect the extent of drug absorption and thus modify systemic bioavailability. Drug interaction may also occur due to change in gastric or urinary pH. For example, the bioavailability of a drug which is predominantly absorbed in gastric pH may be reduced due to concomitant administration of antacids.

Instability of the drug

The drug itself may have instability in the GI tract either due to chemical instability in acidic environment or due to extent of metabolism via enzymes in gut. This instability can have impact on bioavailable fraction of the drug.

- **Pharmaceutical factors**

  Pharmaceutical factors like particle size, chemical formulation, the inclusion of inert fillers and the outer coating of the tablet influence the dissolution of tablets and capsules. In these circumstances, proprietary or generic preparations of the same drug may have different dissolution characteristics and thus produce a range of plasma concentrations after oral administration. At one time, differences in the potency of digoxin tablets suspected from clinical observations were eventually traced to variations in the dissolution of different preparations of the drug. Similarly, toxic effects were produced by diphenylhydantoin (phenytoin) tablets when an excipient (calcium sulphate) was replaced by lactose. In these conditions, dissolution was more rapid, resulting in faster and more extensive absorption, and higher blood levels of the drugs. Manufacturing process may also affect the bioavailability, for example tablets with more hardness may show less bioavailability.

Methods of Improving Bioavailability

There are three major approaches in overcoming the bioavailability problems.

1. *The pharmaceutical approach:* It involve modification of formulation manufacturing process or the physicochemical properties of drugs without changing the chemical structure (Table 1.1).
2. *The pharmacokinetic approach:* In which the pharmacokinetics of the drug is altered by modifying its chemical structure.
3. *The biological approach:* In this approach the route of drug administration may be changed such as changing from oral to parenteral.

Various methods have been investigated for improvement in bioavailability. Table 1.3 gives a summary of all these methods.

Table 1.3 Methods of improving bioavailability

Methods	Mechanism involved	Methodology	Examples
Use of co-solvent	Increase in solubility of drug	Addition of co-solvent ethanol, propylene, glycol, glycerin	Analgesic syrups of paracetamol
Hydrotrophy method	Addition of large amounts of a second solute results in an increase in the aqueous solubility of another solute	Adding hydrotropic agents like urea, nicotinamide etc.	Paracetamol
By addition of polar group	Increasing water solubility by increasing hydrogen bonding and interaction with water	Addition of polar group in the structure of drug (carboxylic acid and amine)	--
Use of solid solution	Improving solubility by preparing sol-gel form of the drug	Fusion, melting	Succinic acid
Solid dispersion	Decreasing the drug's particle size changes the microenvironment of the drug particle which increases the dissolution rate and absorption	Prepared by fusion, solvent evaporation,	Paracetamol-urea
Eutectic mixture	When exposed to water the soluble carrier dissolves leaving the drug in micro crystalline state which solubilize rapidly	Fusion	Paracetamol-camphor
Micronization	Increasing the effective surface area of drug by decreasing particle size	By spray drying and by use of fluid energy mill	Griesiofulvin and several steroidal and sulpha drugs

Table 1.3 Contd...

Methods	Mechanism involved	Methodology	Examples
Use of surfactants	By promoting wetting and penetration of dissolution fluid into the drug	Addition of suitable surfactants (polysorbate)	Spironolactone is a drug whose bioavailability is increased by this method
Alternation of pH of solvent	Changing the pH of drug in solution	Salt formation, addition of buffer	Buffered tablets of aspirin
Use of metastable polymorphs	Metastable forms show better solubility than stable form	Converting the stable form to metastable form	Using B form of chlorom-phenicol than A and C forms
Solvates formation	Powder of submicron size having increased surface area show the improved solubility	Freeze drying of solute with organic solvent	Benzene solvate
Selective absorption on insoluble carrier	Weak physical interaction between adsorbate and adsorbant through hydration and swelling of clay in aqueous media improves solubility	Use of highly active adsorbant, clay like bentonite	Indomethacin, Prednisone
Cyclodextrin complexation	Inclusion of hydrophobic groups of drug in the core of cyclodextrin cavity and thereby improving solubility	Formation of drug Complex with cyclodextrin (α, β, γ) or its derivatives	Meloxicam, phenytoin,
Phospholipid complexation	Drug-Lipid complexes improve amorphous nature of drug in the complexes and being amphiphilic in nature the complex show improved solubility and dissolution	The phospholipid complexes of drug without the presence of covalent bond are formed.	aceclofenac, aspirin, curcumin, silybin etc.

Bioavailability Study Characteristics

With recently introduced products properly conducted bioavailability studies should have been performed before the product is allowed to be marketed. However, products which were approved sometime ago may not have been tested as thoroughly. It is therefore helpful to be able to evaluate the testing which may have been undertaken.

The evaluation of a drug product bioavailability study involves the consideration of various factors. Some are:

1. **Drug**
   (a) The drug substance in each product must be the same
   (b) Bioavailability studies are conducted to compare two or more products
   (c) Different chemical substances cannot be compared
   (d) Compare the drug products with the same drug in each dosage form

2. **Drug product**
   (a) Comparison is made between two or more similar products containing exactly the same chemical substance.
   (b) Different dosage form can be compared when they contain same drug.

3. **Subjects**
   (a) Health
   (i) Subjects of similar kinetic characteristics have taken, so major variations are not introduced.
   (ii) Medical examination will be used to confirm their medical state.
   (iii) For some drugs there may be special disease state which causes exclusion of volunteers.

   (b) Age
   Age can have a significant effect on drug pharmacokinetic.
   Subject between the ages of 18-35 year are preferred.

   (c) Weight
   To better match the subjects with normal weights are preferred.

   (d) Enzyme status
   Smokers or subjects taking certain drug having altered enzyme activity or having drug-drug interaction may be excluded from the study. If these subjects are included, their effect adds complications to study. Therefore, an attempt is usually made to minimize these factors.

(e) Number
Usually 20-20 subjects are used.

(f) Assay
Same assay method should be used far all phases. Assay method should be sensitive and specific.

(g) Design
Usually Cross over design is used.

Bioavailability Studies

Bioavailability studies are designed to determine either an absolute BA (relative to an IV formulation) or relative BA (with an alternate reference dosage form with good absorption characteristics). They can be used to compare different route of administration.

Ex: oral versus iv, ip versus im.

The bioavailability study should be carried out in patient for whom the drug is intended to be used. Because of the following advantages-

- The patient will be benefitted from the study
- Reflects better the therapeutic efficacy of the drug
- Drug absorption in disease states can be evaluated
- Avoids the side effects of the drug to healthy one

There are some drawbacks of using patient volunteer for study like:

- Disease state, other drugs etc. modify the drug absorption,
- Establishing a standard set of conditions necessary for bioavailability study is difficult with patients as volunteer

So healthy patients are taken for bioavailability study to avoid inter subject variability.

Study are performed in young healthy male adult, age 20-40 and body weight within narrow range of ±10%, under restricted dietary and fixed activity condition.

Note: Drug wash out period for a minimum of ten biological half lives must be allowed for between any two studies in the same subject

Measurement of Bioavailability

It is divided into two categories:

1. Pharmacokinetic method

(a) Plasma level time studies
(b) Urinary excretion studies
2. Pharmacodynamic method
    (a) Acute pharmacologic response
    (b) Therapeutic response

Plasma Level Time Studies

Principle: The method is based on the assumption that two dosage forms that exhibit super imposable plasma level time profiles in a group of subjects should result in identical therapeutic activity (and they would be termed as bioequivalent). These studies cab be single dose or multiple dose studies (Table 1.4).

Single Dose Study

Following steps are involved in a single dose study.

- Collection of serial blood samples for period of 2-3 biological half lives after drug administration.
- Analysis for drug concentration.
- Making a plot of plasma concentration versus time of sample collection.
- Obtain plasma level time profile by this plot.

Note:

- *For IV dose sampling should start within 5 minutes of drug taken. At least 3 sample point should be taken*
- *For oral at least 3 sample point*

FDA Guidelines on Collection of Blood Samples

1. When comparison of the test product and the reference material is to be based on blood concentration time curves, unless some other approach is more appropriate for valid scientific reasons, blood samples should be taken with sufficient frequency to permit an estimate of both:

    (i) The peak concentration in the blood of the active drug ingredient or therapeutic moiety, or its metabolite(s), measured; and

    (ii) The total area under the curve for a time period at least three times the half-life of the active drug ingredient or therapeutic moiety, or its metabolite(s), measure

2. In a study comparing oral dosage forms, the sampling times should be identical.
3. In a study comparing an intravenous dosage form and an oral dosage form, the sampling times should be those needed to describe both:
    (i) The distribution and elimination phase of the intravenous dosage form; and
    (ii) The absorption and elimination phase of the oral dosage form.
4. In a study comparing drug delivery systems other than oral or intravenous dosage forms with an appropriate reference standard, the sampling times should be based on valid scientific reasons.

Table 1.4 Single dose verses multiple dose study

Type of Study	Advantages	Disadvantages
Single Dose Study	<ul><li>Easy to conduct.</li><li>Offer less exposure to drug.</li><li>Less tedious.</li></ul>	<ul><li>Dose does not give any idea of drug/metabolites.</li><li>Difficult to predict the steady state characteristics of the drugs.</li></ul>
Multiple Dose Study*:	<ul><li>Easy to predict the peak and valley characteristics of drug</li><li>Fewer blood samples requirements</li><li>Less sensitive analytical method</li><li>Performed in patients because of the therapeutic benefits to the patients</li><li>Small inter subject variability</li><li>Better evaluation of the performance</li><li>Nonlinearity in pharmacokinetics, easily detected</li></ul>	<ul><li>Difficult to control</li><li>Highly tedious</li><li>Time consuming</li><li>Drugs having long half lives require longer period to achieve steady state,</li><li>Exposes the subject to more drug</li></ul>

* For this study the drug should be administered for 5-6 elimination half lives before collecting the blood.

Basic Pharmacokinetic Parameters of Plasma level time Studies

Pharmacokinetics provides a mathematical basis to assess the time course of drugs and their effects in the body. It enables the following processes to be quantified:

Absorption, Distribution, Metabolism, and Excretion.

These pharmacokinetic processes often referred to as ADME; determine the drug concentration in the body when medicines are prescribed. A fundamental understanding of these parameters is required to design an appropriate drug regimen for a patient.

The effectiveness of a dosage regimen is determined by the concentration of the drug in the body. Ideally, the concentration of drug should be measured at the site of action of the drug; that is, at the receptor. However, owing to inaccessibility, drug concentrations are normally measured in whole blood from which serum or plasma is generated. Other body fluids such as saliva, urine and cerebrospinal fluid (CSF) are sometimes used. It is assumed that drug concentrations in these fluids are in equilibrium with the drug concentration at the receptor.

Upon oral (or IV) administration, when plasma concentration of drug is plotted against the time, a plasma level time profile curve (Fig. 1.2) can be plotted. A plasma level time profile curve shows the following pharmacokinetic parameters, which should be studied to assess the bioavailability.

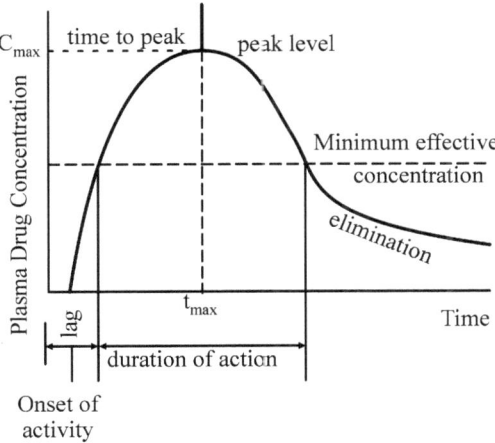

Fig. 1.2 A plasma level time profile curve of a orally administered drug.

Various parameters which should be reported as per FDA guidelines in a BA study are as followed:

AUC_{0-t}, $AUC_{0-\infty}$, Cmax, Tmax, λz, and $t_{1/2}$.

Area under the Concentration vs Time Curve (AUC)

Area under the curve of plasma concentration of a drug versus the time after single-dose administration. This denotes the bioavailability.

$$BA = AUC_{oral}/AUC_{iv}$$

AUC $_{0-t}$

It is area under the plasma concentration-time curve from 0 hr to the last quantifiable concentration to be calculated using the trapezoidal rule (Fig. 1.3).

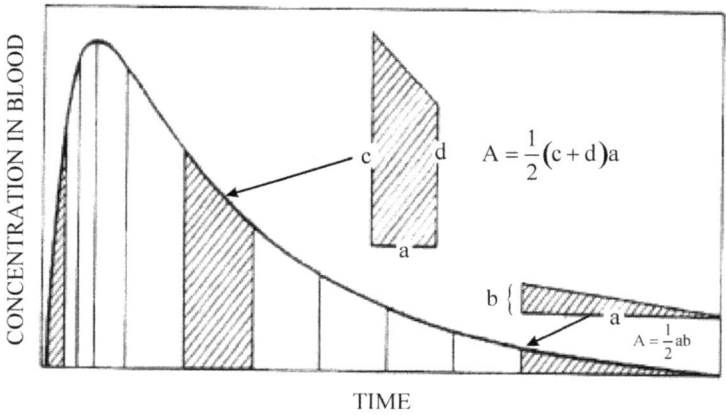

Fig. 1.3 AUC estimated by numerical integration techniques; for example, trapezoidal rule (smaller rectangular areas are integrated) as shown.

$AUC_{0-\infty}$

Area under the plasma concentration-time curve from zero to infinity is calculated as the sum of AUC_{0-t} plus the ratio of the last measurable concentration to the elimination rate constant.

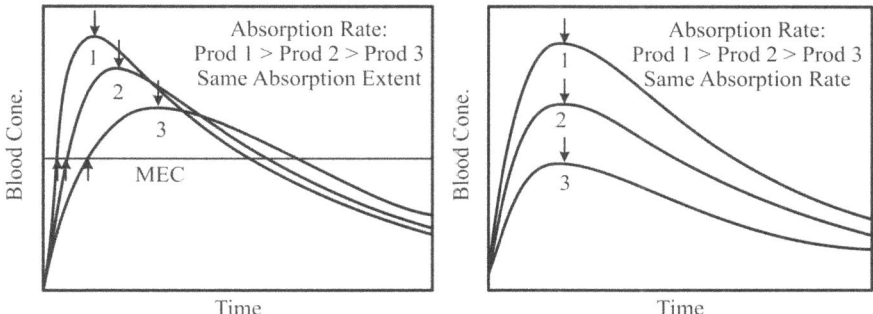

Fig. 1.4 AUC in understanding bioavailability.

- Rate of drug absorption mainly affects the time to onset of action (↑), as well as timing and magnitude of maximal effect (↓).
- Extent of absorption affects maximal effect and overall exposure as measured by area under the blood concentration-time curve (AUC).

Maximum Concentration (Cmax)

This is the maximum drug concentration achieved in systemic circulation following drug administration.

Time of Cmax (Tmax)

It is the time required to achieve the maximum drug concentration in systemic circulation.

Terminal or elimination rate constant (λ_z)

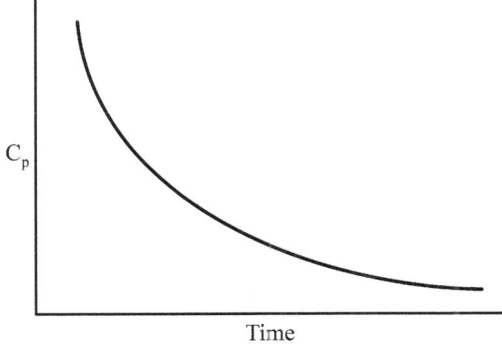

Fig. 1.5 Plasma concentration (Cp) versus time profile of a drug (one-compartment model).

Consider a single IV bolus injection of drug X (see Fig. 1.5). As time proceeds, the amount of drug in the body is eliminated. Thus the rate of elimination can be described (assuming first-order elimination) as:

$$dX/dt = -kX$$

Hence

$$X = X_0 \exp(-kt)$$

where X = amount of drug X, X_0 = dose and k = first-order elimination rate constant.

Half-life ($t_{1/2}$)

The time required to reduce the plasma concentration to one half its initial value is defined as the *half-life* ($t_{1/2}$)

$$t_{1/2} = 0.693/k \qquad \text{(for first order reaction)}$$

where, k = first-order elimination rate constant.

Multiple Dose Study

Some drugs may be used clinically on a single-dose basis, although most drugs are administered continually over a period of time. When a drug is administered at a regular dosing interval (orally or IV), the drug accumulates in the body and the serum concentration will rise until steady-state conditions have been reached, assuming the drug is administered again before all of the previous dose has been eliminated (see Fig. 1.6).

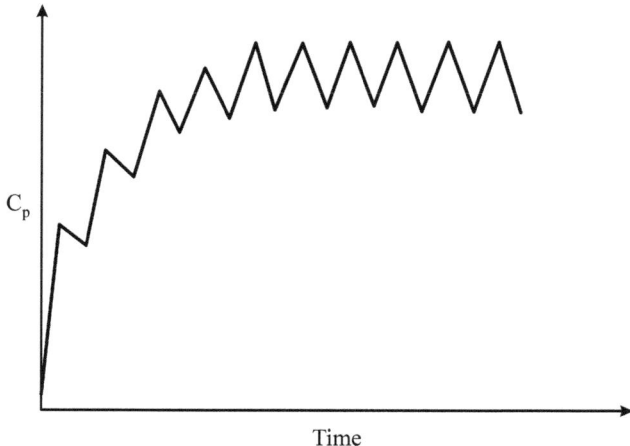

Fig. 1.6 Time profile of multiple IV doses.

At steady state the rate of drug administration is equal to the rate of drug elimination. At steady state the plasma concentrations of the drug (C^{ss}_p) at any time during any dosing interval, as well as the peak and trough, are similar. The time to reach steady-state concentrations is dependent on the half-life of the drug under consideration.

Following steps are involved in a multiple dose study

- Administration of drug for at least 5 biological half lives (administration of at least 5 doses) to reach steady state.
- Collection of blood sample at the end of previous dose interval.
- 8-10 sampling after administration of next dose.

Steady state plasma concentrations $C^{ss}_p = \dfrac{D}{\tau \times CL}$

where **D** is dose, τ is dosing interval and CL is Clearance

$$\text{Bioavailability} = \frac{[AUC]_{test} \; D_{std} \; T_{test}}{[AUC]_{std} \; D_{test} \; T_{std}}$$

§ 320.27 FDA Guidelines on the design of a multiple-dose *in vivo* bioavailability study

(a) Basic Principles

1. In selected circumstances it may be necessary for the test product and the reference material to be compared after repeated administration to determine steady-state levels of the active drug ingredient or therapeutic moiety in the body.
2. The test product and the reference material should be administered to subjects in the fasting or nonfasting state, depending upon the conditions reflected in the proposed labeling of the test product.
3. A multiple-dose study may be required to determine the bioavailability of a drug product in the following circumstances:
    (i) There is a difference in the rate of absorption but not in the extent of absorption.
    (ii) There is excessive variability in bioavailability from subject to subject.
    (iii) The concentration of the active drug ingredient or therapeutic moiety, or its metabolite(s), in the blood

resulting from a single dose is too low for accurate determination by the analytical method.

(iv) The drug product is an extended release dosage form.

(b) Study Design

1. A multiple-dose study should be crossover in design, unless a parallel design or other design is more appropriate for valid scientific reasons, and should provide for a drug elimination period if steady-state conditions are not achieved.
2. A multiple-dose study is not required to be of crossover design if the study is to establish dose proportionality under a multiple-dose regimen or file of a new drug product, a new drug delivery system, or a extended release dosage form.
3. If a drug elimination period is required, unless some other approach is more appropriate for valid scientific reasons, the drug elimination period should be either:
   (i) At least five times the half-life of the active drug ingredient or therapeutic moiety, or its active metabolite(s), measured in the blood or urine; or
   (ii) At least five times the half-life of decay of the acute pharmacological effect.

(c) Achievement of steady-state conditions

Whenever a multiple-dose study is conducted, unless some other approach is more appropriate for valid scientific reasons, sufficient doses of the test product and reference material should be administered in accordance with the labeling to achieve steady state conditions.

(d) Collection of blood or urine samples

1. Whenever comparison of the test product and the reference material is to be based on blood concentration time curves at steady state, appropriate dosage administration and sampling should be carried out to document attainment of steady state.
2. Whenever comparison of the test product and the reference material is to be based on cumulative urinary excretion-time curves at steady state, appropriate dosage administration and sampling should be carried out to document attainment of steady state.
3. A more complete characterization of the blood concentration or urinary excretion rate during the absorption and

elimination phases of a single dose administered at steady-state is encouraged to permit estimation of the total area under concentration-time curves or cumulative urinary excretion-time curves and to obtain pharmacokinetic information, e.g., half-life or blood clearance, that is essential in preparing adequate labeling for the drug product.

(e) Steady-state parameters

1. In certain instances, e.g., in a study involving a new drug entity, blood clearances at steady-state obtained in a multiple dose study should be compared to blood clearances obtained in a single-dose study to support adequate dosage recommendations.

2. In a linear system, the area under the blood concentration-time curve during a dosing interval in a multiple dose steady-state study is directly proportional to the fraction of the dose absorbed and is equal to the corresponding "zero to infinity" area under the curve for a single-dose study. Therefore, when steady-state conditions are achieved, a comparison of blood concentrations during a dosing interval may be used to define the fraction of the active drug ingredient or therapeutic moiety absorbed.

3. Other methods based on valid scientific reasons should be used to determine the bioavailability of a drug product having dose-dependent kinetics (non-linear system).

Various parameters which should be reported as per FDA guidelines in a BA (multiple dose) study are as followed: $AUC_{0\text{-tau}}$, Cmin, Tmax, C_{min} and C_{pd}

$AUC_{0\text{-}\tau}$

Area under the plasma concentration-time curve from time zero to time tau over a dosing interval at steady state ($AUC_{0\text{-}\tau)}$, where tau is the length of the dosing interval.

$AUC_{0\text{-}\tau\,(ss)}$

Area under the plasma concentration-time curve over one dosing interval in multiple dose study at steady state.

Time of Cmax (Tmax)

It is the time required to achieve the maximum drug concentration in systemic circulation.

Cmin

This is the minimum drug concentration achieved in systemic circulation following multiple dosing at steady state.

Cpd

This is the pre dose concentrations determined immediately before a dose is given at steady state.

Urinary Excretion Studies

Principle: The urinary excretion of unchanged drug is directly proportional to the plasma concentration of drug.

The study is particularly useful for drugs extensively excreted unchanged in the urine.

Example: thiazides, sulphonamides, urinary antiseptics, hexamine etc.

Method

- Collection of urine at regular interval for a time span equal to 7 biological half lives.
- Analysis of unchanged drug in the collected sample.
- Determination of the amount of drug excreted in each interval.

Note: At each sample collection total emptying of bladder is necessary to avoid errors resulting from addition of residual amount to the next urine.

A curve of drug excretion rate against the time is plotted and following parameters are studied in urinary excretion studies:

1. $(dx\ u/dt)max$ = maximum urinary excretion rate
2. $(tu)max$ = time for maximum excretion rate
3. Xu = cumulative amount of drug excreted in urine.

Bioavailability

$$F = \frac{Xu_{oral}\ D_{iv}}{Xu_{iv}\ D_{oral}}$$

$$Fr = \frac{Xu_{test} \ D_{std}}{Xu_{std} \ D_{test}}$$

With multiple dos study:

$$Fr = \frac{Xu, \ SS_{test} \ D_{std} \ T_{test}}{Xu, \ SS_{std} \ D_{test} \ T_{std}}$$

where,

Xu, ss = amount of drug excreted unchanged during single dosing interval at steady state

Acute Pharmacologic Response

It may include measurement of one or more of the following pharmacological reponses:
- Change in ECG or EEG reading.
- Pupil diameter etc are related to time course of a given drug.
- Bioavailability can be then determined by plotting the pharmacologic effect- time curve as well as dose response graph.
- Require measurement of response at least 3 biological half lives of drug.

Disadvantages
- Variable pharmacologic response.
- Accurate correlation between measured response and drug available is difficult.

Measurement of an acute pharmacological effect: When comparison of the test product and the reference material is to be based on acute pharmacological effect-time curves, measurements of this effect should be made with sufficient frequency to demonstrate a maximum effect and a lack of significant difference between the test product and the reference material. **(21CFR (320.27 f) FDA)**

Therapeutic Response

Principle: Observing the clinical response to a drug formulation given to patient suffering from disease for which it is intended to be used. But the method is associated with the fact that the response observed is often too improper.

Pharmacodynamic studies are not recommended for orally administered drug products when the drug is absorbed into the systemic circulation and a pharmacokinetic approach can be used to assess systemic exposure and establish BA/BE. However, in those instances where a pharmacokinetic approach is not possible, suitably validated pharmacodynamic methods can be used to demonstrate BE. *FDA*

Bioequivalence Studies (Comparative Bioavailability Studies)

According to the FDA Orange Book (Approved Drug Products with Therapeutic Equivalence Evaluations), test and reference products are said to be bioequivalent, if the rate and extent of absorption of the test drug do not show a significant difference from the rate and extent of absorption of the reference drug, when administered at the same molar dose, of the therapeutic ingredient under similar experimental conditions in either single dose or multiple doses.

Bioequivalence studies are designed to compare dug products. The objective is to determine if these products are bioequivalent. The dosage forms should be similar, especially the route of administration. For example, tablet versus tablet, or may be tablet versus capsule, given orally. These studies may be necessary before a generic period may be marketed. In general a relative bioavailability is determined which may be close to 100%.

Types of Equivalence

Equivalence is a relative term that compares drug products with respect to a specific characteristic or function or to a defined set of standards. There are several types of equivalences.

Chemical Equivalence

It indicates that two or more drug products contain the same labeled drug substance as an active ingredient in the same amount.

Pharmaceutical Equivalence

Pharmaceutical equivalent means drug products that contain identical amounts of the identical active drug ingredient, i.e., the salt or ester of the same therapeutic moiety, in identical dosage forms, but not necessarily containing the same inactive ingredients.

- Central Drug Standard Control Organization (*CDSCO), India.*

"Drug products are considered pharmaceutical equivalents if they contain the same active ingredient(s), are of the same dosage form, route of administration and are identical in strength or concentration (*e.g., chlordiazepoxide hydrochloride, 5 mg capsules*). Pharmaceutically equivalent drug products are formulated to contain the same amount of active ingredient in the same dosage form and to meet the same or compendial or other applicable standards (i.e., strength, quality, purity, and identity), but they may differ in characteristics such as shape, scoring configuration, release mechanisms, packaging, excipients (including colors, flavors, preservatives), expiration time, and, within certain limits, labeling." *-FDA CDER 2004*

Pharmaceutical equivalents are the same drug entity, the same type of dosage form, the same dose and meet the same compendial requirements. For example Aspirin Tablets, U.S.P. of a particular strength. Although the U.S.P. monograph includes dissolution and chemical assay requirements there are no bioavailability requirements (at least not in U.S.P. XX). Thus all Aspirin U.S.P. tablets of a particular dose would be pharmaceutical equivalents. Capsules of aspirin would not and neither would tablets of a different dose. Dosage forms containing different salt forms, esters or other chemical form are not pharmaceutical equivalents.

Pharmaceutical Alternatives

Pharmaceutical alternatives are drug products that contain identical therapeutic moiety or its precursor but not necessarily, in the same amount or dosage form or as the same salt or ester.

- CDSCO, India.

"Drug products are considered pharmaceutical alternatives if they contain the same therapeutic moiety, but are different salts, esters, or complexes of that moiety, or are different dosage forms or strengths (*e.g., tetracycline hydrochloride, 250 mg capsules vs. tetracycline phosphate complex, 250 mg capsules; quinidine sulfate, 200 mg tablets vs. quinidine sulfate, 200 mg capsules*). Data are generally not available for FDA to make the determination of tablet to capsule bioequivalence. Different dosage forms and strengths within a product line by a single manufacturer are thus pharmaceutical alternatives, as are extended release products when compared with immediate- or standard-release formulations of the same active ingredient."

- FDA CDER 2004

Pharmaceutical alternatives are drug products that can provide the same therapeutic moiety. Different dosage forms, doses and even salts can be pharmaceutical alternatives.

Therapeutic Equivalence

Therapeutic equivalents are the drug products that contain the same active substance or therapeutic moiety, and clinically show the same efficacy and safety.

- CDSCO, India

Drug products are considered to be therapeutic equivalents only if they are pharmaceutical equivalents and if they can be expected to have the same clinical effect and safety profile when administered to patients under the conditions specified in the labeling.

- FDA CDER 2004

Thus, pharmaceutical equivalents that have been shown to be bioequivalent (and the same by other determinations of clinical effect and safety profile) are therapeutic equivalents. Therapeutic equivalents would be expected to produce identical drug concentration time profiles and therapeutic response when administered under the same conditions. This is not the same as two pharmacologically similar (equivalent) compounds that may produce the same therapeutic response in some individuals ("e.g., propoxyphene hydrochloride vs. pentazocine hydrochloride for the treatment of pain").

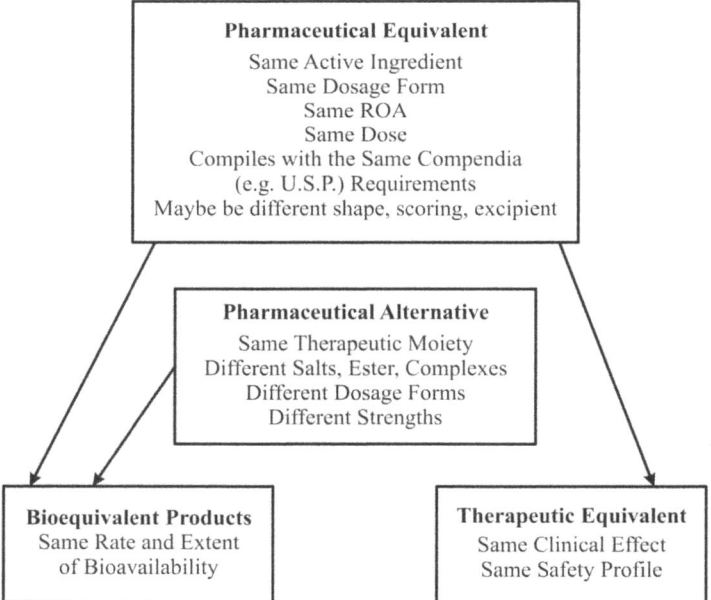

Fig. 1.7 Summary of bioavailability definitions.

Bioequivalence

It is a relative term which denotes that the drug substance in two or more identical dosage forms, reaches the systemic circulation at the same relative rate and to the same relative extent i.e. their plasma concentration-time profiles will be identical without significant statistical differences.

Bioequivalence of a drug product is achieved if its extent and rate of absorption are not statistically significantly different from those of the reference product when administered at the same molar dose.

- CDSCO, India.

Bioequivalent Drug Products means pharmaceutical equivalents or pharmaceutical alternatives whose rate and extent of absorption do not show a significant difference when administered at the same molar dose of the therapeutic moiety under similar experimental conditions, either single dose or multiple dose.

Some pharmaceutical equivalents or pharmaceutical alternatives may be equivalent in the extent of their absorption but not in their rate of absorption and yet may be considered bioequivalent because such differences in the rate of absorption are intentional and are reflected in the labeling, are not essential to the attainment of effective body drug concentrations on chronic use, or are considered medically insignificant for the particular drug product studied as Therapeutic Equivalents.

Bioequivalence is defined in as "the absence of a significant difference in the rate and extent to which the active ingredient or active moiety in pharmaceutical equivalents or pharmaceutical alternatives becomes available at the site of drug action when administered at the same molar dose under similar conditions in an appropriately designed study."

-21CFR 320.1 (FDA)

Bioequivalence (BE) means the absence of a greater –than-allowable difference between the systemic bioavailability of a test product and that of a reference product.

Reasons for Bioequivalence Requirements

The FDA may decide to require bioavailability studies for a variety of reasons including:
- Results from clinical studies indicate that different drug products produce different therapeutic results.

- Results from bioavailability studies indicate that different products are not bioequivalent.
- Drug has a narrow therapeutic range.
- Low solubility and/ or large dose.
- Absorption is considerably less than 100%.
- Bioequivalence studies assess *in vivo* impact of changes to the dosage form/process after pivotal studies commence to ensure product on the market is comparable to that upon which the efficacy is based

Biowaivers

The term biowaiver is applied to a regulatory drug approval process when the dossier (application) is approved based on evidence of equivalence other than through *in vivo* equivalence testing.

WHO Expert Committee on Specifications for Pharmaceutical Preparations (40th Report 2006)

Under certain circumstances, product quality BA and BE can be documented using *in vitro* approaches (21 CFR 320.24(b) and 21 CFR 320.22(d)). For highly soluble, highly permeable, rapidly dissolving, and orally administered drug products, documentation of BE using an *in vitro* approach (dissolution studies) is appropriate based on the biopharmaceutics classification system. This approach may also be suitable under some circumstances in assessing BE during the IND period, for NDA and ANDA submissions, and in the presence of certain post approval changes to approved NDAs and ANDAs.

Diagrams depicting the products eligible (revised criteria) for the biowaiver procedure under the HHS-FDA guidance and those eligible according to the WHO "Multisource document" are presented in Fig. 8 (WHO Expert Committee on Specifications for Pharmaceutical Preparations, 40th Report, 2006).

Thus, the eligibility criteria (Fig. 1.8) according to WHO (40th Report, 2006) are:

1. **The BCS classification** (according to the revised criteria) of the API.
2. **Risk assessment:** only if the risk of an incorrect biowaiver decision and an evaluation of the consequences (of an incorrect, biowaiver-based equivalence decision) in terms of public health and risks to individual patients is outweighed by the potential

benefits accrued from the biowaiver approach, the biowaiver procedure may be applied.

(a)   according to FDA

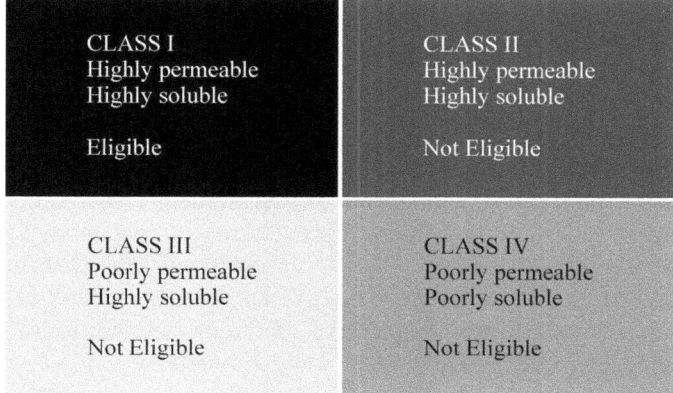

(b)   according to WHO

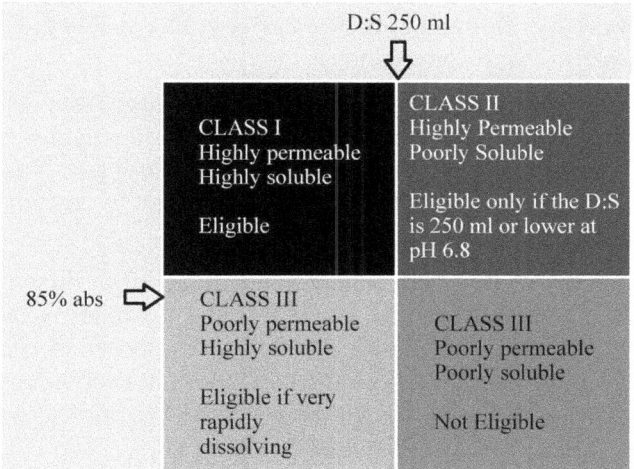

Fig. 1.8 Eligibility for the biowaiver procedure based on solubility and permeability characteristics of the active pharmaceutical ingredient.

3. **Dissolution requirements** for the pharmaceutical product:
   - very rapidly dissolving (release of > 85% of the labelled amount of drug in 15 minutes) in standard media at pH 1.2, 4.5 and 6.8, at a rotational speed of 75 rpm in the paddle apparatus or 100 rpm in the basket apparatus (applies to pharmaceutical

products containing Class III Active Pharmaceutical Ingredients or APIs);
- rapidly dissolving (release of > 85% of the labelled amount of drug in 30 minutes) in standard media at pH 1.2, 4.5 and 6.8, at a rotational speed of 75 rpm in the paddle apparatus or 100 rpm in the basket apparatus (applies to pharmaceutical products containing Class I APIs and/or Class II APIs which are weak acids and meet the 250 ml dose: solubility requirement at pH 6.8).

Dissolution testing is also used to assess batch-to-batch quality, where the dissolution tests, with defined procedures and acceptance criteria, are used to allow batch release. USFDA recommends that dissolution testing is also used to provide process control and quality assurance, and assess whether further BE studies relative to minor post-approval changes be conducted, where dissolution can function as a signal of bioinequivalence. *In vitro* dissolution characterization is encouraged for all product formulations investigated (including prototype formulations), particularly if *in vivo* absorption characteristics are being defined for the different product formulations. Such efforts may enable the establishment of an *in vitro-in vivo* correlation.

If an appropriate dissolution method has been established, and the dissolution results indicate that the dissolution characteristics of the product are not dependent on the product strength, then dissolution profiles in one medium are usually sufficient to support waivers of *in vivo* testing.

A simple model independent approach for dissolution profile comparison uses a difference factor (f_1) and a similarity factor 1 (f_2) to compare dissolution profiles. The difference factor (f_1) calculates the percent (%) difference between the two curves at each time point and is a measurement of the relative error between the two curves:

$$f_1 = [\{\sum_{t=1}^{n} | R_t - T_t |\} / \{\sum_{t=1}^{n} R_t\}] \times 100$$

where n is the number of time points, R_t is the dissolution value of the reference t (pre-change) batch at time t, and T_t is the dissolution value of the test (post-change) batch t at time t.

US FDA recommends that the f_2 test be used to compare profiles from the different strengths of the product. The similarity factor (f_2) is a logarithmic reciprocal square root transformation of the sum of squared error and is a measurement of the similarity in the percent (%) dissolution between the two curves. An f_2 value (similarity factor) > 50 indicates a sufficiently similar dissolution profile such that further *in vivo* studies are not needed. The similarity factor f_2 is to be computed using the equation:

$$f_2 = 50 \times \log [\{1 + (1/n) \sum_{t=1}^{n} (R_t - T_t)^2\}^{-0.5} \times 100]$$

where R_t and T_t are the cumulative percentage of the drug dissolved at each of the selected n time-points of the comparator (reference) and multisource (test) product respectively.

(If the comparator and multisource products are very rapidly dissolving, i.e. at least 85% dissolution in 15 minutes or less, in all media (pH 1.2, 4.5 and 6.8 buffer), using the recommended test method, a profile comparison is not necessary.)

Bibliography

- Abdou H. M. Theory of dissolution and Theoretical concepts for the release of a drug from a dosage form. In *Dissolution, Bioavailability and Bioequivalence*, Gennaro, A., Migdalof, B., Hassert, G. L., Medwick, T., Eds.; Mack Publishing Company: Easton, PA, 1989; pp 11-52.

- Bolton S. Correlation in Pharmaceutical Statistics: Practical and Clinical Applications, 2nd ed., Marcel Dekker Inc., New York, 1991; 211-245. Florence, A. T.; Attwood, D. Properties of the solid state. In *Physicochemical Principles of Pharmacy*, 2nd ed.; Florence, A. T., Attwood, D., Eds.; Macmillan Press: Basingstoke, Hants., England, 1988;

- Central Drug Standard Control Organization (CDSCO), Govt. of India, Guidelines for Bioavailability and Bioequivalence Studies in 2005.

- Emami J. J Pharm Pharmaceut Sci 9 (2): 169-189, 2006.

- FDA guidance for industry on *Waiver of In vivo Bioavailability and Bioequivalence Studies for Immediate Release Solid Oral Dosage Forms Based on a Biopharmaceutics Classification System.*

- Food and Drug administration; Code of Federal regulation Title 21, Part 320, Bioavailability and Bioequivalence Requirements, Section 320 33(C) 2003.

- Gibaldi M. Gastrointestinal absorption – Physicochemical considerations. In *Biopharmaceutics and Clinical*

Pharmacokinetics, 4th ed.; Gibaldi, M., Lea and Febiger: Malvern, PA, 1991; pp 40-60.
- Meyer M. C. Bioavailability of drugs and bioequivalence. In: Encyclopedia of Pharmaceutical Technology" Vol. 2. (Swarbrik J., and Boylon C., Eds) 1998 New York, Marcel Dekker Inc. 33-58.
- Multisource (generic) pharmaceutical products: guidelines on registration requirements to establish interchangeability (WHO Technical Report Series, No. 937, Annex 7)
- Shargil L., and Yu, "Applied Biopharmaceutics and Pharmacokinetics" 2nd edition. Appleton Century Crofts Norwalk, CT, 1985: 193-203.
- US FDA, FDA Guidance for Industry: Bioavailability and Bioequivalence Studies for Orally Administered Drug Products, 2003.
- WHO Expert Committee on Specifications for Pharmaceutical Preparations, 40th Report, 2006.
- Semalty A, Cyclodextrin and phospholipid complexation in solubility and dissolution enhancement: A critical and meta-analysis, Expert Opinion on Drug Delivery, 2014, 11(8):1255-72.

CHAPTER 2

Dissolution Study

Introduction

In vitro dissolution testing serves as an important tool for characterizing the biopharmaceutical quality of a product at different stages in its lifecycle. In early drug development *in vitro* dissolution properties are supportive for choosing between different alternative formulations for further development and for evaluation of active ingredients/drug substances.

Dissolution testing is an official test recommended by all pharmacopoeias for evaluating drug release of solid and semisolid dosage forms.

Dissolution tests were first developed to quantify the amount and extent of drug release from solid oral dosage forms including immediate/sustained release tablets and capsules. Drug absorption from a solid dosage form after oral administration depends on the release of the drug substance from the drug product, the dissolution or solubilization of the drug under physiological conditions, and the permeability across the gastrointestinal tract. *In vitro* dissolution may be relevant to the prediction of *in vivo* performance. (1) assess the lot-to-lot quality of a drug product; (2) guide development of new formulations

In-vitro dissolution testing has been widely used as quality control measures for solid oral dosage form drug products. Recently, it has also been employed as a useful tool to forecast *in vivo* performance of drug products and to ascertain the need for *in vivo* comparative bioavailability and bioequivalence studies. The concept of dissolution was first given by Noyes and Whitney they suggested that the dissolution rate was controlled by a layer of saturated solution that forms instantly around a solid particle.

Dissolution is defined as the process by which a known amount of drug substance goes into solution per unit of time under standardized conditions.

Goals of Dissolution Testing

The primary goal of dissolution testing is to be used as a qualitative tool to provide measurements of the bioavailability, batch-to-batch consistency and to signal potential problems with *in vivo* bioavailability.

The bioavailability and bioequivalence data obtained as a result of dissolution testing can be used to guide the development process toward product optimization, as well to ensure continuing product quality and performance of the manufacturing process. In addition dissolution is a requirement for regulatory approval for product marketing and is a vital component of the overall quality control program.

Need of Dissolution Testing

- To help assure lot-to-lot uniformity
  USP requirement applies even if there is no correlation with *in vivo* data because it is a very discriminating and useful control over manufacturing variables.
- To guide formulation development
- To help establish stability/expiration dates
- To demonstrate to FDA that products after scaleup and post-approval changes are bioequivalent to the originally approved product.
- When correlated with *in vivo* data, dissolution may be used instead of human biostudies.
- Used without *in vivo* correlation for minor changes.

Basic Concept of Dissolution

The dissolution of a solid substance can be described in two steps. In the first step the molecules are released from the surface to the surrounding dissolution media. This creates a saturated layer, called the stagnant layer, adjacent to the solid surface. Thereafter, the drug diffuses into the bulk of the solvent from regions of high drug concentration to regions of low drug concentration. The rate of drug dissolution at a specific time can be described with the Modified Noyes-Whitney's equation

$$\frac{dx}{dt} = \frac{A.D.K}{h} Cs - \frac{xd}{V}$$

where dx/dt is the dissolution rate, A is the surface area of the particle available for dissolution, D is the diffusion rate constant, K is the oil water partition coefficient, h is the thickness of the stagnant layer surrounding the particle, Cs is the saturation solubility of the drug, Xd is the amount dissolved of drug at time t and V is the volume of the dissolution media.

The dissolution rate is influenced both by the physicochemical properties of the substance and by the prevailing physiological conditions in the GI tract (Table 2.1), which varies between the fasted and fed state as well as within and between subjects. Formulation strategies intended to alter these properties have been employed to increase the dissolution rate of low soluble drugs. These include micronisation, nano-suspensions, lipid-formulations, microemulsions, and the use of complexing agents such as cyclodextrins.

Table 2.1 List of the physicochemical and the physiological properties that can influence drug dissolution in the GI tract.

Factor	Physicochemical properties	Physiological properties
Surface area of drug (A)	Particle size, wettability	Surfactants in gastric juice and bile
Diffusion coefficient of the drug (D)	Molecular size	Viscosity of luminal contents
Stagnant layer thickness (h)		Motility patterns and flow rate
Solubility (Cs)	Hydrophilicity, crystal structure, solubilization	pH, buffer capacity, bile and food composition
Amount of drug already dissolved (Xd)		Permeability
Volume of solvent available (V)		Secretion, co-administered fluids

Basic Theories of Dissolution (Dissolution Models)

Dissolution of a solute is a multistep process involving heterogeneous reactions/interactions between the phases of the solute-solute, solute-solvent, solvent-solvent, and at the solute-solvent interface. As one of the most commonly known mass transfer rate processes, the component heterogeneous reactions may broadly be categorized into (i) diffusion or convective transport of the solute from the interface to the bulk phase; and (ii) the rate of solute liberation and transport from and across the interfacial boundaries.

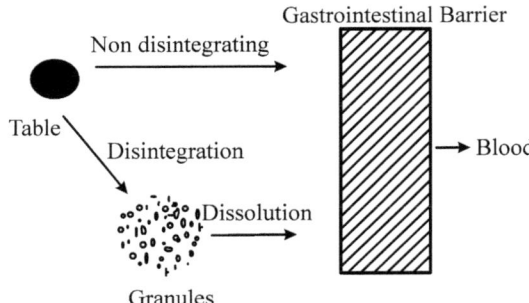

Fig. 2.1 Schematic diagram of the dissolution process.

Various theories have been developed to define the dissolution process. Diffusion layer model, surface renewal theory, and limited solvation theory are the three of the pioneering theories in the field. Table 2.2 concisely depicts the principal mathematical equations associated with the theories and highlights key points regarding the theory. Major theories of dissolution are as followed.

- Diffusion layer Model (Film Theory)
- Penetration or Surface Renewal Theory (Danckwerts' Model)
- Interfacial Barrier Model (Double Barrier Mechanism or Limited Solvation Theory)

The **Diffusion layer theory**, the simplest model describing dissolution, makes use of a single crystal in a nonreactive environment. The initial step in solution of the solid (solute or crystal) at the interface is usually very rapid and results in the formation of a saturated stagnant layer around the particle (Fig. 2.2). This is contrasted by the second diffusion step that is slow and becomes the rate-limiting step in the dissolution process. In particular, the Noyes-Whitney equation (eq 3 in Table 2.2) illustrates that one of the main factors determining the rate of dissolution is drug solubility. From this it is understood that *in vivo* the dissolution process may become the rate-limiting step if the rate of solution is much slower than the rate of absorption. This may be the case when the drug in question has a very low solubility at both gastric and intestinal pH.

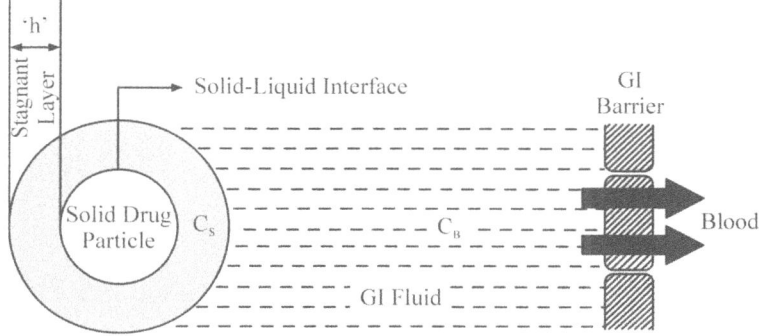

Fig. 2.2 Diffusion layer model.

The **surface renewal theory** assumes an equilibrium at the solute-solution interface is attained and that the rate limiting step in the dissolution process is mass transport. The model is thought of as being continually exposed to fresh dissolution medium. The agitating medium consists of numerous eddies or packets into which the solute diffuses and is carried to the bulk medium. Due to the turbulence at the surface of the solute, there is no boundary layer and therefore no stagnant film layer. In other words the surface is continually being replaced with fresh medium (Fig. 2.3).

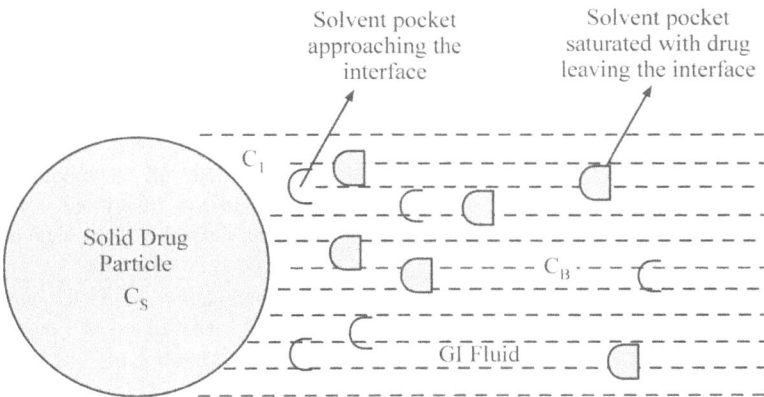

Fig. 2.3 Surface renewal model.

The **Interfacial barrier model or limited solvation theory** predicts that a crystal undergoes dissolution through an interfacial process in the dissolving medium (Fig. 2.4). The true surface area of the crystal must be considered since each face of the crystal may have a different interfacial barrier. Hence each surface may provide a different contribution to the dissolution process. Table 2.2 summarizes all the fundamental theories and their expressions.

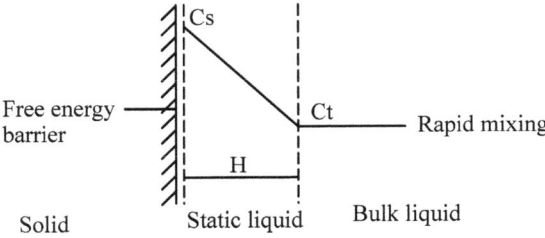

Fig. 2.4 Interfacial barrier model.

Table 2.2 Summary of fundamental dissolution theories.

Theory	Equation	Associated conditions/basis
Diffusion Layer		
Fick's First Law	$J_{ix} = -D_i (\partial c_i/\partial x)$ (1)	Considers diffusion only under steady-state conditions.
Fick's II Law	$\partial c/\partial t = D (\partial^2 c/\partial x^2)$ (2)	Used when drug concentration decreases with time; hence, considers non-steady state conditions.
Noyes & Whitney	$dc/dt = K (c_s - c_t)$ (3)	Description of drug dissolution based on constant surface area.
Brunner & Tolloczko	$dc/dt = KS (c_s - c_t)$ (4)	Manipulation of Noyes-Whitney's eq 3 by incorporation of surface area term S. Proposed the formation of a stagnant layer around the dissolving particle, a layer through which solute diffuses through into the bulk
Nernst-Brunner	$dc/dt = kDS/vh (c_s - c_t)$ (5) If $c_t \ll c_s$; $dc/dt = kDS/vhc_s$ (6) If v and S are constant; $dc/dt = K$ (7)	Manipulation of Fick's first law and expansion of eq 4 by incorporation of a diffusion coefficient D, stagnant layer thickness h, and volume of dissolution medium v.

Table 2.2 contd...

Theory	Equation	Associated conditions/basis
Diffusion Layer		
Penetration or Surface Renewal Theory	$V dc/dt = dW/dt = S(\gamma D)^{1/2}(cs - ct)$ (8)	Assumes solid-solution equilibrium is achieved at the interface and that mass transport is the rate-limiting step in the dissolution process.
Interfacial Barrier Model / Limited solvation	$G = k_i(cs - ct)$ (9)	An intermediate drug concentration less than saturation may exist at the interfacial barrier between the solid surface and solvent. Different faces of a crystal may have different interfacial barriers and therefore make different contributions to the dissolution process

Jix: flux (mg/cm² s⁻¹); Di: diffusion coefficient; $\partial c_i/\partial x$: concentration gradient; $\partial c/\partial t$ or dc/dt: drug dissolution rate; K: first-order dissolution constant; cs: equilibrium drug concentration; ct: drug concentration at time t; k: dissolution constant; S: surface area; v: volume of dissolution medium; h: thickness of stagnant layer; h: thickness of diffusion layer; γ: interfacial tension; G: dissolution rate per unit area; k_i: effective interfacial transport constant.

Official Dissolution Test Apparatus

In *U.S. Pharmacopeia* (USP), seven dissolution test apparatus are mentioned, while Indian Pharmacopoeia (IP) provides only two apparatus.

Various dissolution test apparatus official in USP are given in table 2.3 (Fig. 2.5). The most commonly employed dissolution test methods are (1) the basket method (Apparatus 1) and (2) the paddle method (Apparatus 2). The basket and the paddle methods are simple, robust, well standardized, and used worldwide. These methods are flexible enough to allow dissolution testing for a variety of drug products.

Table 2.3 USP official dissolution test apparatus

Apparatus No.	Description	General Application
1	Rotating Basket	Oral IR and MR
2	Rotating Paddle	Oral IR and MR
3	Reciprocating Cylinder	Oral MR
4	Flow Through Cell	Oral MR
5	Paddle over disk	Transdermal DS
6	Cylinder	Transdermal DS
7	Reciprocating Holder	Transdermal DS or non-disintegrating oral MR

*IR = Immediate release, MR = Modified Release, DS= Delivery System

44 Essentials of Pharmaceutical Technology

For this reason, the official in vitro dissolution methods described in USP, Apparatus 1 and Apparatus 2 should be used unless shown to be unsatisfactory. The in vitro dissolution procedures, such as the reciprocating cylinder (Apparatus 3) and a flow-through cell system (Apparatus 4) described in the USP may be considered if needed. Dissolution methodologies and apparatus described in the USP can generally be used either with manual sampling or with automated procedures.

I.P. Dissolution Test apparatus are of two types paddle type (Type I) and basket type (Type II). The specifications of I.P. Dissolution Test apparatus are given in Fig. 2.6.

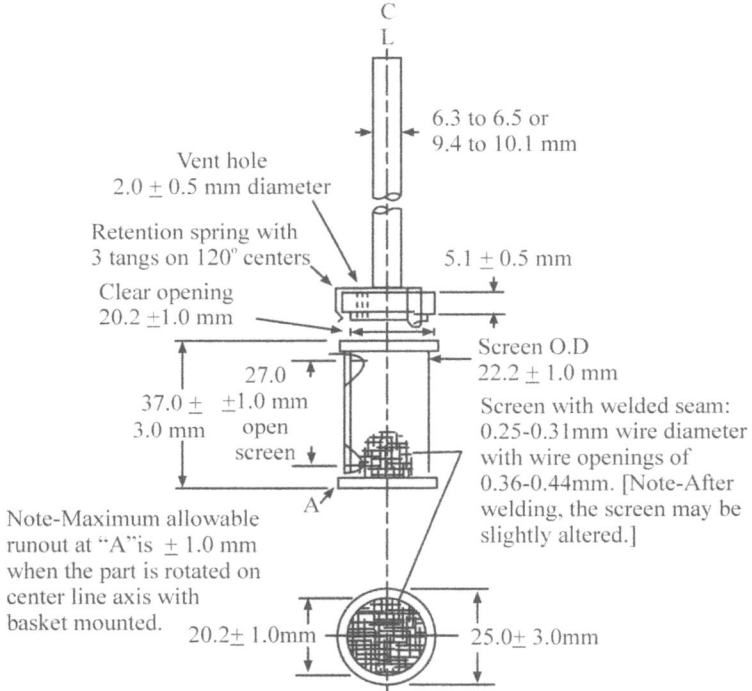

(I) Rotating Basket

Dissolution Study   45

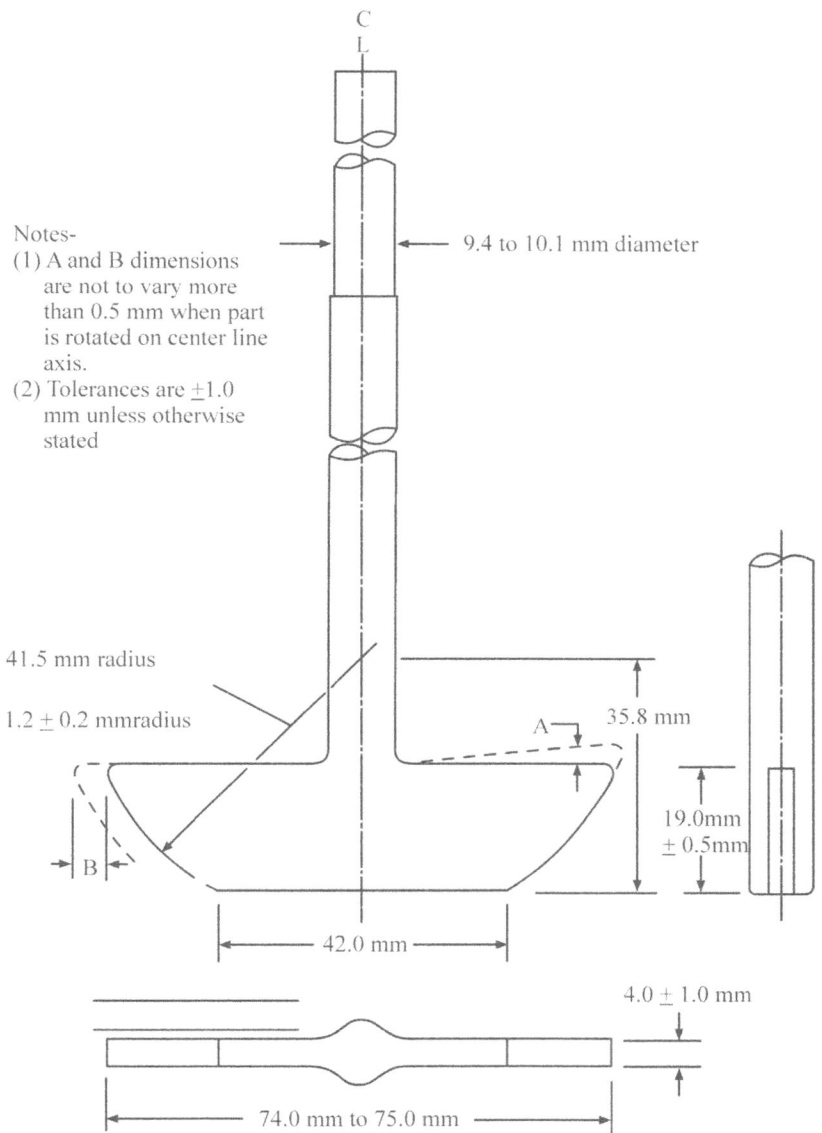

Notes-
(1) A and B dimensions are not to vary more than 0.5 mm when part is rotated on center line axis.
(2) Tolerances are ±1.0 mm unless otherwise stated

(II) Rotating paddle

46   Essentials of Pharmaceutical Technology

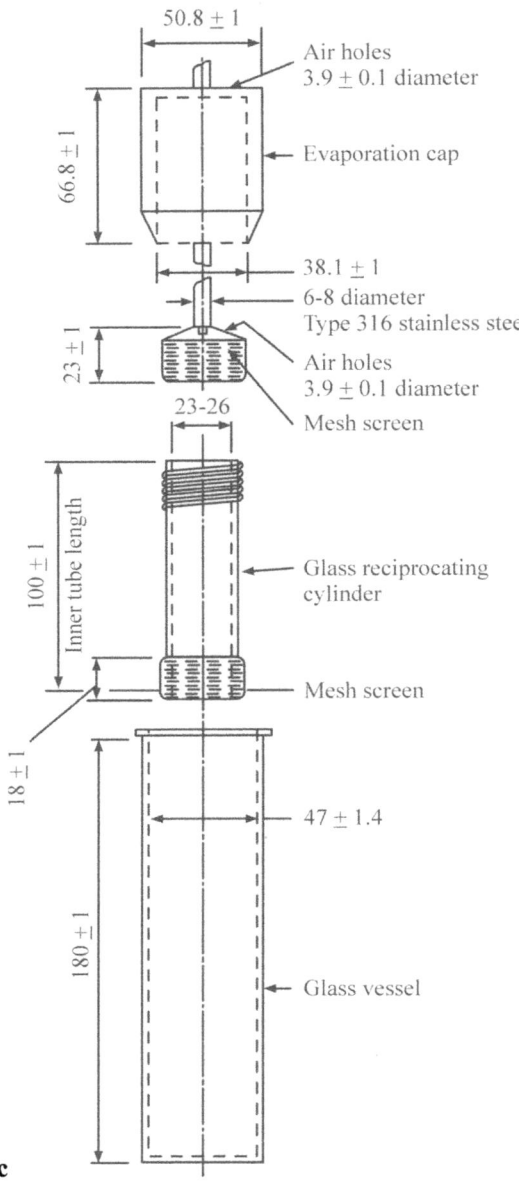

(III) Reciprocaring Cylinder

Dissolution Study 47

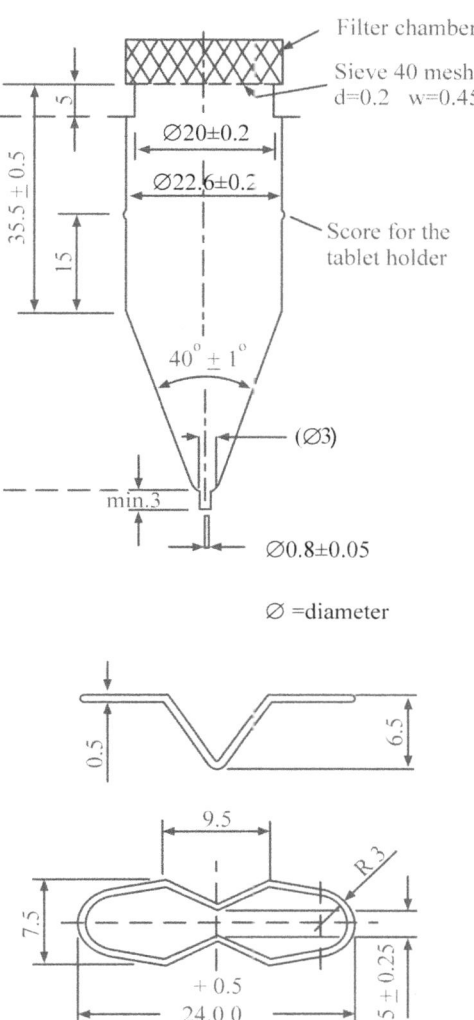

Flow through cell type 1

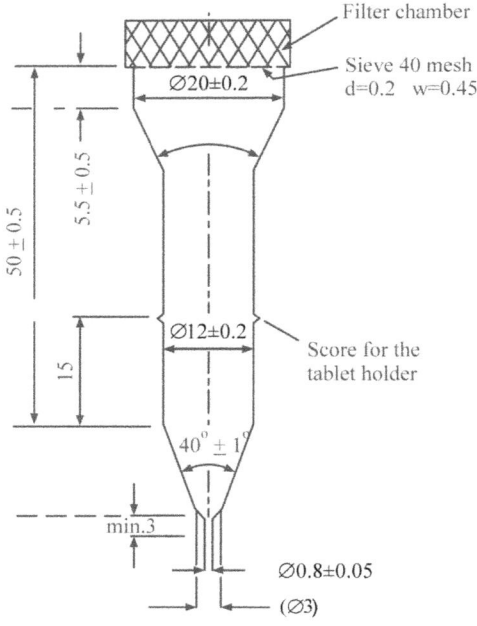

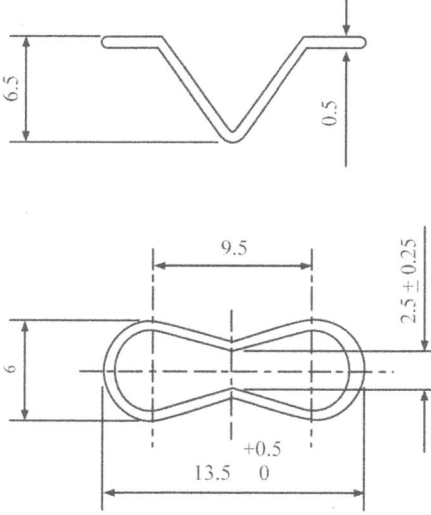

(IV) Flow through cell type 2

Dissolution Study   49

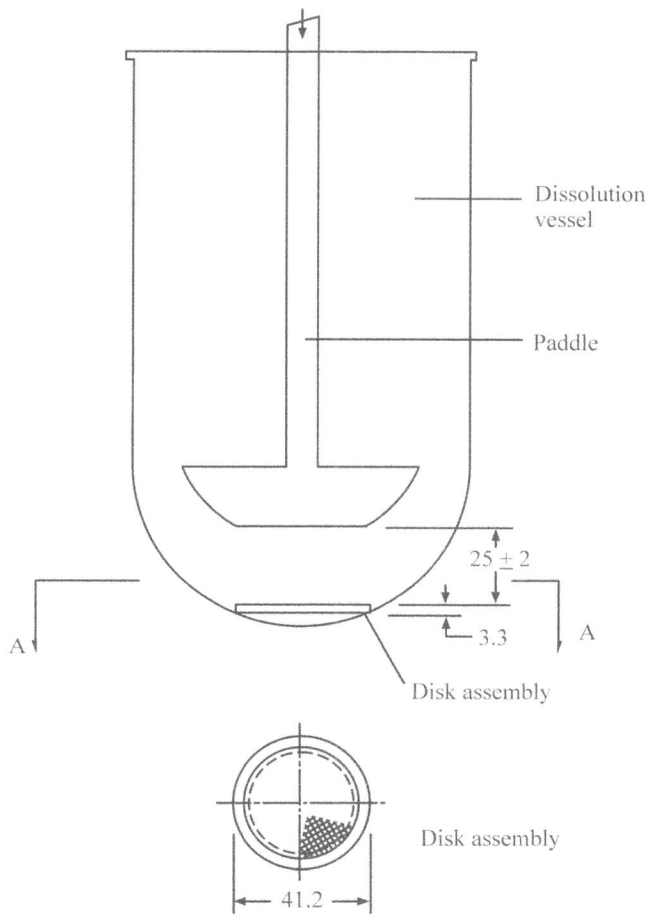

(V) Paddle over disk

50 Essentials of Pharmaceutical Technology

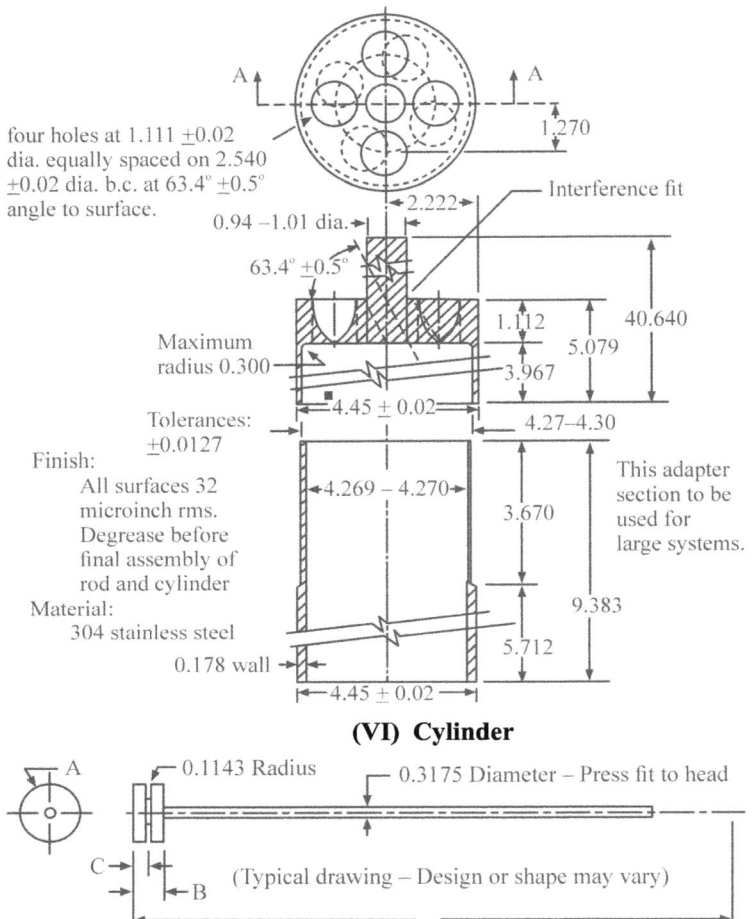

(VI) Cylinder

Dimensions are in centimeters

	HEAD				ROD		O-RING
System[a]	A (Diameter)	B	C	Material[b]	D	Materal	(not shown)
1.6cm2	1.428	0.9525	0.4750	SS/VT	30.48	SS/P	Parker 2-113-V884-75
2.5cm²	1.778	0.9525	0.4750	SS/VT	30.48	SS/P	Parker 2-116-V884-75
5cm²	2.6924	0.7620	0.3810	SS/VT	8.890	SS/P	Parker 2-022-V884-75
7cm²	3.1750	0.7620	0.3810	SS/VT	30.48	SS/P	Parker 2-124-V884-75
10cm²	5.0292	0.6350	0.3505	SS/VT	31.01	SS/P	Parker 2-225-V884-75

aTypical system sizes
bSS/VT=Either stainless steel or virgin Teflon
cSS/P=Either stainless steel or Plexiglas

(VII) Rciprocating Holder

Fig. 2.5 USP Dissolution test apparatus.

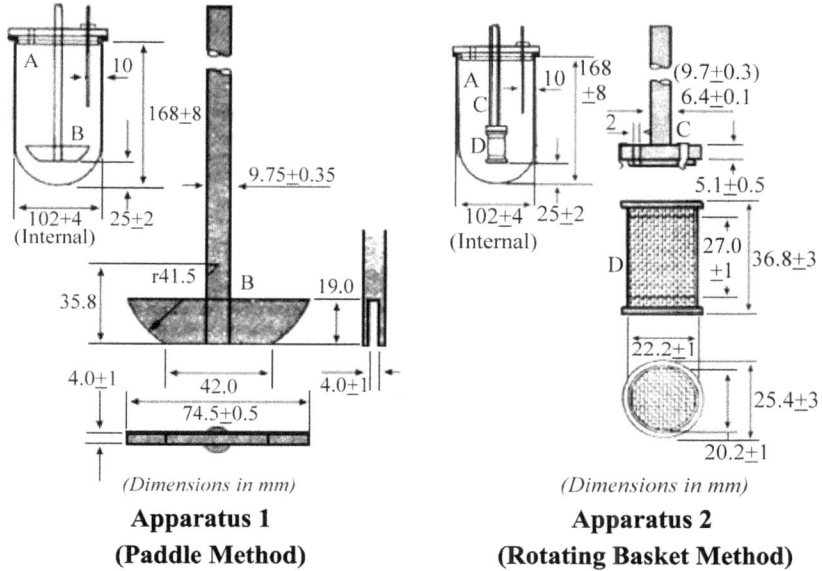

(Dimensions in mm)   (Dimensions in mm)
Apparatus 1   **Apparatus 2**
(Paddle Method)   **(Rotating Basket Method)**

Fig. 2.6 I P. Dissolution test apparatus.

Unofficial/Unconventional Dissolution Test Apparatus

Apart from official test apparatus, various scientists have developed different kinds of dissolution test apparatus, which have been summarized in Table 2.4. The unofficial test apparatus are classified as natural convection and forced convection models, on the basis of mode of agitation of dissolution medium.

Table 2.4 Unofficial/Unconventional dissolution test apparatus

A. Natural Convection Models	
Static disc method	It is used for non disintegrating tablets. Whole, slow release or enteric coated tablets of KCl was placed in pots containing 10 ml of dissolution fluid.
Sintered filter method	It employs a dissolution model with a sintered glass funnel. Dissolution medium moves past the dosage form in the filter funnel under gravity.

Table 2.4 contd. .

B. Forced Convectional Model	
Beaker method	250 ml of 0.1N HCl at 37 ^{0}C in 400 ml beaker is used as dissolution medium. Agitation is provided by means of a 3 blade polyethylene steroids, 5 cm in dia. And caused to rotate at 60 rpm. Samples are removed at known time intervals and assayed for the drug content.
Rotating disc method	For nondisintegrating tablets or disc. Tablet were not removed after compression, one face was made flush with die surface, other end of die was sealed with cork, immersed in dissolution medium and stirred at 150 rpm
Rotating bottle method	A sample of sustained release product is placed in 90 ml cylindrical screw capped bottles, 60 ml of fluid is added in each and bottles are rotated slowly end over end on a temperature controlled water bath at 37 ^{0}C. A bottle is withdrawn after half an hour for initial analysis and others rotated for remaining test period.
Rotating basket method	Original apparatus is based on beaker method. The tablet is placed in 10 mesh screen basket which is suspended below a 3 blade 5 cm stirrer.
Stationary basket method	Utilizing cylindrical stainless steel mesh basket in a Lucite frame. This is mounted rigidly in a 3 lt beaker containing 2 lt of dissolution medium. A 'T' shaped glass stirring rod, rotates at 150 rpm placed at temperature controlled bath at 37± 1^{0}C. The test tablet is dropped in to basket and filtered samples of the dissolution fluid are taken at suitable time interval
Oscillating tube method	It is official in USP, is a modified disintegration test apparatus, a 30 or 40 mesh screen, is employed in place of 10 mesh screen.
Dialysis method	A tablet was placed in dissolution medium on one side of dialysis membrane and the cell wall rotated in a water bath at 15 rpm, sample were removed from distal chamber at appropriate time interval. In this method membrane should have a short equilibrium time and adequate physical strength to retain solid particles.
C. Miscellaneous methods	
FDA method	In this method more precise control of changes in the medium with time have been proposed for better simulation of biological situation in GIT. Ten ml of fluid is pumped and circulated at 37 ^{0}C through passed the dosage form, held in an inert matrix. 50 ml of this menstrum is removed for analysis at each hour and replaced by 50 ml of simulated intestinal fluid. Process is continued for the duration of the period over which dosage form is expected to last.

Table 2.4 *contd...*

Tape method	A weighed quantity of article is dusted on a pressure sensitive tape mounted on a frame and the whole assembly is inserted into a beaker, dissolution of drug into the stirred dissolution medium is monitored by the removal of sample of drug at known time interval.
Flow through dissolution cell	In this method, dissolution medium is made to circulate through a dissolution cell which contain the tablet resting on a fine wire screened to a reservoir and then back to dissolution chamber.

Dissolution Medium

Generally dissolution testing should be carried out under physiological conditions, as far as possible. However, it is not recommended to attempt to strictly mimic the physiologic gastrointestinal environment (composition of gastric or intestinal fluid) but to choose the testing conditions as far as is reasonable, based on the physicochemical characteristics of drug substance, within the range which a drug or dosage form could experience after oral administration.

Reasonable mimicking of physiological conditions to carry out dissolution testing allows interpretation of dissolution data with regard to *in vivo* performance of the product. The volume of the dissolution medium is generally 500, 900 or 1000 mL. Sink conditions are desirable but not mandatory. An aqueous medium with pH range 1.2 to 6.8 (ionic strength of buffers the same as in USP) should be used. To simulate intestinal fluid (SIF), a dissolution medium of pH 6.8 should be employed. A higher pH should be justified on a case-by-case basis and, in general, should not exceed pH 8.0. For low pH in the acidic range HCl should be used (0.1N HCl for pH 1). If, in a certain case, artificial gastric juice without enzymes (pH 1.2) is advantageous, this should be demonstrated. In the pH-range of 4.5 to 8.0 USP buffer solutions are recommended, as summarized in Table 2.5.

The use of simulated gastric juice (with pepsin) may be appropriate for gelatin capsules. To simulate gastric fluid (SGF), a dissolution medium of pH 1.2 should be employed without enzymes. The need for enzymes in SGF and SIF should be evaluated on a case-by-case basis and should be justified. Recent experience with gelatin capsule products indicates the possible need for enzymes (pepsin with SGF and pancreatin with SIF) to dissolve pellicles, if formed, to permit the dissolution of the drug. Use of water as a dissolution medium also is discouraged because test conditions such as pH and surface tension can vary depending on the source of water and may change during the dissolution test itself, due to the influence of the active and inactive ingredients. For water insoluble or sparingly water soluble drug products, use of a surfactant such as sodium lauryl sulfate is recommended. The need for and the amount of the surfactant should be justified. Use of a hydro alcoholic medium is discouraged. An IR drug product is characterized as a rapid dissolving when no less than 85% of the labeled amount of the drug substance dissolves within 30 minutes using USP Apparatus I at 100 rpm or USP Apparatus II at 50 rpm in a volume of 900 mL or less of each of the recommended media:

Table 2.5 Recommended dissolution media

Medium	Proposed Concentration
0.1N hydrochloric acid	3.636 g of HCl, corresponding to 8.3 ml hydrochloric acid 37% (m/m) per 1000 ml of aqueous solution
Buffer solution pH 4.5	*Acetate buffer solution pH 4.5:* 2.99 g of sodium acetate trihydrate and 1.66 g of glacial acetic acid are dissolved in water to 1000 ml or *Phosphate buffer solution pH 4.5:* 13.61 g monobasic potassium phosphate is dissolved in 750 ml of water. After adjusting the pH to 4.5 with 0.1N hydrochloric acid or 0.1N sodium hydroxide, water is added to make 1000 ml
Simulated intestinal fluid without pancreatin pH 7.5	250 ml of a solution containing 6.8 g monobasic potassium phosphate + 190 ml of 0.2N sodium hydroxide + water to make 1000 ml
0.05M phosphate buffer solution of pH 5.8 to 8.0	50 volumes of 0.2M monobasic potassium phosphate solution + specified volume of 0.1N sodium hydroxide + water to 200 volumes

Source: FIP Guidelines for Dissolution Testing of Solid Oral Products

The basket and paddle method can be used for performing dissolution tests under multimedia conditions (e.g., the initial dissolution test can be carried out at pH 1.2, and, after a suitable time interval, a small amount of buffer can be added to raise pH to 6.8). Alternatively, if addition of an enzyme is desired, it can be added after initial studies (without enzymes).

Use of Apparatus 3 allows easy change of the medium. Apparatus 4 can also be adopted for a change in dissolution medium during the dissolution run. Certain drug products and formulations are sensitive to dissolved air in the dissolution medium and will need deaeration. In general, capsule dosage forms tend to float during dissolution testing with the paddle method. In such cases, it is recommended that a few turns of a wire helix (USP) around the capsule be used. The apparatus suitability tests should be carried out with a performance standard (i.e., calibrators) at least twice a year and after any significant equipment change or movement. However, a change from basket to paddle or vice versa may need recalibration. The equipment and dissolution methodology should include the product related operating instructions such as deaeration of the dissolution medium and use of a wire helix for capsules. Validation of automated procedures compared to the manual procedures should be well documented. Validation of determinative steps in the dissolution testing process should comply with the set standards for analytical methodology.

Agitation

In general, mild agitation conditions should be maintained during dissolution testing to allow maximum discriminating power and to detect products with poor in vivo performance. Using the basket method, the common agitation (or stirring speed) is 50-100 rpm; with the paddle method, it is 50-75 rpm (Shah et al., 1992). Apparatus 3 and 4 are seldom used to assess the dissolution of immediate release drug products.

Validation

Validation of the dissolution apparatus/methodology should include (1) the system suitability test using calibrators; (2) deaeration, if necessary; (3) validation between manual and automated procedures; and (4) validation of a determinative step (i.e., analytical methods employed in quantitative analysis of dissolution samples).

This should include all appropriate steps and procedures of analytical methods validation.

Correlation of Dissolution with Bioavailability
(*In Vitro In Vivo* Correlation)

Correlation of in vitro rate of Dissolution with in vivo Bioavailability is termed as *in vitro in vivo* correlation (IVIVC). Methodologies of determination of bioavailability have already been discussed in chapter 1.

After performing in vitro (dissolution) and in vivo (bioavailability) studies the next immediate step is to judge how much, up to which extent and in which manner they are related. This is done by performing IVIVC.

The therapeutic efficacy of pharmaceutical formulations is governed by factors related to both the in vitro dissolution characteristics of the drug and its in vivo bioavailability. This inherent interdependency within the drug-patient biosystem is the major concern that underlines the *in vitro in vivo* correlation studies. The dissolution rate of a specific dosage form is, essentially, an arbitrary parameter, that is very dependent on the methodology utilized in generating the data. Changes in the type of apparatus, dissolution medium, agitation speed, etc. can modify dramatically the dissolution pattern.

So, until a carefully designed correlation is established between *in vitro* dissolution and *in vivo* bioavailability, the bioavailability implications of dissolution should never be accepted on faith.

Definitions

The term correlation is frequently employed within the pharmaceutical and related sciences to describe the relationship that exists between variables. Mathematically, the term correlation means interdependence between quantitative or qualitative data or relationship between measurable variables and ranks. From biopharmaceutical standpoint, correlation could be referred to as the relationship between appropriate in vitro release characteristics and in vivo bioavailability parameters. Two definitions of IVIVC have been proposed by the USP and by the FDA.

The establishment of a rational relationship between a biological property, or a parameter derived from a biological property produced by a dosage form, and a physicochemical property or characteristic of the same dosage form.

United State Pharmacopoeia (USP)

IVIVC is a predictive mathematical model describing the relationship between an in vitro property of a dosage form and a relevant in vivo response. Generally, the in vitro property is the rate or extent of drug dissolution or release while the in vivo response is the plasma drug concentration or amount of drug absorbed.

Food and Drug Administration (FDA)

Role of IVIVC

IVIVC can be used in the development of new pharmaceuticals to reduce the number of human studies during the formulation development. The main objective of an IVIVC is to serve as a surrogate for in vivo bioavailability and to support biowaivers. IVIVCs could also be employed to establish dissolution specifications and to support and/or validate the use of dissolution methods. This is because the IVIVC includes in vivo relevance to in vitro dissolution specifications. It can also assist in quality control for certain scale up and post-approval changes (SUPAC), for instance, to improve formulations or to change production processes.

Correlation Levels

Five correlation levels have been defined in the IVIVC FDA guidance and USP. The concept of correlation level is based upon the ability of the correlation to reflect the complete plasma drug level-time profile which will result from administration of the given dosage form.

Level A Correlation

This level of correlation is the highest category of correlation and represents a point-to-point relationship between in vitro dissolution rate and in vivo input rate of the drug from the dosage form. Generally, percent of drug absorbed may be calculated by means of model dependent techniques such as Wagner-Nelson procedure or Loo-Riegelman method or by model-independent numerical deconvolution. These techniques represent a major advance over the single-point approach in that these methodologies utilize all of the dissolution and plasma level data available to develop the correlations and will be discussed more in detail later in this article.

The purpose of Level A correlation is to define a direct relationship between in vivo data such that measurement of in vitro dissolution rate alone is sufficient to determine the biopharmaceutical rate of the dosage form. In the case of a level A correlation, an in vitro dissolution curve can serve as a surrogate for in vivo performance. Therefore, a change in manufacturing site, method of manufacture, raw material supplies, minor formulation modification, and even product strength using the same formulation can be justified without the need for additional human studies. It is an excellent quality control procedure since it is predictive of the dosage form's in vivo performance.

Level B Correlation

A level B IVIVC utilizes the principles of statistical moment analysis. In this level of correlation, the mean in vitro dissolution time (MDT_{vitro}) of the product is compared to either mean in vivo residence time (MRT) or the mean in vivo dissolution time (MDT_{vivo}). MRT, MDT_{vitro} and MDT_{vivo} will be defined throughout the manuscript where appropriate. Although a level B correlation uses all of the in vitro and in vivo data, it is not considered to be a point-to point correlation, since there are a number of different in vivo curves that will produce similar mean residence time values. A level B correlation does not uniquely reflect the actual in vivo plasma level curves. Therefore, one can not rely upon a level B correlation alone to justify formulation modification, manufacturing site change, excipient source change, etc. In addition in vitro data from such a correlation could not be used to justify the extremes of quality control standards.

Level C Correlation

In this level of correlation, one dissolution time point (t50%, t90%, etc.) is compared to one mean pharmacokinetic parameter such as AUC, tmax or Cmax. Therefore, it represents a single point correlation and doses not reflect the entire shape of the plasma drug concentration curve, which is indeed a crucial factor that is a good indicative of the performance of modified-release products. This is the weakest level of correlation as partial relationship between absorption and dissolution is established. Due to its obvious limitations, the usefulness of a Level C correlation is limited in predicting in vivo drug performance. The usefulness of this correlation level is subject to the same caveats as a Level B correlation in its ability to support product and site changes as well as justification of quality control standard extremes. Level C correlations can be useful in the early stages of formulation development when pilot formulations are being selected. While the information may be useful in formulation development, waiver of an in vivo bioequivalance study (biowaiver) is generally not possible.

Multiple-level C Correlation

A multiple level C correlation relates one or several pharmacokinetic parameters of interest (Cmax, AUC, or any other suitable parameters) to the amount of drug dissolved at several time points of the dissolution profile. A multiple point level C correlation may be used to justify a biowaiver, provided that the correlation has been established over the entire dissolution profile with one or more pharmacokinetic parameters of interest. A relationship should be demonstrated at each time point at the same parameter such that the effect on the in vivo performance of any change in dissolution can be assessed. If such a multiple level C correlation is achievable, then the development of a level A correlation is also likely. A multiple Level C correlation should be based on at least three dissolution time points covering the early, middle, and late stages of the dissolution profile.

Level D correlation

Level D correlation is a rank order and qualitative analysis and is not considered useful for regulatory purposes. It is not a formal correlation but serves as an aid in the development of a formulation or processing procedure.

Biopharmaceutical Classification System

The Biopharmaceutical Classification System (BCS) is a scientific framework for classifying drug substances based on their aqueous solubility and intestinal permeability (described in chapter 1). In the following text the BCS shall be further discussed in terns of its relationship with IVIVC.

$$\text{Formulated Drug} \xrightarrow{K_d} \text{Solubilized Drug} \xrightarrow{K_p} \text{Absorbed Drug}$$

where K_d = dissolution rate; which is a function of solubility (including food), drug product quality attributes

K_p = permeability rate; which is a major function of API molecular structure and shows minor dependence on salt form, food, excipients, etc.

As shown above, three fundamental factors including dissolution, solubility and intestinal permeability govern the rate and extent of drug absorption from solid oral dosage forms. The Biopharmaceutical Classification System (BCS), which was proposed by Amidon et al. in 1995, classifies drugs into four different groups, depending on their solubility and permeability (Table 2.6).

Table 2.6 Biopharmaceutical classification system of drugs

Class	Solubility	Permeability
I	High	High
II	Low	High
III	High	Low
IV	Low	Low

The intention of the system was to set up a theoretical basis for correlating the *in vitro* dissolution profiles with *in vivo* bioavailability of drugs. BCS is also a fundamental guideline for determining the conditions under which IVIVCs are expected (Table 2.7).

Table 2.7 IVIVC expectations for immediate release products based on BCS

Class	Solubility	Permeability	Absorption rate control	IVIVC expectations for Immediate release product
I	High	High	Gastric emptying	IVIVC expected, if dissolution rate is slower than gastric emptying rate, otherwise limited or no correlations
II	Low	High	Dissolution	IVIVC expected, if in vitro dissolution rate is similar to *in-vivo* dissolution rate, unless dose is very high.
III	High	Low	Permeability	Absorption (permeability) is rate determining and limited or no IVIVC with dissolution.
IV	Low	Low	Case by case	Limited or no IVIVC is expected

It is also used as a tool for developing the in-vitro dissolution specification. The BCS can be employed as a tool to develop a strategy for improving the bioavailability of new chemical entities. Additionally, the system provides information about whether a compound's BA is solubility or permeability limited.

With this framework, when certain criteria are met, the BCS can be used as a drug development tool to help sponsors justify requests for biowaivers.

(a) **Solubility:** The solubility of a drug in the BCS is based on the highest dose strength in an IR product. A drug substance is considered *highly soluble* when the highest strength is soluble in 250 mL or less of aqueous media over the pH range of 1.0-7.5; otherwise the drug substance is considered poorly soluble. The volume estimate of 250 mL is derived from typical bioequivalence study protocols that prescribe the administration of a drug product to fasting human volunteers with a glass of water.

(b) **Permeability:** The permeability classification is based directly on the extent of intestinal absorption of a drug substance in humans or indirectly on the measurement of the rate of mass transfer across the human intestinal membrane. A drug substance is considered *highly permeable* when the extent of intestinal absorption is determined to be 85% or higher. Otherwise the substance is considered to be poorly permeable.

(c) **Dissolution:** An IR drug product is characterized as a *rapid dissolving* when no less than 85% of the labeled amount of the drug substance dissolves within 30 minutes using USP Apparatus I at 100 rpm or USP Apparatus II at 50 rpm in a volume of 900 mL or less of each of the following media:

- 0.1N HCl or Simulated Gastric Fluid USP without enzymes
- pH 4.5 buffer
- pH 6.8 buffer or Simulated Intestinal Fluid USP without enzymes

(However FIP recommends 4 dissolution media as given in Table 2.5)

The BCS guidance document (August 2000) recommends that sponsors may request biowaivers for highly soluble and highly permeable drug substances (Class I) in IR solid oral-dosage forms that exhibit rapid *in vitro* dissolution, provided the following conditions are met:

- the drug must be stable in the gastrointestinal tract
- excipients used in the IR solid oral-dosage forms have no significant effect on the rate and extent of oral drug absorption
- the drug must not have a narrow therapeutic index
- the product is designed not to be absorbed in the oral cavity.

Thus for BCS Class I drug substances, demonstration of rapid *in vitro* dissolution using the recommended test methods would provide sufficient assurance of rapid *in vivo* dissolution, thereby ensuring human *in vivo* bioequivalence. The potential benefit from this FDA guidance is not only lowering expenditures associated with bioavailability / bioequivalence studies but more critically expediting the development of new chemical entities for the marketplace, entities that will ultimately be of benefit to the health of the public.

The classification deals with drug dissolution and absorption model and considers the key parameters controlling drug dissolution and absorption as a set of dimensionless numbers: the absorption number, the dissolution number, and the dose number (described in chapter 1).

Bibliography

- Abdou HM, Theory of dissolution and Theoretical concepts for the release of a drug from a dosage form. In *Dissolution, Bioavailability and Bioequivalence*, Gennaro A., Migdalof B., Hassert G. L., Medwick T., Eds.; Mack Publishing Company: Easton, PA, 1989; pp 11-52.
- Amidon GL, Lennernas H, Shah VP, Crison JR, *Pharm Res.* 1995, 12:413-420.
- Bolton S. Correlation in Pharmaceutical Statistics: Practical and Clinical Applications, 2nd ed., Marcel Dekker Inc., New York, 1991; 211-245.
- CDER, *Waiver of in vivo bioavailability and bioequivalence studies for immediate release solid oral dosage forms based on a biopharmaceutics classification system*.2000, Food and Drug Administration.
- Devane J. *Pharm. Tech.* 1998; Nov:68-80 .
- Dressman JB, Amidon GL, Reppas C., and Shah VP, *Pharm Res.*, 1998;15:11-22.
- Dressman JB, Karmer J, *Pharmaceutical Dissolution Testing*, 2005, Taylor and Francis, New York.
- Dressman JB, Reppas C. *Eur J Pharm Sci.* 2000, 11(2):S73-80.
- Dressman JB, Amidon GL, Reppas C, Shah VP, *Pharm. Res.* 1998, *15*, 11-22.
- Emami J, J Pharm Pharm Sci 2006; 9 (2): 169-189.
- FDA, 1995, Center for Drug Evaluation and Research, *Guidance for Industry: Immediate Release Solid Oral Dosage Forms. Scale-up and Post-Approval Changes: Chemistry, Manufacturing and Controls, In Vitro Dissolution Testing, and In Vivo Bioequivalence Documentation* [SUPAC-IR], November 1995.
- FIP Guidelines for Dissolution Testing of Solid Oral Products, Vancouver, 1997.

- Fleischer D, Li C, Zhou Y, Pao LH, and Karim A. *Clin Pharmacokinet.*, 1999; 36:233-254.
- Florence AT, Attwood D, Properties of the solid state. In *Physicochemical Principles of Pharmacy*, 2nd ed.; Florence AT, Attwood D, Eds.; Macmillan Press: Basingstoke, Hants., England, 1988; pp 21-46.
- Gibaldi M. Gastrointestinal absorption – Physicochemical considerations. In *Biopharmaceutics and Clinical Pharmacokinetics*, 4th ed.; Gibaldi, M., Lea and Febiger: Malvern, PA, 1991; pp 40-60.
- Goldberg AH, Higuchi, WI, Ho. NF, Zographi G, *J. Pharm. Sci.* 1967, 56, 1432-1437.
- *IVIVC*; Center for Drug Evaluation and Research (CDER) at the Food and Drug Administration (FDA): Washington, D.C., 1996.
- Martinez MN Amidon GL, *Pharmacokinet. Pharmacodyn.* 2002; 42:620-643.
- Meyer MC, Straughn AB, Jarvi EJ, *et al. Pharm Res.* 1992; 9:1612-1616.
- Moore JW and Flanner HH., *Pharm Tech*, 1996; 20 (6):64-74.
- Nernst W, and Brunner EZ. *f Physik Chemie.* 1904; 47:52-110.
- Pernarowski M (1974) Dissolution Methodology, in Leeson LJ and Carstensen JT (Eds.): Dissolution Technology. APhA, Washington, DC, 73.
- Pillay V, Fassihi R. *J Pharm Sci*, 1999, 88,9,*843*-51.
- Shah VP, et al., *J Pharm Sci*, 1992; 81:500-503.
- Shah VP, et al., *Pharm Res,* 1989; 6:612-618.
- Shah VP, Skelly JP, Barr WH, Malinowski H, and Amidon GL, *Pharm Tech,* 1992; 16(5):35-40.
- Shah VP, et al., *Int J Pharm.,*1995; 125:99-106.
- Shah VP; Tsong Y; Sathe P; Liu JP. *Pharm. Res.* 1998, *15*, 889-896.
- Shargel L. and Yu, A.B.C. Applied biopharmaceutics and pharmacokinetics, 4th Edition, Appleton and Lange, Stamford, Connecticut, 1999.
- Siewert M., 1995, "FIP Guidelines for Dissolution Testing of Solid Oral Products," *Pharm. Ind.* 57:362-369.

- Skelly JP, GL, Amidon WH, Barr LZ, Benet JE, Carter JR, Robinson VP Shah, and A. Yacobi *in vitro* and *in vivo* testing and correlation for Oral Controlled/Modified-Release Dosage Forms . Pharmaceutical Research 1990, 975-982.
- US FDA, CDER, Guidance for Industry, Bioavailability and Bioequivalence Studies for Orally Administered Drug Products — General Considerations, *March 2003.*
- US FDA, CDER, Guidance for Industry, Dissolution Testing of Immediate Release Solid Oral Dosage Forms, August 1997.
- *USP 23-NF18*; United States Pharmacopoeial Convention, Inc.: Rockville, MD, 1995.
- Wagner JG, *J. Pharm. Sci.* 1969, *58*, 1253-1257.
- Yacobi A., *Pharm Res*; 1990; 7:975-82.
- Yu L.X., Amidon G.L., et al. *Pharm Res.* 2002; 19:921-923.
- Semalty A, Expert Opinion on Drug Delivery, 2014, 11(8): 1255-72.

CHAPTER 3

Tablets and Tablet Coating

Introduction

Pharmaceutical tablets are solid, flat or biconvex dishes, unit dosage form, prepared by compressing a drug or a mixture of drugs, with or without diluents.

Tablets dosage form is one of a most preferred dosage form all over the world. They vary in shape and differ greatly in size and weight, depending on amount of medicinal substances and the intended mode of administration. It is the most popular dosage form and 70% of the total medicines are dispensed in the form of Tablet.

Tablets may be swallowed whole or being chewed. Some are dissolved or dispersed in water before administration. Some are put in oral cavity, where the active ingredient is liberated at a predetermined rate. Implants or pesseries may also be presented in form of tablet.

Advantages of Tablet Dosage Forms

Tablet has a number of advantages, one of the major advantage over capsule, is that tablet is an essentially tamperproof doses form. Types and general properties of tablets are given in Table 3.1 and 3.2, respectively. Other potential advantages of tablets are as followed:

- These are the unit dosage forms which offer the greatest flexibility (with respect to doses) of all oral doses forms.
- Its cost is lowest of all oral dosage forms.
- These are the lightest and most compact of all oral doses forms.
- These are in general the easiest and cheapest to package and ship of all oral doses forms.
- Product identification is simplest and cheapest, requiring no additional processing steps.
- These may provide the greatest ease of swallowing with least tendency for "hang-up' above stomach, especially when coated, provided that tablet disintegration is not excessively rapid.
- These are better suited to large scale production than other unit oral forms.
- These have best combined properties of chemical, mechanical, and microbiological stability of all the oral forms.
- Objectionable odor and bitter taste can be masked by coating technique.
- Generally more stable than liquids with longer expiration dates.
- Release rate of the drug from tablet can be tailored to meet pharmacological requirements.

Disadvantages

- Disintegration and dissolution is required before drug is available for absorption.
- Solids having irritant effect on GIT mucosa poses problems for formulation into tablets.
- Some drugs resist compression into dense compacts, owing to their amorphous nature or flocculent, low-density character.
- Drugs with poor wetting, slow dissolution properties or any combination of this type of feature may be difficult or impossible to formulate and manufacture as a tablet.

- Bitter-tasting drugs, drugs with an objectionable odor, or drugs that are sensitive to oxygen or atmospheric moisture may require encapsulation or entrapment prior to compression, or the tablet may require coating. In such cases, capsule may offer the best and lowest cost approach.

Table 3.1 Types of tablets

According to drug release rate from the tablet (USP classification)
A-Immediate-release tablet:
• Disintegrating tablet (conventional or plain tablet)
• Chewable tablets
• Effervescent tablets
• Sublingual and Buccal tablets
• Lozenges
B- Modified-release tablet

Types of Tablets

A. Immediate-release tablet

The tablet is intended to be released rapidly after administration, or the tablet is dissolved and administered as solution.

Disintegrating tablet

Disintegrating tablet is the most common type of tablets that is intended to be swallowed and to release the drug in a relatively short time thereafter, by disintegration and dissolution (fast and complete drug release in vivo). It includes normally the following type of excipient; filler (with low dose drug), disintegrant, binder, glidant, lubricant and antiadherent.

Tablet disintegration may be affected by; Choice of the excipient, Production conditions during manufacture, Conventional tablet may be single layer or multilayer. Multilayer tablets are prepared by repeated compression of powders and are made primarily to separate incompatible drugs from each other.

Chewable tablets

Chewable tablets are to be chewed and thus mechanically disintegrated in the mouth, so that no disintegrant is included in its composition. Flavoring, sweetening and coloring agents are important. Sorbitol and mannitol are common examples of fillers in chewable tablets, (mannitol has negative heat of solution which results in cooling affect and also has sweetening action as previously mentioned under mannitol as filler).

Advantages of chewable tablets
- Provide quick and complete disintegration of the tablet and thus obtain a rapid drug effect after swallowing and dissolution.
- Easy administration, especially for infants and elderly people.
- Could be administered when water is not available.
- Examples for chewable tablets are; Chewable Aspirin tablets (for children in the treatment of rheumatoid and to prevent clot formations in adults), Chewable Antacid tablets

Effervescent Tablets

Effervescent tablets are dropped into a glass of water before administration during which CO_2 is liberated. This facilitates tablet disintegration and drug dissolution; the tablet disintegration should be complete within few minutes (Effervescence is a special mechanism for disintegration). CO_2 is created by the reaction between carbonate or bicarbonate and a weak acid such as citric acid or tartaric acid.

Advantages of Effervescent Tablets
- To obtain rapid drug action, for example analgesics and antacids. Effervescent Paracetamol tablet (analgesic) Effervescent antacid tablets
- To facilitate drug intake, for example vitamins, Vitamin C Effervescent tablets

Effervescent tablets often include a flavor and a colorant. Effervescent tablets are prepared by direct compression or dry granulation. Effervescent tablets should be protected from moisture, so that a special package is needed; each tablet is completely covered with aluminum foil and kept in a water-proof container, often including a desiccant. Effervescent tablets may be packed in blister packs. Effervescent tab package – Examples: analgesics and antacids.

Sublingual and Buccal Tablets

They are used for drug release in mouth followed by systemic uptake of the drug. A rapid systemic drug effect can thus be obtained without first-path liver metabolism, because the drug diffuses into the blood, directly through tissues under the tongue in case of sublingual tablets and through oral mucosa in case of buccal tablets.

Sublingual tablets are placed under the tongue. For example, Nitroglycerin sublingual tablet exerts its action within two minutes for rapid relief of "Angina pectoris" attack, because the sublingual area is rich in blood supply. Nitroglycerine suffers from first-pass metabolism if taken orally.

Also other cardiovascular drug, barbiturates, and vitamins are prepared as sublingual tablet dosage form. Vitamin B12 Sublingual tablet Buccal tablets are placed in the side of the cheek for absorption through oral mucosa.

Note: Buccal tablets may be also prepared for their local application. The sublingual area is rich in blood supply.

Lozenges

They are tablets that dissolve slowly in the mouth and so release the drug dissolved in the saliva. Lozenges may be used for local medications in the mouth or throat, e.g. local anesthetics, antiseptics and antibiotics and for systemic drug uptake.

Compressed lozenges are made by using tablet machine with large and flat punches, with high pressure is applied to produce hard tablets, so that they dissolve slowly in the mouth. No disintegrant is included in compressed lozenges composition. Other additives (binder and filler) must have pleasant taste or feeling during dissolution. Hard candy lozenges, e.g. Halls®, may be made by molding into a hard candy lozenges using candy making machine, for thermostable drugs. Warm, highly conc. flavored syrup is used as a base and the lozenges are formed by molding and drying.

B. Modified-Release Tablets

According to the USP/NF the term *'modified release dosage forms'* is defined as "one for which the drug release characteristics of time course and/or location are chosen to accomplish therapeutic objectives not offered by the conventional dosage forms. Modified release dosage forms may be classified into two types.

- **Extended-release dosage forms:** It is defined as the one that allows at least a twofold reduction in the dosing frequency as compared to that of conventional (immediate release) dosage form.

For example: controlled release or sustained release tablets (Fig. 3.1).

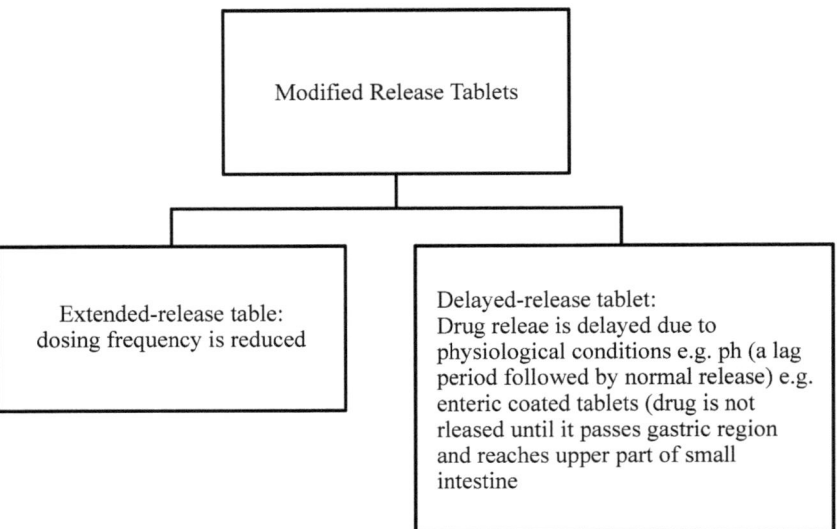

- **Delayed release dosage forms:** It is defined as the dosage form that releases a discrete portion or portions of drug at a time (or times) other than promptly after administration. Enteric coated tablets are the example of delayed release dosage forms (Fig. 3.1).

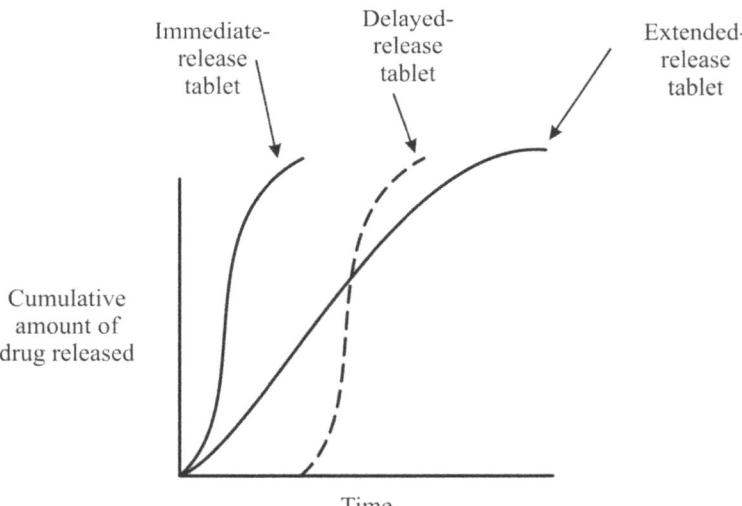

Fig. 3.1 A plot of cumulative amount of drug release Vs Time.

Table 3.2 General properties of tablet dosage forms

- A tablet should have elegant product identity while free of defects like chips, cracks, discoloration, and contamination
- Should have sufficient strength to withstand mechanical shock during its production, packaging, shipping and dispensing.
- Should have the chemical and physical stability to maintain its physical attributes over time.
- The tablet must be able to release the medicinal agents in predictable and reproducible manner.
- Must have a chemical stability over time so as not to follow alteration of the medicinal agents.

Manufacture of the Tablet

The tablet manufacturing involves two important steps:

- Step1: Blending of drug with excipients and;
- Step 2: Forcing tableting blend into a closed compartment (die cavity) followed by (powder or granules) compression (by punches)

In the tablet pressing process, the main guideline is to ensure that the appropriate amount of active ingredient is in each tablet. Important technical properties of powders must be controlled to ensure success of tableting operation such as, homogeneity, good flowability, good compressibility, cohesiveness, and avoidance of sticking to the die surface or punch tips. If a sufficiently homogenous mix of the components can't be obtained with simple blending processes, the ingredients must be granulated prior to compression to assure an even distribution of the active compound in the final tablet.

Two basic techniques are used to granulate powders for compression into a tablet: wet granulation and dry granulation.

Powders that can be mixed well don't require granulation and can be compressed into tablets through direct compression.

Direct Compression

This method is used when the ingredients can be blended and placed in a tablet press to make a tablet without any of the ingredients having to be pre-processed. This requires the active ingredient(s) to have appropriate physical and chemical properties, such as good compatibility and low stickiness. Direct compression is often preferred because of its simplicity and relatively low cost, but may not always be technically feasible. Granulation is the process of combining particles together by creating bonds between them. There are several different methods of granulation. The most popular, which is used by over 70% of formulation in tablet manufacture is wet granulation. Dry granulation is another method used to form granules.

Wet Granulation

Wet granulation is a process of using a liquid binder to lightly agglomerate the powder mixture. The amount of liquid has to be properly controlled, as over-wetting will cause the granules to be too hard and under-wetting will cause them to be too soft and friable. Aqueous solutions have the advantage of being safer to deal with than solvent based systems.

Procedure

- Step 1: The active ingredient and excipients are weighed and mixed.
- Step 2: The wet granulate is prepared by adding the liquid binder/adhesive to the powder blend and mixing thoroughly. Examples of binders/adhesives include aqueous preparations of cornstarch, natural gums such as acacia, and cellulose derivatives such as methyl cellulose, gelatin, and povidone.
- Step 3: Screening the damp mass through a mesh to form pellets or granules.
- Step 4: Drying the granulation. A conventional tray-dryer or fluid-bed dryer are most commonly used.
- Step 5: After the granules are dried, they are passed through a screen of smaller size than the one used for the wet mass to create granules of uniform size.

Low shear wet granulation processes use very simple mixing equipment, and can take a considerable time to achieve a uniformly mixed state. High shear wet granulation processes use equipment that mixes the powder and liquid at a very fast rate, and thus speeds up the manufacturing process. Fluid bed granulation is a multiple step wet granulation process performed in the same vessel to pre-heat, granulate, and dry the powders. It is used because it allows close control of the granulation process.

Dry Granulation

Dry granulation processes create granules by light compaction of the powder blend under low pressures. The compacts so-formed are broken up gently to produce granules (agglomerates). This process is often used when the product to be granulated is sensitive to moisture and heat. Dry granulation can be conducted on a tablet press using slugging tooling or on a roll press called a roller compactor. Dry granulation equipment offers a wide range of pressures to attain proper densification and granule formation. Dry granulation is simpler than wet granulation, therefore the cost is reduced. However, dry granulation often produces a higher percentage of fine granules, which can compromise the quality or create yield problems for the tablet. Dry granulation requires drugs or excipients with cohesive properties, and a 'dry binder' may need to be added to the formulation to facilitate the formation of granules. The detailed processing of direct compression, dry granulation and wet granulation is shown in Fig. 3.2

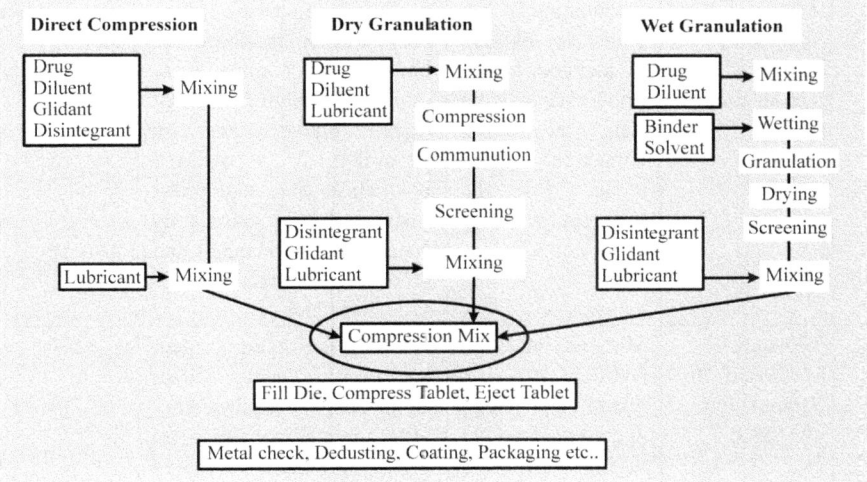

Fig. 3.2 Processing of direct compression, dry granulation and wet granulation.

Recently many advanced granulation techniques have been developed to prepare better quality granules with time and cost effectiveness as compared to conventional techniques (Table 3.3).

Table 3.3 Advanced techniques in Granulation

Technique	Description	Advantages	Limitations
Steam Granulation	Modification of wet granulation; steam is used as a binder in place of water	Higher distribution uniformity, higher diffusion rate into powders, more favourable thermal balance during drying step, more spherical granules with large surface area hence show increased dissolution rate of the drug from granules, shorter processing time so tableting speed in higher for each batch, environmentally friendly (instead of organic solvent water vapour is used, no health hazards to operators, compliance to regulatory guidelines like ICH for presence of trace.	unsuitable for thermolabile drugs; special equipment needed; unsuitable for binders which need water and not the water vapour for activation.
Melt Granulation / Thermoplastic Granulation	Granulation is done by addition of meltable binder (binder is in solid state at room temperature but melts in the temperature range of 50 – 80°C).	no need of drying phase (since dried granules are obtained by cooling it to room temperature); need of liquid binder can be controlled; reduced production and equipment costs; useful for granulating water sensitive material and producing SR granulation or solid dispersion	not suitable for thermolabile substances
Moisture Activated Dry Granulation (MADG)	Minimal moisture addition, distribution and agglomeration. No drying step is required. Water distribution is via high shear mixer, or low-shear mixer with highly atomized water spray	Tablets show better content uniformity than direct compression; require very little granulating fluid; no drying required; prepared granules show excellent flowability and uniformity, and can be used for controlled release tablets.	-

Table 3.3 *contd...*

Technique	Description	Advantages	Limitations
Moist Granulation Technique (MGT)	Works on the principle of MADG. A small amount granulating fluid is added to activate dry binder and to facilitate agglomeration. Then a moisture absorbing material likeMicrocrystalline Cellulose (MCC) is added to absorb any excess moisture.	All advantages as mentioned in MADG; addition of MCC helps to skip the drying step; for developing a controlled release formulation	-
Thermal Adhesion Granulation Process (TAGP)	Used for preparing direct tableting; performed under low moisture content or low content of pharmaceutically acceptable solvent by subjecting a mixture containing excipients to heating at a temperature in the range from about 30°C to 130°C in a closed system under mixing by tumble rotation until the formation of granules.	Less water or solvent used than that of traditional wet granulation; granules show good flow properties and binding capacity to form tablets of low friability, adequate hardness and have a high uptake capacity for active substances whose tableting is poor.	-
Foam Granulation	Liquid binders are added as aqueous foam.	Requires less binder and water than wet Granulation; no adverse effects on granulate, tablet, or drug dissolution; no plugging problems (due to no use of spray nozzles); less binder required for Immediate Release; no overwetting; suitable for water sensitive formulations' granulation; reduced drying and	-

Table 3.3 *contd...*

Technique	Description	Advantages	Limitations
		manufacturing time; uniform distribution of binder throughout the powder bed	
Extrusion-spheronization (ES)	Extrusion (forming a raw material into a product of uniform shape and density by forming it through an orifice or die under controlled conditions) followed by spheronization (a rapid and flexible process where wet extruded mass is converted to small spheres) through multi step processing	Relatively dense; uniform size and shape; Optimum flow and handling characteristics; More reproducible packing into small containers; Minimum surface area to volume ratio; Easy mixing of non-compatible products; Elimination of dust; Improved hardness and friability; useful for making dense granules for controlled-release solid oral dosage forms with a minimum amount of excipients;	high pressure can generate excessive friction and heat; not suitable for thermolabile products; Cleaning of the granulating system set up is troublesome; expensive set up.
Continuous twin screw wet granulation (cTSWG)	Advanced technique of ES; Preblend of crystalline poorly soluble API and amorphous polymer is charged into Twin screw granulator	Continuous process; Cost effective, space saving, easy scale up, less granulation liquid required; dry sieving required only; better control on size and porosity of granules; Improvement in compressibility, flow ability, wettability and homogeneity over mixer granulation and roller compaction	Cleaning is critical, charges and heat problem still be there.

Tablet Manufacturing

Tablets are prepared by forcing particles (drug and excipients) into a closed compartment (die cavity) followed by (powder or granules) compression (by punches), to allow the particles to cohere into a porous solid mass (tablet).

Tablet machine

A standard tablet compression machines consist of following components (Fig. 3.3)

- **Hopper**: for storing the material for compressing.

- **Feed frame**: for distributing the materials into the dies.
- **Dies**: for controlling the size and the shape of the tablet.
- **Punches**: for compressing the materials within the dies.

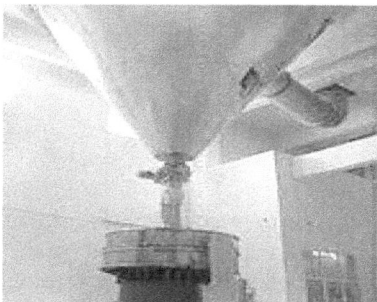

Hopper

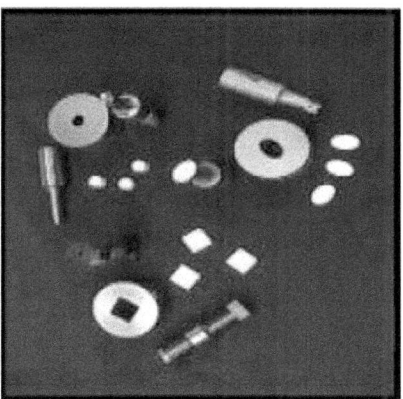

Dies: for controlling the size and the
shape of the tablet

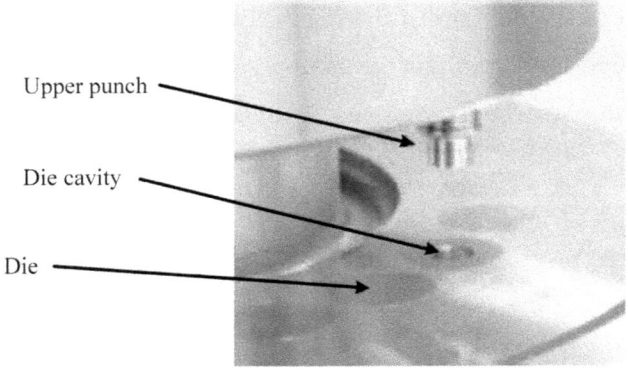

Fig. 3.3 Schematic diagram of hopper, dies and upper punch.

A tablet compression machine compresses a powder in the dies and ejects them in the form of tablets (Fig. 3.4). The basic steps in compaction cycle are given in Table 3.4. The tablet presses may be of various types (Table 3.5).

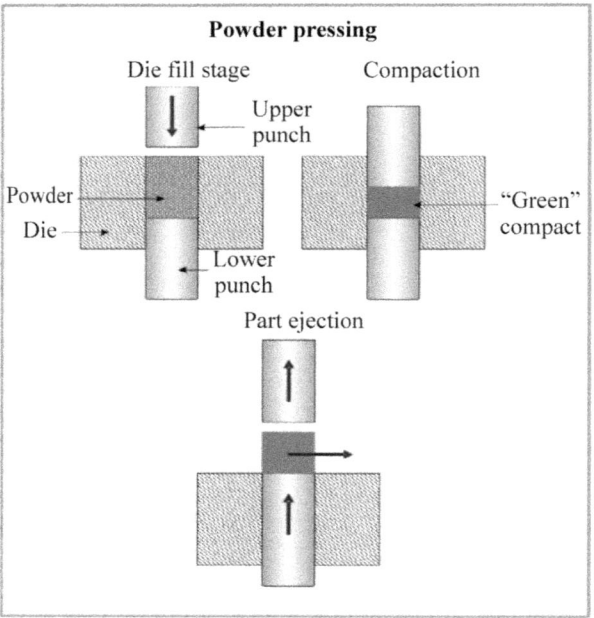

Fig. 3.4 Compaction cycle of tablet compression machines.

Table 3.4 Stages in tablet formation "Compaction cycle"

- Die filling
- Fill weight adjustment
- Tablet compaction

.

- Tablet ejection.

Die Filling

Flow of powder (or granules) of the drug and excipients from a hopper into the die. N.B. the die is closed at its lower end by the lower punch.

Fill weight adjustment

Using vibration fill weight adjustment

Compaction

The upper punch descends powder is compressed until a tablet is formed.

N.B. lower punch may be stationary or moving upward in the die. After maximum applied force is reached, the upper punch leaves the die by moving upward.

Tablet ejection

The lower punch rises up until its tip reaches the die top. The tablet is subsequently removed by a pushing device.

Table 3.5 Types of tablet press

They differ in their rate of production
- Single-punch press: It is composed of one die and one pair of punches (up to 100 tab/ min).
- Rotary tablet press: It contains ≥ 60 dies (10,000 Tabet/min).
- Hydraulic press: For research work (computerized).

Tablet Compaction

Tablet formation is one of the most complex process which involves the volume reduction of a blend of particles/granules (compression) followed by consolidation (into a defined solid dosage form/ tablet). For volume reduction granules/powder is placed in a die and then a set of punches reduce the volume by pressing the powder. A typical complete tablet manufacturing cycle consists of the four steps: (I) Die filling, (ii) fill weight adjustment, (iii) Tablet compaction and (iv) Tablet ejection (from the die). The process of compaction can be described by a set of events or phases (Fig. 3.5). The initial volume reduction of particles leads to their rearrangement which in turn results into a closer packing structure.

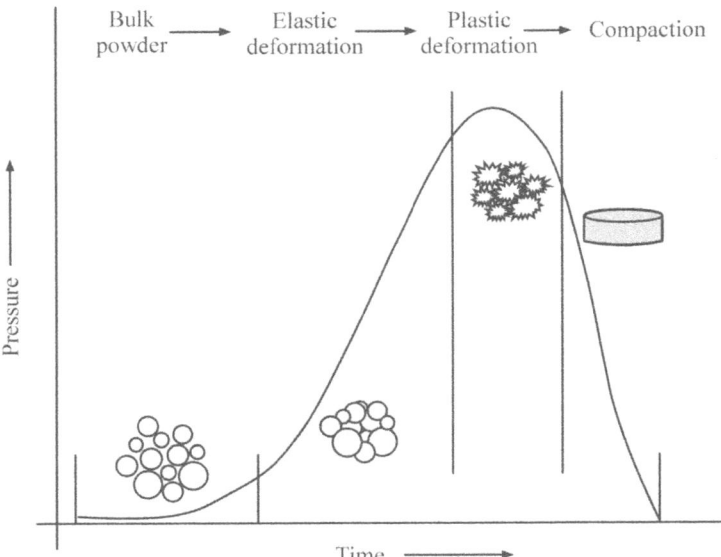

Fig. 3.5 Punch and die stress vs. time

The particle rearrangement occurs only upto a certain point where the packing characteristics of the particles and interparticulale friction does not allow further rearrangement. The further reduction beyond this point in compact volume results in the elastic (reversible), viscoelastic and plastic (irreversible) deformation of the particles. Apart from these, particle fragmentation (or breakage) results into smaller particles. This again contributes in further decrease of the compact volume. The smaller particles formed by fragmentation can undergo deformation when the volume is further reduced. These processes finally lead to the formation of interparticulate bonds because the particles' surfaces are brought closer to each other (by the overall effect of these processes). These bonds may later break. which facilitates further compression. Overall, the process of compaction of a powder include following steps:

1. Particle rearrangement
2. Elastic, viscoelastic and plastic deformation of particles
3. Fragmentation of particles
4. Formation of interparticulatc bonds

Materials like sodium chloride, starch, and microcrystalline cellulose (MCC) consolidate by predominantly plastic deformation. On the other hand, materials like sucrose, crystalline lactose and Encompress undergo fragmenting. However, all materials possess some degree of elastic, viscoelastic, plastic, and brittle characteristics. Factors like temperature and compaction rate govern the predominate type of volume reduction mechanism for a specific material. In general, the condition of lower temperature and faster loading during compression is expected to promote consolidation by fragmentation.

The type of bonds during tablet formation may be of following types:

1. Mechanical interlocking (between irregularly shaped particles)
2. Interparticulate attraction force s (e.g., intermolecular force s, such as Van der Waal forces. electrostatic forces. and hydrogen bonding)
3. Solid bridges (due to melting)

In tableting, compact formation occurs due to interparticulate attraction that arises in part from intermolecular bonding forces that act over very short distances. As the powder bed is consolidated and the particles start to deform around each other, this leads to a mechanical interlocking of the particles and this also increases the number of contact points between the particles. The dominant interaction force between solid surfaces in the Van der Waals force of attraction and hydrogen bonding may occur intra and inrermolecularly.

The bulk volume reduction during compression/compaction is a complex process involving several events: (I) transitional repacking/filling the voids between granules, (ii) deformation at contact points, (iii) fragmentation and/or plastic deformation of granules, (iv) filling of voids between primary particles (v) fragmentation and/or plastic deformation of primary particles, and (vi) bonding/formation of a compact.

Athy-Heckel Equation in analysis of compaction

The Heckel equation is among the most popular methods used in pharmaceutical research to determine the volume reduction mechanism during compression. It is based on the assumption that powder compression follows first-order kinetics; with the interparticulate voids as the reactants and the densification of the powder as the product.

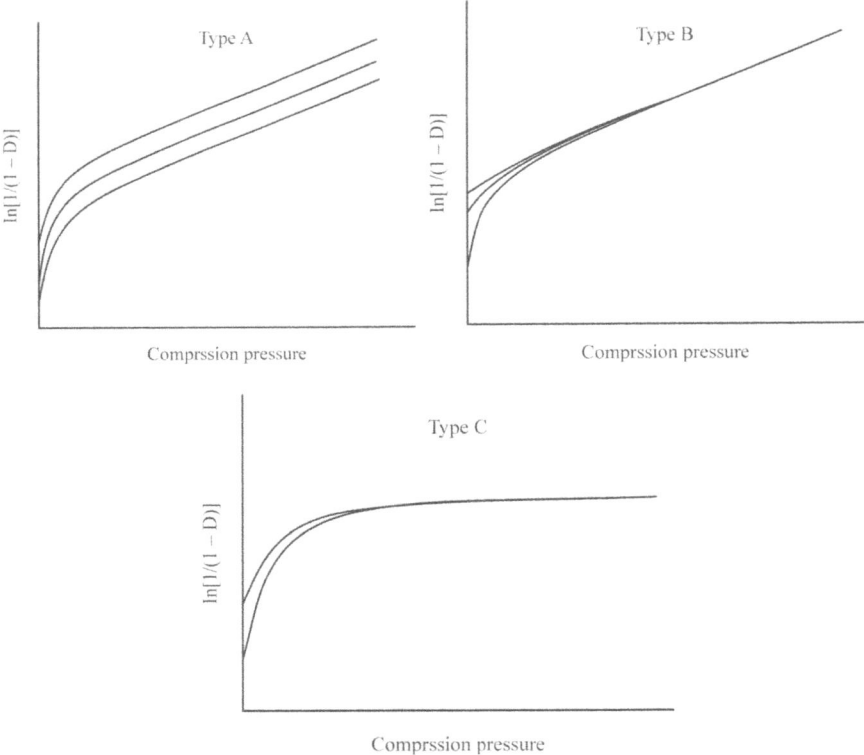

Fig. 3.6 Three phases of particle deformation shown by a typical Heckel plot (adapted from Augsburger LL, Hoag SW (Eds), Pharmaceutical Dosage Forms: Tablets, Volume 1, III Edn, Informa healthcare, 2008)

According to the relationship, the degree of compact densification with increasing compression pressure is directly proportional to the porosity. The main utility of Heckel plots arises from their ability to identify the predominant deformation behavior of the material. The relationship is mostly used to distinguish between substances that consolidate by fragmentation and those that consolidate by plastic deformation.

Empirical evidence shows that materials with low mean yield pressures undergo plastic deformation, whereas, tableting materials with high mean yield pressure have a tendency to be brittle and consolidate via fragmentation. Based on Heckel plots and the compaction behavior of materials can be classified into three types, A (MCC, corn starch, maize starch), B (lactose and di calcium phosphate), and C (Fig. 3.6).

Inspite of several criticism Heckel relationship is still the most common method of studying the compression behavior of pharmaceutical powders/granules in R&D and F&D of pharmaceutical solids. Other compaction analyses include Kawakita equation, mechanical analysis, 3D viscoelastic analysis, Hiestand tableting indices etc.

Tablet Excipients

An excipient is an inactive substance used as a carrier for the active ingredients of a medication. In addition to the drug, tablets contain a number of inert materials, known as additives or excipients. The selection of excipients is done on the basis nature of drug, nature of other excipients, compatibility with drug and other excipients and the desired release or performance characteristics of tablet (Table 3.6). They are classified according to the part they play in the finished tablet.

1. ***The Primary group*** contains excipients that help in imparting satisfactory compression characteristics to the formulation. These include; diluents, binders, glidants and lubricants.

2. ***The secondary group*** helps to give additional desirable physical characteristics to the finished tablet. These include; disintegrants, coloring, flavoring and sweetening agents.

   - *Filler (or diluent)*: Diluent adds bulk to make the tablet with practical size for compression and to be easily handled. Tablets weigh normally at least 50 mg, therefore a low dose of a potent drugs (e.g. Dexamethasone 0.5 mg/Tablet, Levothyroid Tablet 0.05 mg/Tablet) requires addition of a filler to increase the bulk volume of the powder and hence the size of the tablet. Examples of Diluents are Glucose (hygroscopic, reducing sugar), Sodium chloride (freely soluble, used in solution tablets), Sucrose (hygroscopic, sweet taste), Mannitol (chewable tablet, freely soluble in water, cool taste), Microcrystaline Cellulose (excellent compression property, highly stable and disintegrating property).

   - *Binder:* A binder, is added to hold the tablet together after it has been compressed, stopping it from breaking down into its separate ingredients. The binders most commonly used are from natural sources e.g. Aacacia mucilage, Glucose, Gelatin, providone (PVP), Starch mucilage.

- *Disintegrant*: Disintegrants, such as starch help the tablet to break down into small fragments, when it is ingested. This helps the medicine to dissolve and be taken up by the body so that it can act more quickly.
- *Glidant*: The glidants improve the flowability of the tablet granules or powder by reducing the friction between particles, preventing formation of lumps e.g. Talc, Corn starch, Colloids silicates.
- *Antiadherent*: The antiadherents stop the powder from sticking to the equipment as the tablet is being made. Exp- Talc, Magnesium stearate, Starch derivatives
- *Lubricant*: Lubricants ensure that the tablet has a smooth surface. They reduce the friction occurs between the walls of the tablets and the walls of the die cavity when the tablet is ejected e.g. Talc, Steric acid, magnesium stearate
- *Flavor*: Flavoring agents help to make the tablet taste better.
- *Colorant*: Colors are added to help you to recognize your tablet and to make it easier to take your medicine correctly.

Table 3.6 Selection of diluents

Based on the experience of the manufacturer as well as on the cost of the diluent and its compatibility with the other tablet ingredients, the proper diluent could be chosen. • Calcium salts can not be used as fillers for Tetracycline products because calcium interferes with the absorption of Tetracycline from GIT. • When drug shows low water solubility, it is recommended that water soluble diluents be used to avoid possible bioavailability problems. • The combination of amine bases and salts with Lactose in presence of alkaline lubricant results in discoloration upon ageing.

Tablet Defects

Tablet manufacturing is a complex process which needs the optimization of each sub process and in-process quality control measures for producing a defect free tablet batch. From mixing of drug and excipients for preparing tablet blend to compression of the blend in tablet press many elements are critical and if they are not taken care of various defects occur in tablets. Fig. 3.7 and Table 3.7 provide various kinds of tablet defects along with their causes and remedies.

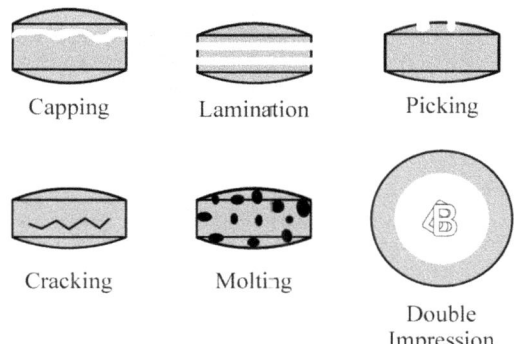

Fig. 3.7 Tablet defects

Table 3.7 Causes and remedies of tablet defects

Tablet Defect	Causes	Remedy
Capping Partial or complete separation of top or bottom crowns of a tablet from the main body of tablet **Lamination** Separation of tablet in two or more distinct layers	• Air entrapment in the granules • Rapid decompression • Deep concave punches • Use of too dry granulation tends to cap or laminate for lack of cohesion • Incorrect setup at the press	• **Precompression-** Slowing the rate of tableting or reducing the final compression pressure. • Use of flat punches • Maintenance of optimum moisture in the processing of granulation • Use of special durable dies with tungsten carbide insert
Picking Surface materials from a tablet that is sticking to the punch and being removed from the tablet surface is *picking*. **Sticking** It refers to tablet materials adhering to the die wall.	• Adhesion of materials to the punch faces • Over-wetting the tablets, by under-drying, or by poor tablet quality. • Tablet material sticking to the punch tips with engraving or embossing	• Use of large lettering on punches with small diameters • Reformulation of tablets to large size • Plating of the punch faces with chromium • Addition of colloidal silica to the granules as polishing agents • Use of more or new binder to increase cohesiveness of tablets • Addition of more high melting point lubricants/ reduction of low m.p. lubricants

Table 3.7 *contd...*

86   Essentials of Pharmaceutical Technology

Tablet Defect	Causes	Remedy
Mottling It is an unequal distribution of colors on a tablet with light and dark areas on tablet surface.	• Use of a drug whose color differs from tablet excipients • Use of a drug whose dehydration products are colored • Migration of dyes to the surface of a granulation during drying	• Changing the Solvent system • Reduction of drying temperature • Dispersing a dry color additive during powder binding steps.
Weight Variation Variation of tablet weight beyond the acceptable limits	• Non uniform granule size and size distribution • Poor Flow through the feed frame • Punch variation • Poor design of the granulation hopper • Poor mixing	• Addition or increase of a glidant like talcum, colloidal silica. • Use of vibrators attached to the hopper • Use of well-designed hopper
Double Impression Faulty engraving by punches with monogram or engraving	• Slight rotation of punch after precompression	• using non-rotating cam track

Evaluation of Tablets

Various official and un-official tests for evaluation of tablets are mentioned in Table 3.8.

Tablet 3.8 Evaluation of tablets

Official test
• Dissolution
• Content uniformity (weight variation)
• Disintegration
Unofficial test
• Mechanical strength
   • Tensile strength
   • Friability Test for Tablets
• Tablet size and shape
• Thickness
• Average weight

Dissolution

The dissolution test measures the amount of time required for certain percentage of the drug substance in a tablet to go into solution under a specified set of conditions. It describes a step towards physiological availability of the drug substance, but it is not designed to measure the safety or efficacy of the tablet being tested. It provides *in vitro* control procedure to eliminate variation among production batches. The dissolution medium must be aqueous and the pH of the medium should be controlled and should simulate *in vivo* conditions. The dissolution medium should be 0.1M HCl and pH 6.8 buffer to simulate the biological extremes. The possible role of bile salts in absorption of highly insoluble drugs suggests the inclusion of physiological concentrations of sodium taurocholate in the mildly acid or alkaline media. Studies have shown that low agitation must be used (i.e. in the order of 50 rpm) and that the tablet must not be subjected to abrasion in keeping with the mild agitation in the gastrointestinal tract.

Dissolution Test (U.S.P.)

Two main set of apparatus are official in USP and IP for dissolution testing of tablets. However there are total five dissolution apparatus official in USP (See Chapter of Dissolution testing).

Apparatus-1: A single tablet is placed in a small wire mesh basket attached to the bottom of the shaft connected to a variable speed motor. The basket is immersed in a dissolution medium (as specified in monograph) contained in a 100 ml flask. The flask is cylindrical with a hemispherical bottom. The flask is maintained at $37 \pm 0.5\ ^0C$ by a constant temperature bath. The motor is adjusted to turn at the specified speed and sample of the fluid are withdrawn at intervals to determine the amount of drug in solutions.

Apparatus-2: It is same as apparatus-1, except the basket is replaced by a paddle. The dosage form is allowed to sink to the bottom of the flask before stirring. For dissolution test U.S.P. specifies the dissolution test medium and volume, type of apparatus to be used, rpm of the shaft, time limit of the test and assay procedure for. The test tolerance is expressed as a % of the labeled amount of drug dissolved in the time limit.

Dissolution testing and Interpretation can be done in three stages:

Stage 1: Six tablets are tested and are acceptable if all of the tablets are not less than the monograph tolerance limit (Q) plus 5% if fail

Stage 2: Another six tablets are tested. The tablets are acceptable

Take 6 tablets, test individually, Avg. weight 12 tablets is greater or equal to but no one less than (Q-15) %

If the average of the twelve is greater than or equal to Q and no unit is less than (Q-15) % if fail

Stage 3: Another 12 tablets are tested. The tablets are acceptable if the average of all 24 tablets is greater than or equal to Q and if no more than 2 tablets are less than (Q-15) %

Content Uniformity (Weight Variation)

The content uniformity test is used to ensure that every tablet contains the amount of drug substance intended with little variation among tablets within a batch. The content uniformity test has been included in the monographs of all coated and uncoated tablets and all capsules intended for oral administration with the size range of the dosage form 50 mg or smaller sizes. Tablet monographs with a content uniformity requirement do not have weight variation requirements. For content uniformity test, representative samples of 30 tablets are selected and 10 are assayed individually. At least 9 must assay within ±15% of the declared potency and none may exceed ± 25%.

Tablet Disintegration

For a drug to be absorbed from a solid dosage form after oral administration, it must first be in solution, and the first important step toward this condition is usually the break-up of the tablet; a process known as disintegration. The disintegration test is a measure of the time required under a given set of conditions for a group of tablets to disintegrate into particles which will pass through a 10 mesh screen. Generally, the test is useful as a quality assurance tool for conventional dosage forms. The disintegration test is carried out using the disintegration tester which consists of a basket rack holding 6 plastic tubes, open at the top and bottom, the bottom of the tube is covered by a 10-mesh screen. The basket is immersed in a bath of suitable liquid held at 37 °C, preferably in a 1 L beaker. For compressed uncoated tablets, the testing fluid is usually water at 37 ° C but some monographs direct that simulated gastric fluid be used. If one or two tablets fail to disintegrate, the test is repeated using 12 tablets. For most uncoated tablets, the BP requires that the tablets disintegrate in 15 minutes (although it varies for some uncoated tablets) while for coated tablets, up to 2 hours may be required. The individual drug monographs specify the time disintegration must occur to meet the Pharmacopoeial standards.

Mechanical Strength of Tablets (Hardness)

The mechanical strength of a tablet provides a measure of the bonding potential of the material concerned and this information is useful in the selection of excipients. An excessively strong bond may prevent rapid disintegration and subsequent dissolution of a drug. Weak bonding characteristics may limit the selection and/or proportion of excipients, such as lubricants, that would be added to the formulation.

The mechanical properties of pharmaceutical tablets are quantifiable by the friability, hardness or crushing strength, crushing strength-friability values, tensile strength and brittle fracture Index.

Friability Test for Tablets

Friction and shock are the forces that most often cause tablets to chip, cap or break. The **friability test** is closely related to tablet hardness and is designed to evaluate the ability of the tablet to withstand abrasion in packaging, handling and shipping. It is usually measured by the use of the Roche friabilator. A number of tablets are weighed and placed in the apparatus where they are exposed to rolling and repeated shocks as they fall 6 inches in each turn within the apparatus. After four minutes of this treatment or 100 revolutions, the tablets are weighed and the weight compared with the initial weight. The loss due to abrasion is a measure of the tablet friability. The value is expressed as a percentage. A maximum weight loss of not more than 1% of the weight of the tablets being tested during the friability test is considered generally acceptable and any broken or smashed tablets are not picked up. Normally, when capping occurs, friability values are not calculated.

Tensile Strength

A non-compendial method of measuring the mechanical strength of tablets that is now widely used is the tensile strength. This is the force required to break a tablet in a diametral compression test. The radial tensile strength, T, of the tablets can be calculated from the equation:

$$T = 2F / p d H \quad \ldots\ldots(1)$$

where F is the load needed to break the tablet, and d and H are the diameter and thickness respectively. Several precautions must be taken when using the equation. Various factors e.g. test conditions, deformation properties of the material, adhesion conditions between compact and its support and tablet shape may influence the measurements of the tensile strength.

Some authors have suggested the determination of axial tensile strength because of the sensitivity of the radial tensile strength measurements to crack propagation variations. The axial tensile strength (T_x) can be calculated from the following relationship:

$$T_x = 4F/pd^2 \qquad \ldots\ldots(2)$$

Tensile strength has been used in combination with indentation hardness to evaluate tableting performance of materials. The indentation hardness is a time-dependent property used to measure the plastic yield of a material. It can be determined by either static methods (e.g. the Brinell, Vickers and Rockwell hardness tests) or the dynamic methods. The static indentation methods involve the formation of a permanent indentation on the surface of the material tested and the hardness is determined by means of the load applied and the size of the indentation formed. In the dynamic indentation tests, either a pendulum is allowed to strike from a known distance or an indenter is allowed to fall under gravity unto the surface of the test material. The hardness is then determined from the rebound height of the pendulum or the volume of the resulting indentation. Using an apparatus consisting of a steel sphere pendulum acting as an indenter, estimated the hardness (i. e. the mean deformation pressure) of compacted materials by dividing the energy consumed during the impact by the volume of indentation.

Tablets Size and Shape

The shape and dimensions of compressed tablets are determined by the type of tooling during the compression process. At a constant compressive load, tablets thickness varies with changes in die fill, particle size distribution and packing of the powder mix being compressed and with tablet weight, while with a constant die fill, thickness varies with variation in compressive load.

Thickness

The thickness of individual tablets may be measured with a micrometer, which permits accurate measurements and provides information of the variation between tablets. Tablet thickness should be controlled within a ±5% variation of a standard value. Any variation in thickness within a particular lot of tablets or between manufacturer's lots should not be apparent to the unaided eye for consumer acceptance of the product. In addition, thickness must be controlled to facilitate packaging.

Average Weight

The physical dimensions of the tablet along with the density of the material in the tablet formulation and their proportions, determine the weight of the tablet. The USP has provided limits for the average weight of uncoated compressed tablets. These are applicable when the tablet contains 50 mg or more of the drug substance or when the latter comprises 50% or more, by weight of the dosage form. Twenty tablets are weighed individually and the average weight is calculated. The individual tablet weights are then compared to the average weight. Not more than two of the tablets must differ from the average weight by not more than the percentages stated in Table 3.9. No tablet must differ by more than double the relevant percentage. Tablets that are coated are exempted from these requirements but must conform to the test for content uniformity if applicable.

Table 3.9 Weight variation requirements

Average weight	Permissible Percent Difference
130 mg or less	10
More than 130 mg through 324 mg	7.5
More than 324 mg	5

Tablet Coating

Many a times tablets are prepared as coated tablets. Various different kinds of tablet coating are done for various purposes. The main purposes of coating are given as below.

- Protection of the drug from the surrounding (environment) (air, light and moisture) and thus improve stability.
- Modifying drug release, as in enteric coating and extended-release formulation.
- Masking unpleasant taste or odour of the drug.
- Improving product appearance and helping in brand identification.
- Facilitating rapid identification by the manufacturer, the pharmacist and the patient (mostly colored).
- Increasing the mechanical strength of the product.
- Masking batch differences in the appearance of raw materials.

Types of Tablet Coating Processes

Tablet coatings are of following types (Table 3.9).

Table 3.10 Types of tablet coating processes

- **Film coating:** The most popular today. It involves the deposition, usually by spraying method, of a thin uniform film of a polymer formulation surrounding a tablet.
- **Sugar coating:** It involves successive application of sucrose-based coating formulations to tablet cores, in suitable coating equipment. Water evaporates from the syrup leaving a thick sugar layer around each tablet. Sugar coats are often shiny and highly colored.
- **Compression coating** (less popular)
  Although less popular, it gained increased interest in the recent years for creating modified-released products. It involves the compaction of granular materials around a preformed tablet core using specially designed tableting equipment. Compression coating is a dry process.
- **Gelatin-coated tablets** e.g. Gelcap, is a capsule shaped compressed tablet coated with gelatin layer.

Film Coating

It involves the deposition, usually by spraying method, of a thin uniform film of a polymer formulation surrounding a tablet. Film coating provides an alternative means of masking the taste of the medicament and providing protection against adverse climatic conditions without significantly altering the tablet weight or size. Film coatings are a mixture of solids and liquids. For many years, the liquid component of coatings was a volatile solvent, such as alcohol or other quick-drying substances like methylene chloride. While solvent-based coatings performed well in many respects, they presented problems in handling, operator safety, recovery, and odor. They could even make the finished tablets smell like solvent, which is not a desirable side effect. Solvent-based coatings are still used in some applications, but water based, or aqueous, coatings have largely replaced them.

Types of Film Coating

1. *Immediate-release (non-functional) film coating*: They do not affect the biopharmaceutical properties of the tablet. They are readily soluble in water.

2. *Modified-release (functional) film coating*: They allow the drug to be delivered in a specific manner; i.e. they affect drug release behavior. Modified release film coatings are sub-classified into;

- *Delayed-release coating (enteric coating)*: Only soluble in water at pH ≥ 5-6. Intended to protect the drug from gastric acidic pH (for acid labile drugs). Used for colonic drug delivery systems.
- *Extended-release coating*: Mostly water-insoluble. Designed to ensure consistent drug release manner over a long period of time (6-12 hr) and thus decreasing dosing regimen and improving patient compliance.

Composition of Film Coating Agents

Film coating formulation/ materials are composed of Polymer, Plasticizer, Colorants, Solvent (vehicle)

Polymer: A film former capable of producing smooth thin films reproducible under the prescribed coating conditions (Table 3.11).

Plasticizer: Affords flexibility and elasticity to the coat and thus provide durability. Examples; Polyethylene glycol (PEG), Polypropylene glycol and coconut oil.

Colorants: Provides an elegant appearance. Ex. Iron oxide pigment, Titanium dioxide and Aluminum lakes.

Solvent (vehicle): Volatile organic solvents may be used to allow good spreadability of the coat components over the tablet and allowing rapid evaporation, but they are expensive and show environmental hazards and solvent residue in the formulation must be investigated (certain limit). Aqueous vehicles are safer, but they show slower evaporation and may affect drug stability.

Table 3.11 Polymers for film coating

Immediate-release coating polymers	Modified-release coating polymers Sugar coating	
	Extended-release coating polymers	Enteric-coating polymers
	They are dissolved in organic solvent or dispersed in aqueous medium	

Table 3.11 Contd...

Immediate-release coating polymers	Modified-release coating polymers Sugar coating	
	Extended-release coating polymers	Enteric-coating polymers
1. Cellulose derivatives: The most widely used of cellulosic polymers is HPMC	1. Cellulose derivatives: Highly substituted cellulosic ether, thus rendering the polymer water-insoluble, e.g. **Ethyl cellulose** (EC).	1. Methacrylic acid copolymers: The presence of carboxylic acid groups renders this class to be insoluble in water at low pH (stomach) but gradually becomes soluble as the pH rises towards neutrality (upper part of the small intestine).
2. Vinyl derivatives: PVP, it has a limited use in film coating because of its inherent tackiness. A copolymer of PVP and vinyl acetate forms better films.		2. Phthalate esters: e.g. Cellulose acetate phthalate (CAP).

Film Coating Equipment

It is possible to use the conventional "coating-pan" and "fluid-bed coating equipment". This procedure involves spraying of the coating liquid (solution or suspension) onto the rotating tablets (in the coating-pan), or tablets held in suspension by column of air (in the fluid-bed coating equipment), followed by drying to remove the solvent, leaving a thin film around each tablet core.

Coating-pan

Tablet coating system combines several components: a coating pan, a spraying system, an air handling unit, a dust collector, and the controls. The tablet coating pan is used for both film coating as well as sugar coating. The coating pan is actually a perforated drum that rotates within a cabinet (Fig. 3.8). The cabinet enables to control airflow, air temperature, air pressure, and the coating application. The spraying system consists of several spray guns mounted on a manifold, a solution pump, a supply tank and mixer, and an air supply. The pump delivers the coating solution to the guns, where it combines with atomizing air to create a fine mist that is directed at the bed of tablets in the coating pan.

Tablets and Tablet Coating   95

The air handling unit heats and filters the air used to dry the coating on the tablets. Depending on the circumstances, it may include a humidifier or dehumidifier. The dust collector extracts air from the coating pan and keeps a slightly negative pressure within the cabinet. The controls enable to orchestrate the operation of all the components to achieve the desired results.

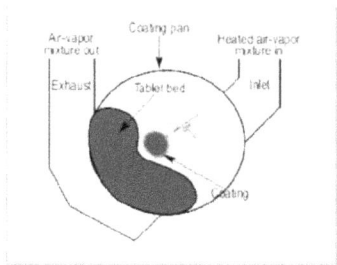 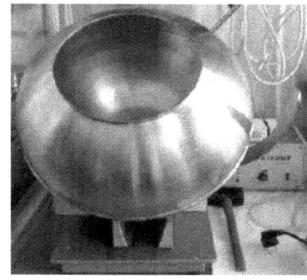

Fig. 3.8 Conventional coating-pan and its working.

Fluidized bed coating

Wurster (1959) first described the application of sugar or film coatings to tablets suspended in an air stream (Fig. 3.9). In that equipment the coating solution is introduced into the fluidizing air stream at the base of a tall vertical tube in which tablets circulate as they are coated. Evaporated solvent and air are removed at the top of the chamber. As the tablets circulate in the air stream they are subjected to considerable abrasive action and for this reason they are compressed with extra firmness on punches which give a well rounded profile.

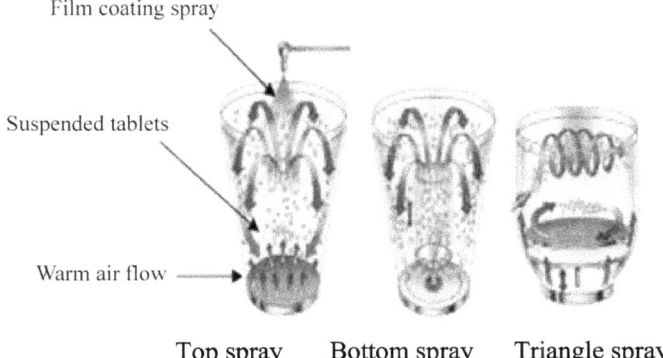

Fig. 3.9 Fluidized bed coating.

Ideal Cures Ltd. manufactures and supplies the full range of tablet film coating systems under the brand name of INSTACOAT, for normal film coating and functional coating. INSTACOAT has a wide range of products available.

It is for film coatings, hydro alcoholic film coatings, tablet-coating films, cellulose film coating systems for various pharmaceutical solid oral dosage forms.

The brief details of various film coating systems and equipments are given in Table 3.12 and 3.13.

Table 3.12 Popular film coating systems

Product	Description	Reconstitution level	Average weight gain
Instacoat Aqua	HPMC based Aqueous System	11 %	2.5 %
Instacoat Sol	HPMC based Organic Solvent System	5%	2.5%
Instacoat Universal	HPMC based Aqueous / Organic / Hydro-Alcoholic System	Aqueous 11 % Organic Solvent - 5% Hydro Alcoholic - 9%	2.5%
Instacoat Aqua -II	Grafted PVA based Aqueous System	20%	2.5%
Instacoat Aqua -III	HPMC based Aqueous System	15%	2.5%
Instacoat - P4	SA based Aqueous System	20%	2.5%
Instacoat Herbo	Customized Polymer based Aqueous/ Organic System	Aqueous 11% to 20 % Organic - 5%	5%
Instacoat Natcol	Aqueous / Organic System with Natural Colourants	Aqueous 11% to 20 % Organic - 5%	5%

Table 3.13 Equipment suitable for film coating

- Accela Cota-Manestry Machine, Liverpool, UK
- Hi-Coater-Freund Company, Japan
- Driacoater-Driam Metallprodukt GmbH, Germany
- HTF/150-GS. Italy
- IDA-Dumoulin, France

Sugar Coating

It involves successive application of sucrose-based coating formulations to tablet cores, in suitable coating equipment. Water evaporates from the syrup leaving a thick sugar layer around each tablet. Sugar coats are often shiny and highly colored. Typically, tablets are sugar coated by panning technique, using traditional rotating sugar-coating pan with a supply of drying air (thermostatically controlled). The pan is automatically rotated, allowing tablets to tumble over each other while making contact with the coating solutions which are gently poured or sprayed, portion wise onto the tablets with warm air blown to hasten drying. Each coat is applied only after the previous coat is dried (Table 3.14).

Table 3.14 Steps for sugar-coating process.

- Sealing of the tablet cores
- Subcoating
- Smoothing
- Coloring
- Polishing
- Printing

Sealing (Waterproofing)

This involves the application of one or more coats of a waterproofing substance in the form of alcoholic spray, such as pharmaceutical Shellac or synthetic polymers, such as Cellulose Acetate Pthallate (CAP). Unless a modified-release feature needs to be introduced, the amount of the sealing coat applied should be carefully calculated so that there is no negative effect on the drug release characteristics in case of immediate release product. Sugar-coatings (Table 3.15) are aqueous formulations which allow water to penetrate directly into the tablet core and thus potentially affecting product stability and possibly causing premature tablet disintegration. This step involves application of many coats of partially or completely water-insoluble polymers enables sugar-coated product to exhibit modified-release pattern (extended release or delayed "enteric"- release characteristics).

Sub coating

Large quantities of sugar-coatings are usually applied to the tablet core (typically increasing the tablet weight by 50- 100%) in order to round off the tablet edge. Much of this material build-up occurs during this stage and is achieved by adding a bulking agent such as Calcium carbonate, to the sucrose solution. Antiadherents e.g. Talc may be added after partial drying to prevent sticking of the tablets together.

Table 3.15 Constituents of coating solutions used for sugar coating

Seal coating	Sub coating	Syrup coating	Polishing solution
PEG 4000	Gelatin	Colorant	Bees wax (white)
Zein/Shellac	Acacia	Sub coating powder	Naphtha
Propylene glycol	Sugar cane powder	Cal. Carbonate	Carnauba wax(yellow)
Oleic acid	Syrup	Cane sugar powder	Paraffin wax
Alcohol	Corn syrup	Syrup	
Methylene chloride	Distilled water	Corn starch	

Smoothing

The subcoating stage results in tablets with rough surfaces. To facilitate the color application (which requires a smooth surface), subcoated tablets are smoothed out by a thick sucrose syrup coating.

Coloring

Color coatings usually consist of thin sucrose syrup containing the requisite coloring materials. (Water-soluble dyes or water-insoluble pigments may be used).

Polishing

After the coloring step, the tablet surfaces tend to be smooth but somewhat dull in appearance. To achieve glossy finish, final stage involving application of waxes (beeswax or carnuba wax) is employed.

Printing

Different tablets could be identified by manufacturer' logo, product name, dosage strength or other appropriate code. For sugar-coated tablets, such identification could be only achieved by printing process using special edible inks.

Table 3.16 gives a comparative view of film and sugar coating.

Compression-coating of tablets

Although less popular, it gained increased interest in the recent years for creating modified-released products. It involves the compaction of granular materials around a preformed tablet core using specially designed tableting equipment. Compression coating is a dry process. Mechanically, it is a complex process, as the tablet may be tilted when transferred to the second die cavity (Fig. 3.10).

The machine described by Whitehouse (1954), the Kilian Prescoter, used preformed cores which were fed into holes on the periphery of a transfer disc and deposited on the lower fill of coating granules as the lower punch dropped in readiness for the top fill. The core was centered by a light tap of the top punch, the top fill deposited and the coating bonded to the core by compression. The force developed during compaction in the presence of a core was sufficient to cause slight deflection of the overload release but failed to do so in the absence of a core. A switch connected to the overload release provided an electrical signal which, when fed to a memory unit, actuated a gate on the collection chute such that coreless tablets were rejected.

Gelatin-coated tablets

A recent innovation is the gelatin-coated tablets. The innovator product, the gelcap, is a capsule shaped compressed tablet coated with gelatin layer. This allows the coated product to be about one-third smaller than a capsule filled with an equivalent amount of powder. The gelatin coating facilitates swallowing. Gelatin coated tablets are more tamper evident than unsealed capsule.

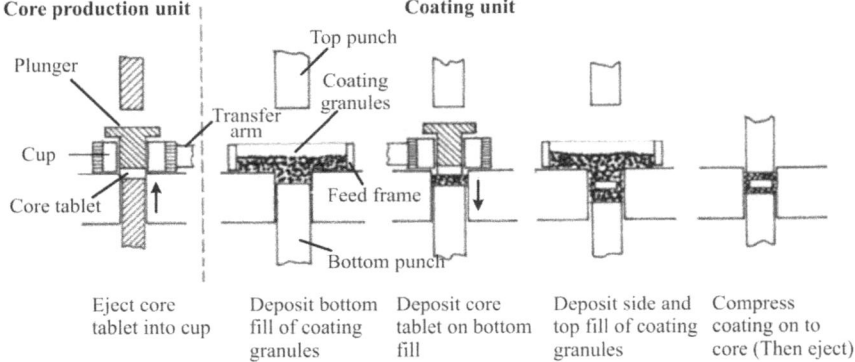

Fig. 3.10 Compression coating of tablet.

Table 3.16 Comparative features of film and sugar coatings

Features	Film coating	Sugar coating
Tablet appearance	Retains original contour usually not shiny	Rounded with high degree of polish and highly colored
Weight increase due to coating materials	2-3% (because of a thin coat).	50-100%
Logo or breaklines	Possible during tablet compression by tablet punches	Break-lines are not possible; logo is only achieved by printing.
Number of stages required	Usually single stage	Multiple stages
Typically batch coating time	1.5-2 hrs	≥ 8 hrs
Functional coating	Easily adaptable for modified-release	Mostly for immediate release tablets, unless specials treatment during the sealing stage

Bibliography

- Alderborn G. In: Aulton ME (Editor), Pharmaceutics: The science of dosage form design. 2nd Edn., 2002, Churchil Livingstone, New York, 397-430.
- Amidon GL, Lennernas H, Shah VP, Crison JR. *Pharm Res*, 1995; 12:413-420.

- Banker GS and Anderson NR, Tablets. In : *The Theory and Practice of Industrial Pharmacy*. Lachman, L., Lieberman, H. A. and Kanig, J. L. (Eds.) 3 rd Edition.,1986, Lea & Febiger, Philadelphia, pp. 301-303.
- David ST. and Augsburger, L. L. *J. Pharm. Sci.,* 1977;66: 155-159.
- Fell JT. and Newton , J. M. *J. Pharm. Sci.,* 1970;59: 688-691.
- Florence AT. and Halbert, GW. Formulation. In: Comparative medicinal chemistry: The rational design, mechanistic study and therapeutic application of chemical compound. Hansch C, Sammes PG. and Taylor J. B. (Eds), 1990, Vol. 6. 1 st Edition. Pergamon Press Plc. Oxford , UK . pp. 567-592.
- Guyot-Hermann; The disintegration and disintegrating agent; S.T.P. Pharmaceutical Science: 1992;2(6): 445-462.
- Hiestand EN. and Smith, D. P. *Powder Technol.,*1984; 38: 145-159.
- Hoag SW, Dave VS, Moolchandani V, Compression and Compaction (In); Augsburger LL, Hoag SW (Eds), Pharmaceutical Dosage Forms: Tablets, Volume 1, III Edn, Informa healthcare, 2008.
- Itiola OA. and Pilpel, N. *J. Pharm. Pharmacol.,* 1986; 38: 81-86.
- Itiola OA. and Pilpel, N. *Pharmazie,* 1996; 51: 997-998.
- Kotike MJ, Rudnik EM, In: Banker GS, Rhodes CT (Eds). Modern Pharmaceutics, 4th Edn., Marcel Dekker Inc., New York, 2005, pp- 287-334.
- Levy G, Leonards J. R. and Procknel J. A. *J. Pharm. Sci.,* 1965; 54: 1719-1722.
- Levy G. *J. Pharm. Sci.,* 1961;50: 388-392.
- Odeku OA. and Itiola OA. *Trop. J. Pharm. Res* . 2003;2 (1): 147-153.
- Siewert M., Dressman J., Brown C. K. and Shah V. P. FIP/AAPS Guidelines to Dissolution/ *in vitro* release testing of novel/special dosage forms. *AAPS PharmSciTech,* 2003; 4 (1) Article 7.

CHAPTER 4

Capsules

Introduction

Capsules are solid dosage forms in which the drug substance is enclosed in either a hard or soft soluble container or shell of a suitable form of gelatin. The medication may be a powder, a liquid or a semisolid mass.

Capsules are usually intended to be administered orally by swallowing them whole. Occasionally, capsules may be administered rectally or vaginally. Gelatin capsule shells may be hard or soft depending on their composition.

Advantages
- Neat and elegant in appearance.
- Enclosing the medication within capsule shells provides a tasteless, odourless means of administering medication.
- The ready solubility of gelatin at gastric pH provides rapid release of medication in the stomach.

- Since hard gelatin capsules may be compounded by the pharmacist, this dosage form offers physician's greater flexibility in dosages and drug combinations than is available with prefabricated medication.

Disadvantages

- Capsules are not suitable containers for liquids that dissolve gelatin, such as aqueous or hydroalcoholic solutions.
- Very soluble salts, such as bromides or iodides should not be dispensed in capsules, as the rapid release of such materials may cause gastric irritation.

Capsule Production

Capsule production involves various steps shown in Fig. 4.1. Capsule shells of different sizes are prepared in which ingredients and lubricants are filled (manually or by automatic machines) and after their uniformity test they are packed properly.

Capsule shell production

Capsule shells may be hard or soft depending on their composition.

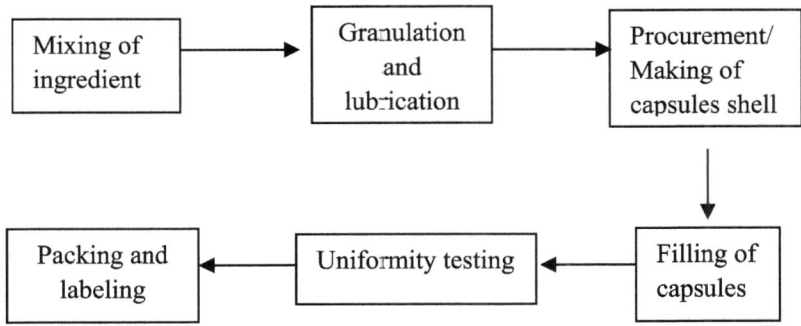

Fig. 4.1 General steps in capsule production.

Raw materials for capsule shell production

Gelatin, colorants and preservatives are used as raw materials in manufacturing of capsule shells.

- **Gelatin**

  It is the major component of the capsule. Gelatin is non-toxic; soluble in biological fluids at body temperature, and it is a good film-forming material. Solutions of high concentration, 40% w/v, are mobile at 50°C as compare to other polymers like agar.

  There are two main types of gelatin:

  Type A: produced by acid hydrolysis of animal skins.

  Type B: produced by basic hydrolysis of bovine bones.

  The two types can be differentiated by their isoelectric points (7.0 – 9.0 for type A and 4.8-5.0 for type B) and by their viscosity and film forming characteristics.

- **Colorants**

  Two types of colorants are used: water soluble dyes (e.g. erythrosine) and pigments (e.g. iron oxides, titanium dioxide)

- **Preservatives**

  When preservatives are employed, parabens are often selected

Hard gelatin capsules

The hard gelatin capsule has been conventionally used as a dosage form for prescription and over the counter (OTC) drugs and herbal products, which are formulated either as powder or pellets. This has considerably expanded the range of possible formulations utilizing hard gelatin capsules as a simple dosage form for oral drug delivery. It consists of two pieces in the form of cylinders: the shorter piece "cap" and the longer piece "body". The shells consist largely of gelatin, sugar and water.

Capsule shell manufacturing machines

Construction: The manufacturing machines consist of two parts, which are mirror images of each other: on one half the capsule cap is made and on the other the capsule body. The moulds 'pins', are made up of stainless steel and are mounted in sets on metal strips, called 'bars'. There are approximately 40000 mould pins per machine.

Working: Steps involved in manufacturing are as followed (Fig. 4.2).

- The prepared gelatin solution is transferred to a heated holding hopper on the manufacturing machine.
- The level of solution is maintained automatically by a feed from the holding hopper.
- Capsules are formed by dipping sets of moulds, which are at room temperature, 22°C, into this solution.
- A film is formed on the surface of each mould by gelling.
- The moulds are slowly withdrawn from the solution and then rotated during their transfer to the upper level of the machine, in order to form a film of uniform thickness.
- Groups of 'pin bars' are then passed through a series of drying kilns (ovens), in which large volumes of controlled humidity air are blown over them.
- The dried films are removed from the moulds, cut to the correct length, the two parts joined together and the complete capsule delivered from the machine.
- The mould pins are then cleaned and lubricated for the start of the next cycle.

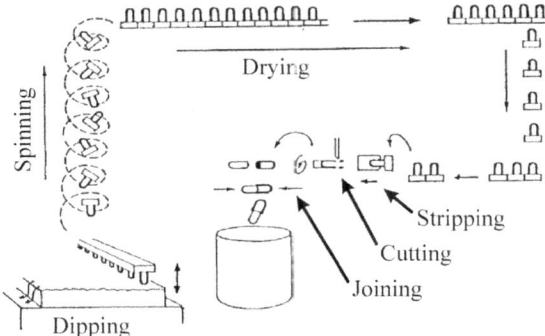

Fig. 4.2 The sequence of two-piece hard gelatin capsule shell manufacture.

Capsule Shell Filling

Capsule shell is typically filled with dry solids (powders, granules, pellets, tablets) and semisolids. Fixed oils and other liquids that do not dissolve gelatin may be filled into hard gelatin capsules with a pipette or calibrated dropper, and then capsules are sealed by moisturizing the lower part of the caps with water. Liquids may often be sorbed onto inert carrier powders to form dry powders suitable for capsule filling.

Methods of Filling Capsules

Capsule filling is done either manually (Fig. 4.3) or by automated operations (industrial method of filling).

- **Manual Filling**

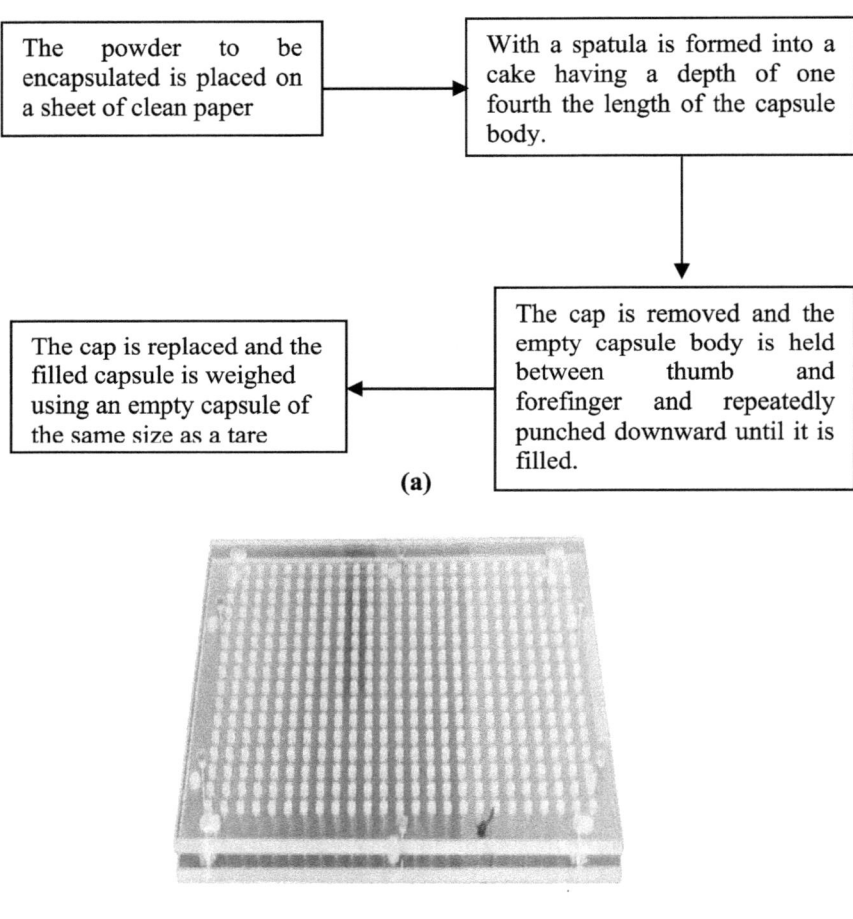

(a) Flow chart of manual filling process; (b) Hand-operated capsule filling machines.

Fig. 4.3 Manual filling of capsules.

This is the cheapest method for producing small batches of hard gelatin capsules. The steps involved are given in the flow chart form in Fig. 4.3.

- **Industrial Filling**

    The industry uses semi-automatic and fully automatic equipment for the large-scale filling of capsules. The semi-automatic machine is capable of filling all capsule sizes from 000 through 5 and attains its maximum rated capacity of 15,000 capsules per hour. Industrial filling is completed by following steps.

    - Removal of caps
    - Filling of the bodies
    - Replacement of caps, and
    - Ejection of filled capsules

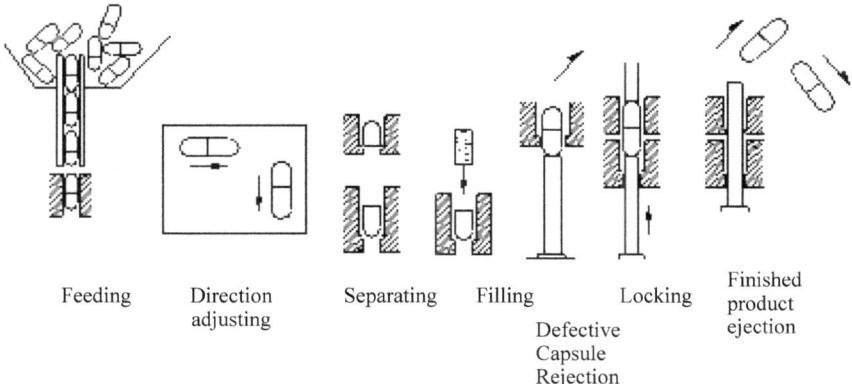

Feeding   Direction adjusting   Separating   Filling   Defective Capsule Rejection   Locking   Finished product ejection

Fig. 4.4 Flow diagram for hard gelatin capsules.

Capsules are delivered into the perforated capsule filling ring. The ring is rotated on a turntable, and a vacuum pulls the bodies into the lower half of the ring, leaving the caps in the upper half of the ring. The top & bottom halves of the filling ring are separated manually, and the cap half of the ring is set aside. The body half of the ring is then moved to another turntable where it is rotated mechanically under a powder hopper. The hopper contains an auger which feeds the powder into the bodies. When the capsule bodies are filled, the cap and body rings are rejoined (Fig. 4.4). As per the fill volume, capsule shells are classified in various size numbers (Table 4.1; Fig 4.5).

The weight of filled drug and excipients blend should be according to the volume of capsule shell and tapped bulk density of powder (filling blend) and this can be expressed as followed.

The fill weight = body volume × powder tapped bulk density

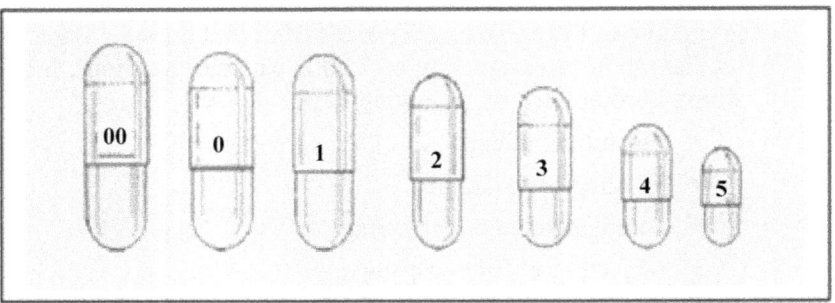

Fig. 4.5 Sizes of hard capsules.

Table 4.1 Capsule sizes and corresponding volume

Size	Volume (cm^3)
000	1.37
00	0.95
0	0.68
1	0.50
2	0.37
3	0.30
4	0.21
5	0.13

Soft Gelatin Capsule

Soft gelatin capsules are becoming a popular dosage form for the administration of liquids, suspensions, pastes, and dry powders in the dietary supplement industry and they differ from hard gelatin capsules in various terms (Table 4.2).

Table 4.2 Comparison of hard and soft gelatin capsules

Characteristics	Hard Gelatin Capsules	Soft Gelatin Capsules
Small batches manufacturing ability	Yes	No
Scale up	Simple and in house	Large quantities of drug substance required and must be outsourced
Fill Temperature	Max. 70 °C	Max. 35 °C
Plasticizer in shell	No	Yes
Risk of drug migration	Low	High for drug soluble in plasticizer
Permeability of shell to oxygen	Low	High due to plasticizer and varies with moisture content
Sensitivity to heat and humidity	Low	High due to plasticizer
Hygroscopic excipients	High concentration must be avoided	Can be tolerated due to presence of plasticizer in shell
Capsule dimension	Constant	May vary

A soft gel capsule is a one-piece, hermetically sealed soft gelatin shell containing a liquid, a suspension or a semisolid; referred to as a fill. They are formed, filled and sealed in one continuous operation, preferably by the rotary die process. Depending on the polymer forming the shell, they can be subdivided into two categories, namely *soft gelatin capsules* and *non-gelatin soft capsules*. The majority of soft capsules are made from gelatin owing to its unique physical properties that make it an ideal excipient for the rotary die process. Other various components of soft gelatin capsules are given in Table 4.3.

Table 4.3 The components of soft gelatin capsules

- Gelatin
- Glycerin or polyhydric alcohol
- Water/moisture
- Preservative
- Colorant
- Markings
- Opaquants
- Flavors may be added and up to 5% sucrose may be included for its sweetness and to produce a chewable shell

Advantages of Soft Gelatin Capsules

- Soft gelatin capsules are easy to swallow, and have the ability to mask odours and unpleasant tastes
- These have an elegant appearance, readily dissolve in the gastric juices of the digestive tract, and they may enhance the bioavailability of the active ingredient. (for example through the use of microemulsions)
- Increased rate of adsorption (solutions)
- High patient compliance, easy to swallow, good taste masking
- These can be used for oils and for semisolid active substances
- Provide dose uniformity for low dose drugs
- Provide the stability to product

Disadvantages

- Soft gelatin capsules are not easily prepared except on a large scale and with specialized equipment.
- These are an expensive dosage form, when compared with direct compression tablets.
- There is a more intimate contact between the shell and its liquid contents than exists with dry-filled hard gelatin

Formulation Consideration

Gabriele Reich described the formulation and physical properties of soft capsules. The specific shell/fill interactions that may occur during manufacture, drying and on storage must be considered in designing formulation strategies for soft gelatin capsule. These interactions control

their rate and extent to achieve a stable product. Two major types of interactions have to be distinguished:
- Chemical reactions of fill components with the gelatin and the plasticizer
- Physical interactions, i.e. migration of fill components in or through the shell and vice versa.

Cross-linking of gelatin leading to solubility problems of the shell is a well-known problem associated with the encapsulation of drugs containing reactive groups such as the aldehyde group. It can be successfully reduced by the use of succinylated gelatin, an approach that is often used for health and nutrition products, and in some countries even for pharmaceutical products.

Esterification and transesterification of drugs with polyols present another unwanted chemical reaction that may occur. Since glycerol is more reactive than other polyols, glycerol-free shell formulations and/or the addition of polyvinyl pyrrolidone to the fill are preferred to reduce this problem. The rate and extent of physical shell/fill interactions depend strongly on the qualitative and quantitative composition of both, the shell and the fill. As a general rule, the water content of the fill should not exceed a critical value of about 5%. Fill formulations simply composed of a lipophilic drug in a lipophilic oily vehicle do not interact with the hydrophilic gelatin capsule shell at any time, i.e. either during production or on storage. The proper choice of the shell composition therefore only depends on the stability of the active ingredient, the capsule size, shape and end use and the anticipated storage conditions. For very soft capsules and those stored at ambient conditions, glycerol is the plasticizer of choice. For more rigid soft gelatin capsules and those intended to be used in hot and humid climates, glycerol/sorbitol blends are preferred.

Compared to lipophilic solutions, fill compositions with hydrophilic components are more challenging to encapsulate, since they are prone to interact with the shell. The most critical period for diffusional exchanges between shell and fill is the manufacturing process, since the moisture content of the initial shells before drying is around 40% and the equilibrium moisture level is only reached after several days. Thus, during manufacture and drying, hydrophilic components of the fill may migrate rapidly into the shell and vice versa, thereby changing the initial composition of both, the shell and the fill. On storage, these processes may continue until equilibrium is reached. As a result, the capsule shells can become brittle or tacky and the fill formulation may be deteriorated, either shortly after production or on storage.

To overcome these problems, the following solutions have been proposed:
- Use of high-Bloom, low-viscosity pigskin or acid bone gelatin to reduce the initial water content in the capsule shell and accelerate the drying process;
- Replacement of glycerol by glycerol/sorbitol or sorbitol/sorbitan blends to minimize diffusion of glycerol-soluble active ingredients into the shell.
- Coating of drug particles to inhibit the browning reaction between active ingredients, such as ascorbic acid and gelatin.

In general an ideal soft capsule gelatin should have the following specifications
- Gel strength: 150-200 Bloom, depending on the gelatin type;
- Viscosity (60°C/6.6 % w/w in water): 2.8-4.5 mPa s, depending on the gelatin type.
- Well-controlled degree of viscosity breakdown;
- Well-defined particle size to allow fast dissolution and deaeration of the molten mass, even at high gelatin concentrations;
- A broad molecular weight distribution to provide a fast setting and the fusion temperature being well below the melting temperature of the plasticized wet film.

Production of Soft Gelatin Capsules
A. Plate process
The plate process involves placing the upper half of a plasticized gelatin sheet over a die plate containing numerous die pockets. Vacuum is applied to draw the sheet in to the die pockets. Filling the pockets with liquor or paste, folding the lower half of gelatin sheet back over the filled pockets, and inserting the "sandwich" under a die press where the capsules are formed and cut out.

B. Rotary die process
Soft gelatin capsules are produced in an encapsulation machine employing a rotary die process. Gelatin and water forms gel mass to which plasticizer is added (e.g. glycerol). Once the gelatin is

fully dissolved then other components, such as colours, opacifier, flavors and preservatives, may be added. The hot gel mass is then supplied to the encapsulation machine through heated transfer pipes by a casting method that forms two separate gelatin ribbons (each approximately 150 mm wide). The ribbons are transported to the die where the liquid fill is injected (Fig. 4.6 and 4.7).

During the casting process the gelatin passes through the sol-gel transition and the thickness of each gel ribbon is controlled to ± 0.1 mm. The two gel ribbons are then carried through rollers to the rotary die encapsulation tooling.

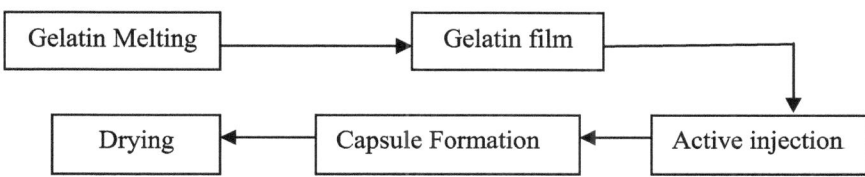

Fig. 4.6 Outline of soft capsule process.

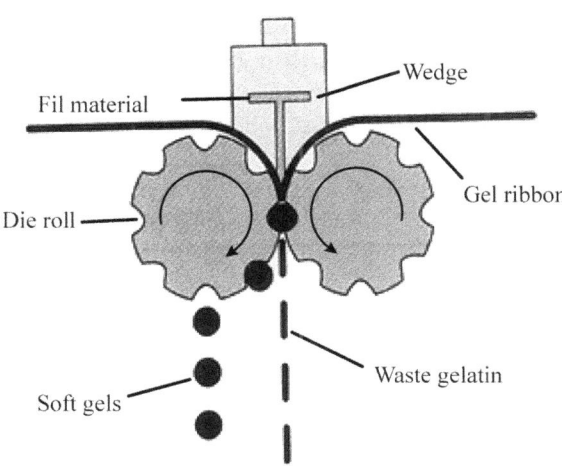

Fig. 4.7 Mechanism of soft gel capsule formation.

Evaluation of Commercial Capsules
Content Uniformity

Thirty capsules are selected and 10 of these are assayed individually. The preparation complies with the test if not more than one individual content is outside the limits of 85-115 % of the average content and none is outside the limits of 75-125% of the average content. The preparation fails to comply with the test if more than three individual contents are outside the limits of 85- 115 % of the average content or if one or more individual contents are outside the limits of 75-125 % of the average content. If 2 or 3 individual contents are outside the limits of 85-115% of the average content but within the limits of 75-125 %, repeat the determination using another 20 capsules. The requirements are met if not more than 3 individual contents of the total sample of 30 capsules are outside the limits of 85-115 % of the average content and none is outside the limits of 75-125 % of the average content (IP and BP method).

Weight Uniformity

This test applies to all types of capsules and it is to be done on 20 capsules. Weigh an intact capsule. Open the capsule without losing any part of the shell and remove the contents as completely as possible. Weigh the shell. The weight of the contents is the difference between the weighing. Repeat the procedure with a further 19 capsules selected at random. Determine the average weight. Not more than two of the individual weights deviate from the average weight by more than the percentage deviation shown in the table below, and none deviates by more than twice that percentage (Table 4.4).

Table 4.4 Limits of percent deviations for weight uniformity (IP/BP)

Average Weight of Capsule Content	Percentage Deviation
Less than 300 mg	10
300 mg or more	7.5

Disintegration

The disintegration test determines whether tablets or capsules disintegrate within a prescribed time when placed in a liquid medium under the prescribed experimental conditions. The capsules are placed in the basket-rack assembly, which is repeatedly immersed 30 times per minute into a thermostatically controlled fluid at 37°C and observed over the time described in the individual monograph.

Dissolution

The dissolution test is carried out using the dissolution apparatus official in both the U.S.P. and N.F. The capsule is placed in a basket formed from 40-mesh stainless steel fabric. A stirrer shaft is attached to the basket, and the basket is immersed in the dissolution medium and caused to rotate at a specified speed. The dissolution medium is held in a covered 1000 ml glass vessel and maintained at 37°C ± 0.5°C by means of a suitable constant temperature water bath. The stirrer speed and type of dissolution medium are specified in the individual monograph.

When capsule shells interfere with the analysis, remove the contents of not less than 6 capsules as completely as possible, and dissolve the empty capsule shells in the specified volume of the dissolution medium. Perform the analysis as directed in the individual monograph. Make any necessary correction. Correction factor should not be greater than 25 % of the stated amount. Acceptance criteria is the same as prescribed for dissolution of tablets (Refer Chapter 3)

Non-Gelatin Soft Capsules

Traditionally, gelatin has been used almost exclusively as shell-forming material of soft capsules. This is due to its legal status and its unique physicochemical properties, namely its oxygen impermeability and the combination of film forming capability and thermo reversible sol/gel formation that favour its use for the industrial soft capsule production especially in the rotary die process. Despite these great advantages, which have been described in detail in the section above on 'Soft gelatin capsules', gelatin has several drawbacks that limit its use for soft capsules:

- The animal source of gelatin can be a problem for certain consumers such as vegetarians or vegans and religious or ethnic groups (Jews, Muslims, Hindus, etc.) who observe dietary laws that forbid the use of certain animal products.
- Since unmodified gelatin is prone to crosslinking when in contact with aldehydes, solubility problems might be expected with certain fill formulations.
- Transparent low-colour capsules are difficult to produce owing to the effect of the intrinsic Maillard reaction on gelatin colour.
- The temperature and moisture sensitivity of gelatin-based soft capsules is an issue that complicates the use of soft gelatin capsules

in very hot and humid regions and requires special packaging and storage conditions to ensure product stability.
- For low-price health and nutrition products, pricing of commercially available gelatin might be an additional problem.

To date, three non-gelatin soft capsule concepts with different process adjustments have reached prototype status: two are based on plant derived hydrocolloids and the third is based on a synthetic polymer.

- Use of a combination of iota carrageenan (12–24% w/w of dry shell) and modified starch, namely hydroxypropyl starch (30–60% w/w of dry shell), as a gelatin substitute.
- Potato starch (45–80% w/w), with a specific molecular weight distribution and amylopectin content, together with a conventional plasticizer such as glycerol (12% w/w), a glidant and a disintegrant.
- Use of polyvinyl alcohol (PVA) and optional use of some other materials, all being film-forming polymers that lack the gelling properties that are necessary for soft capsule production using the conventional rotary die process.

Bibliography

- Augsburger LL, In; Banker GS, Rhodes CT (Eds). Modern Pharmaceutics. 2005 (Vol. 121) Marcel Dekker, Inc. New York, Basel, US, pp 335-79.
- Reich G. In: Fridrun P, Brian J. Eds: Pharmaceutical capsules, II Edn, 2004, Pharma Press, pp- 201-212.
- Brown M. D. (1996). Improvements in or relating to encapsulation. International Patent Application WO 9 735 537.
- Draper P. R., Tanner K. E., Getz J. J., Burnett S. and Youngblood E. (1999). Film forming compositions comprising modified starches and iota-carrageenan and methods for manufacturing soft capsules using same. International Patent Application WO 0 103 677.
- Gullapalli R. P. (2001). Ibuprofen-containing softgels. US Patent 6 251 426.
- Hom F. S., Veresh S. A. and Ebert, W.R. *J. Pharm. Sci.*,1975; 64, 851–857.

- Hutchison K, Ferdinando J. In: Aulton ME (Editor), Pharmaceutics: The science of dosage form design. 2nd Edn., 2002, Churchil Livingstone, New York, pp. 461-72.
- Jones B, In: Aulton ME (Editor), Pharmaceutics: The science of dosage form design. 2nd Edn., 2002, Churchil Livingstone, New York, pp. 449-60.
- Menard R., Tomka I., Engel W. D. and Brocker E.(1999). Process to manufacture starch-containing shaped bodies, mass containing homogenized starch and device to manufacture soft capsules. International Patent Application WO 0 137 817.
- Oppenheim R. C. and Truong H. C. (2002). Discoloration- resistant vitamin composition. US Patent Application 2002 004 069.

CHAPTER 5

Suspensions

Introduction

Suspension is heterogeneous system consisting of two phases. The continuous or external phase is generally liquid or semi solid and the dispersed phase or internal phase is made up of particulate matter that is essentially insoluble in but dispersed throughout the dispersed phase.

Suspension is a dispersion of finely divided insoluble solid particles (disperse phase) in a fluid (dispersion medium). Dispersion medium is mostly aqueous or may be oily liquid, while dispersed phase comprises insoluble solids.

Most pharmaceutical suspension consists of aqueous dispersion medium but in some instance it may be an oily liquid. The particles have diameter for the most part greater than 0.1 µm and some particle and some particles are observed under the microscope to exhibit Brownian movement if the dispersion has low viscosity. Pharmaceutical suspension may be classified into three groups on the basis of routes of administration, particle size, electrokinetic nature of particles, and proportion of solid particles (Table 5.1).

Physical properties of well formulated suspension
- Suspensions should possess good pourability leading to ease of removal of dose from container,
- should have good organoleptic properties,
- should have uniform particle size distribution,
- should be ease of redispersion of settled solid particles,
- should be physically and chemically stable,
- should be resistant against microbial contamination.

Table 5.1 Classification of pharmaceutical suspensions

Based on Routes of Administration	Based on Size of Solid Particles	Based on Electrokinetic Nature of Solid Particles	Based on Proportion of Solid Particles
• Oral suspension • Externally applied suspension • Parenteral suspension	• Colloidal suspension ($< 1\ \mu$) • Coarse suspension ($>1\ \mu$)	• Flocculated suspension • Deflocculated suspension	• Dilute suspension (2 to10%w/v solid) • Concentrated suspension (50%w/v solid)

Advantages of Suspension
- Suspension can improve chemical stability of certain drugs.
  e.g. Procaine penicillin G
- Drug in suspension exhibits higher rate of bioavailability than other dosage forms.
- Duration and onset of action can be controlled.
  E.g. Protamine Zinc-Insulin suspension
- Suspension can mask the unpleasant/ bitter taste of drug.
  e.g. Chloramphenicol.

Disadvantages

- Physical stability, sedimentation and compaction can cause problems.
- It is bulky, sufficient care must be taken during handling and transport.
- It is difficult to formulate.
- Uniform and accurate dose cannot be achieved unless suspension are packed in unit dosage form.

Theories of Suspension

Sedimentation Concept

In dispersions the dispersed particles encounters between themselves as a result of Brownian movement. Depending upon the forces of interactions (electrical forces of repulsion, forces of attraction and forces arising due to salvation) the particles aggregate to form collection of particles. The collisions result in permanent contact of particles known as coagulation leading to the formation of larger aggregates, which sediment out known to exhibit flocculation or if the particles rebound they remain freely suspended and form stable system. These particles sediment according to stokes' law.

According to Stokes' law, the sedimentation velocity is expressed by following equation

$$v = 2r^2 g\,(\rho_s - \rho_l)/9\eta$$

where v is velocity of sedimentation, a is the radius of particles, ρ_s density of solid particles, g is acceleration due to gravity and ρ_l is the density of liquid and η is the viscosity of the dispersion phase.

The equation of stokes' law reflects that larger particles exhibit greater velocity of sedimentation. The velocity of sedimentation is inversely proportional to the viscosity of dispersion medium.

Interfacial Phenomenon

Smaller solid particles are used to disperse in a continuous medium. Smaller particle size and large surface area is associated with a surface free energy making it thermodynamically unstable. Thus the particles possess high energy which leads to grouping together to reduce surface free energy thus leading to formation of floccules. These floccules are held together among themselves and within by weak van-der-waals forces. However in cases where particles are adhered by stronger forces to form aggregates forming hard cake. These phenomena occur in order to make system more thermodynamically stable. In order to achieve a state of stability the system tend to reduce the surface free energy, which may be accomplished by reduction of interfacial tension that is achieved by use of surfactants.

Electrical Double Layer and Zeta Potential

Most surfaces acquire a surface electric charge when they come in contact with aqueous surface. A solid charged surface when in contact with an aqueous medium possesses positive and negative ions. Initially, attraction from the negative ions causes some of the positive ions to form a firmly attached layer around the surface of the colloid; this layer of counter-ions is known as the *Stern layer* (Fig. 5.1). Additional positive ions are still attracted by the negative colloid, but now they are repelled by the Stern layer as well as by other positive ions that are also trying to approach the colloid. This dynamic equilibrium results in the formation of a *diffuse layer* of counterions. They have a high concentration near the surface which gradually decreases with distance, until it reaches equilibrium with the counter-ion concentration in the solution.

In a similar, but opposite, fashion there is a lack of negative ions in the neighborhood of the surface, because they are repelled by the negative colloid. Negative ions are called *co-ions* because they have the same charge as the colloid. Their concentration will gradually increase with distance, as the repulsive forces of the colloid are screened out by the positive ions, until equilibrium is again reached.

The diffuse layer can be visualized as a charged atmosphere surrounding the colloid. The charge density at any distance from the surface is equal to the difference in concentration of positive and negative ions at that point. Charge density is greatest near the colloid and gradually diminishes toward zero as the concentration of positive and negative ions merge together. The attached counter-ions in the Stern layer and the charged atmosphere in the diffuse layer are what we refer to as the *double layer*. The thickness of this layer depends upon the type and concentration of ions in solution.

The double layer is formed in order to neutralize the charged colloid and, in turn, causes an electrokinetic potential between the surface of the colloid and any point in the mass of the suspending liquid. This voltage difference is on the order of millivolts and is referred to as the surface potential. The magnitude of the surface potential is related to the surface charge and the thickness of the double layer.

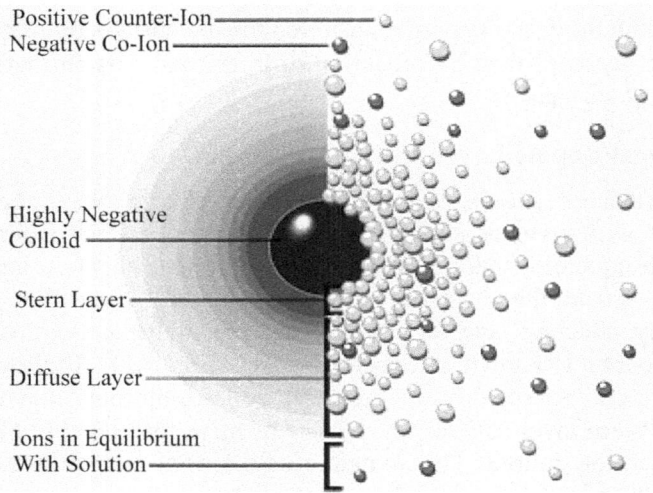

Fig. 5.1 Two ways to visualize the double layer, The left view shows the change in charge density around the colloid. The right view shows the distribution of positive and negative ions around the charged colloid.

As we leave the surface, the potential drops off roughly linearly in the Stern layer and then exponentially through the diffuse layer, approaching zero at the imaginary boundary of the double layer. The potential curve is useful because it indicates the strength of the electrical force between particles and the distance at which this force comes into play.

A charged particle will move with a fixed velocity in a voltage field. This phenomenon is called electrophoresis. The particle's mobility is related to the dielectric constant and viscosity of the suspending liquid and to the electrical potential at the boundary between the moving particle and the liquid. This boundary is called the slip plane and is usually defined as the point where the Stern layer and the diffuse layer meet. The Stern layer is considered to be rigidly attached to the colloid, while the diffuse layer is not. As a result, the electrical potential at this junction is related to the mobility of the particle and is called the *zeta potential*. Although zeta potential is an intermediate value, it is sometimes considered to be more significant than surface potential as far as electrostatic repulsion is concerned. Zeta potential can be quantified by tracking the colloidal particles through a microscope as they migrate in a voltage field.

The Balance of Repulsion and Attraction

The DLVO Theory (named after Derjaguin, Landau, Verwey and Overbeek) is the classical explanation of the stability of colloids in suspension. It looks at the balance between two opposing forces electrostatic repulsion and vander Waals attraction, to explain why some colloidal systems agglomerate while others do not. Electrostatic repulsion becomes significant when two colloids approach each other and their double layers begin to interfere. Energy is required to overcome this repulsion. An electrostatic repulsion curve is used to indicate the energy that must be overcome if the particles are to be forced together. It has a maximum value when they are almost touching and decreases to zero outside the double layer. The maximum energy is related to the surface potential and the zeta potential.

Vander Waals attraction is actually the result of forces between individual molecules in each colloid. The effect is additive; that is, one molecule of the first colloid has a vander Waals attraction to each molecule in the second colloid. This is repeated for each molecule in the first colloid, and the total force is the sum of all of these. An attractive energy curve is used to indicate the variation in vander Waals force with distance between the particles.

The DLVO theory explains the tendency of colloids to agglomerate or remain discrete by combining the vander Waals attraction curve with the electrostatic repulsion curve to form the net interaction energy curve. At each distance, the smaller value is subtracted from the larger to get the net energy. The net value is then plotted and a curve (Fig. 5.2: above if repulsive and below if attractive) is formed. If there is a repulsive section, then the point of maximum repulsive energy is called the energy barrier. The height of the barrier indicates how stable the system is. In order to agglomerate, two particles on a collision course must have sufficient kinetic energy due to their velocity and mass, to "jump over" this barrier. If the barrier is cleared, then the net interaction is all attractive, and as a result the particles agglomerate. This inner region is after referred to as an energy trap since the colloids can be considered to be trapped together by vander Waals forces.

124 Essentials of Pharmaceutical Technology

In many cases we can alter the environment to either increase or decrease the energy barrier, depending upon our goals. Various methods can be used to achieve this, such as changing the ionic environment, or pH, or adding surface active materials to directly affect the charge of the colloid. In each case, zeta potential measurements can indicate the impact of the alteration on overall stability.

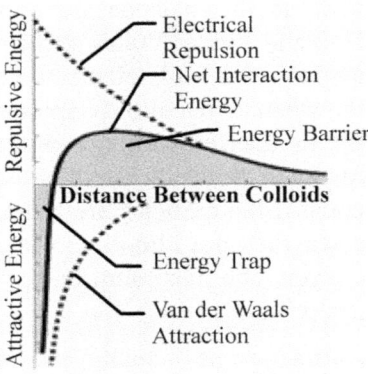

Fig. 5.2 The net interaction curve.

Formulation Consideration

Particle Size Control

It is necessary to ensure that the drug to be suspended is of a fine particle size prior to formulation to ensure slow rate of sedimentation of suspended particles. Large particles, if greater than 5 µm in diameter will also impart a gritty texture to the product, and may cause irritation if injected or instilled into the eyes. The ease of administration of a parenteral suspension may depend upon particle shape and size, and it is quite impossible to block a hypodermic needle with particles over about 25 µm diameter. It is also advantageous to use a suspended drug of a narrow size range because crystals of less than 1 µm diameter will exhibit a greater solubility than larger ones. To prevent crystal growth polymeric colloids or surface active agents are added which adsorbed on to the surface of each particle.

Viscosity of Suspensions

Viscosity of suspensions is of great importance for stability and pourability of suspensions. As we know suspensions have the least physical stability amongst all dosage forms due to sedimentation and cake formation. So as the viscosity of the dispersion medium increases, the terminal settling velocity decreases thus the dispersed phase settle at a slower rate and they remain dispersed for longer time yielding higher stability to the suspension. On the other hand as the viscosity of the suspension increases, it's pourability decreases and inconvenience to the patients for dosing increases. Thus, the viscosity of suspension should be maintained within optimum range to yield stable and easily pourable suspensions. Now a day's structured vehicles are used to solve both the problems. Generally viscosity is measured as a part of rheological studies because it is easy to measure practically. Here, the shear stress and shear rate are directly proportional, and the proportionality constant is the Co-efficient of viscosity. it is denoted by η.

$$\eta = S/D$$

where, S = Shear stress and D = Shear rate. Viscosity has units dynes-sec/cm or g/cm-sec or poise in CGS system. If we plot graph of shear stress verses shear rate (Fig. 5.3), the slope gives the viscosity. The curve always passes through the origin.

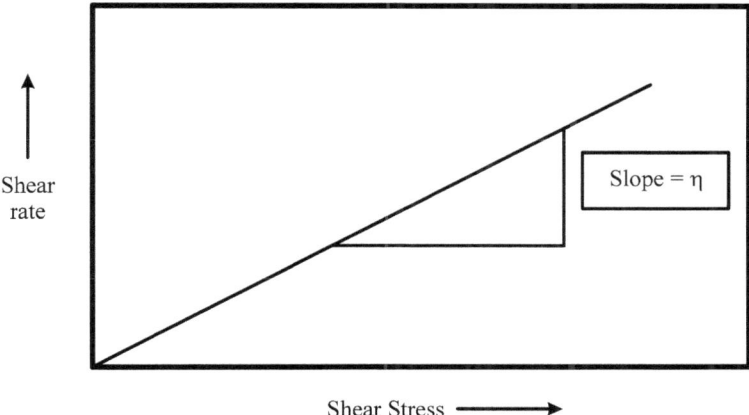

Fig. 5.3 Shear stress verses shear rate for measurement of viscosity.

Formulation of Pharmaceutical Suspensions

The formulator must encounter important problems regarding particle size distribution, specific surface area, inhibition of crystal growth and changes in the polymorphic form. The formulator must ensure that these and other properties should not change after long term storage and do not

adversely affect the performance of suspension. Choice of pH, particle size, viscosity, flocculation, taste, color and odor are some of the most important factors that must be controlled at the time of formulation. Formulation of suspension includes:
- Structured vehicles
- Other components

Structured Vehicles

Structured vehicles are used to formulate the stable suspension so that particles remain deflocculated, with ease of dispersibility with a minimum agitation. Structured vehicle concept is applicable only to deflocculated suspensions, where hard solid cake forms due to settling of solid particles and they must be redispersed easily and uniformly at the time of administration. Structured vehicles are prepared with the help of Hydrocolloids. In a particular medium, they first hydrolyzed and swell to great degree and increase viscosity at the lower concentration. In addition, it can act as a 'Protective colloid' and stabilize charge. Density of structured vehicle also can be increased by: Polyvinylpyrrolidone, Sugars, Polyethylene glycols and by using Glycerin.

Wetting Agents

Some insoluble solids get easily wetted by water, most of them exhibits hydrophobicity and do not get easily wetted by it. Wetting agents are additives which are usually added to decrease this hydrophobicity. These agents generally get adsorbed at the solid-liquid interface and promote wetting of the solid particles by the liquid of the dispersion medium.

- **Surfactants:** Generally, Surfactants possessing HLB values between 7 and 9 have been employed as wetting agents. These orient themselves at solid-liquid interface and decrease the interfacial tension between the particles of the dispersed phase and the dispersed medium. Most surfactants are used at concentration of 0.1 to 0.2%. The minimum concentration that is sufficient to cause wetting should generally be employed since an excess of these agents may cause foaming in the preparation. Examples of surfactants employed for oral preparation include polysorbates, sorbitan, esters, etc; for external preparations, sodium lauryl sulfate, sodium dioctyl sulfosuccinate and quillia extracts can also be used. Ionic as well as non-ionic surfactants may be employed as flocculation agent.

- **Hydrophilic Polymers:** Various hydrophilic colloids such as acacia, bentonite, and colloidal silicon dioxide and cellulose derivatives have also been employed as wetting agents. These act by coating the surface of hydrophobic particles and imparting hydrophilic character to these.
- **Hydrophilic Liquids:** Hydrophilic liquids such as alcohol, glycerol, propylene glycol, are sometimes employed as wetting agents. These penetrate the loose aggregates of solid particles and displace the air from the pores thus facilitating wetting of the particles by the dispersion medium.

Flocculating Agents

These are substances added to cause controlled aggregation of the particles of the dispersed phase in a suspension. Examples of such agents include surfactants, electrolytes and hydrophilic polymers.

- **Electrolytes:** Electrolytes such as sodium salt of acetates, phosphates and citrates have been commonly employed as flocculating agents. These act by neutralizing the surface charge on the particles of the dispersed phase thereby reducing the electrical barrier between them. The effectiveness of the electrolytes as flocculating agents depends on the valance of the ions of these electrolytes. Thus, divalent ions are ten times more effective than the monovalent ions while trivalent ones are thousand times more effective. The concentration of the electrolytes used should be minimum that is required to cause flocculation since an excess may cause reversal of this phenomenon.
- **Polymeric Flocculating Agents:** Their linear branched chain molecules form a gel like network within the system and become absorbed on the surface of dispersed particle thus holding them in a flocculated state. E.g. Starch, alginates cellulose derivatives, carbomers, tragacanth, silicates.

Viscosity Enhancers/ Suspending Agents

They are added with the objective to increase apparent viscosity of the continuous phase thus preventing rapid sedimentation of the dispersed particles. The selection of the type and concentration of a suspending agent depends on sedimentation rate of dispersed particles, pourability and spreadability (Table 5.3). The ideal suspending agent should have a high viscosity at negligible shear i.e., during shelf storage and it should have a low viscosity at high shearing rates i.e., it should be free flowing during agitation, pouring and spreadibility. A suspending agent that is thixotropic as well as pseudoplastic should prove to be useful as it forms a gel on standing and becomes fluid when shaken. They include natural polysaccharides (Gum Acacia, Gum Tragacanth, Guar Gum, Sodiun Alginate, Xanthan Gum and Carrageenan), Semi-synthetic polysaccharides (Sodium Carboxymethylcellulose, Methyl Cellulose, Hydroxyethyl Cellulose, Hydroxypropyl Cellulose, Hydroxypropyl Methyl Cellulose and Microcrystalline Cellulose), Clays (Aluminium Magnesium Silicate, Bentonite and Hectorite) and synthetic agents (Carbomer, Colloidal silicon dioxide). Pseudoplastic substances like tragacanth, sodium alginate and sodium carboxymethyl cellulose show these desirable qualities. In cases of combination use of suspending agents like bentonite and CMC dispersions are both pseudoplastic and thixotropic. The suspending agents which gave highest stability are jota carageenan (having low-temperature gelation characteristics) and MC/CMC (having thixotropic flux).

Table 5.3 Suspending agents and their properties

Suspending agents	Stability pH range	Concentrations used as suspending agent (%)
Sodium alginate	4-10	1–5
Methylcellulose	3-11	1–2
Hydroxyethylcellulose	2-12	1-2
Hydroxypropylcellulose	6-8	1-2
Hydroxypropylmethylcellulose	3-11	1-2
Carboxy methyl cellulose	7-9	1-2
Sodium Carboxy methyl cellulose	5-10	0.1-5
Microcrystalline cellulose	1-11	0.6–1.5
Tragacanth	4-8	1-5
Xanthangum	3-12	0.05-0.5
Bentonite	>6	0.5–5.0
Carageenan	6-10	0.5–1
Guar gum	4-10.5	1-5
Colloidal silicon dioxide	0-7.5	2–4

Miscellaneous

Other additives to be included in the formulation of a suspension are as followed.

- *Buffers and pH adjusting agents*: They are added to stabilize the suspension to a desired pH range.
- *Osmotic agents*: They are added to adjust osmotic pressure comparable to biological fluid.
- *Coloring agents*: They are added to impart desired color to suspension and improve elegance.
- *Preservatives*: They are added to prevent microbial growth.

Flocculated and Deflocculated Suspension

A suspension may be flocculated or deflocculated type depending on the relative magnitudes of force of repulsion, force of attraction between particles.

Flocculated System

In this type of system, the solid particles of dispersed phase aggregate leading to network like structure of solid particles in dispersion medium. The aggregates form no hard cake. These aggregates settle rapidly due to their size as rate of sedimentation is high and sediment formed is loose and easily redispersible. The suspension is not elegant, as dispersed phase tends to separate out from the dispersion medium. Therefore it is desired that flocculation should be carried out in a controlled manner so that a balance exists between the rate of sedimentation and nature of sediment formed and pourability of the suspension.

There are two important steps to formulate flocculated suspension

- The wetting of particles
- Controlled flocculation

The primary step in formulation is that adequate wetting of particles is ensured. Suitable amount of wetting agents solve this problem which is described under wetting agents.

Controlled Flocculation

A deflocculated system with high viscosity to prevent sedimentation would be an ideal formulation. The next stage of formulation process, after the addition of wetting agent, is to ensure that the product exhibit the correct degree of flocculation. Under flocculation will give those undesirable properties that are associated with the deflocculated system. While an over flocculated product will be inelegant and, to minimize settling, the viscosity of the product may have to be so high that any necessary redispersion would be difficult. Controlled flocculation is usually achieved by a combination of particle size control, the use of electrolytes to control zeta potential, and addition of polymers to enable cross linking to occur between particles. Some polymers have advantage of becoming ionized in an aqueous solution, and can therefore act both electrostatically and sterically. These materials are also termed as polyelectrolyte.

Properties of Flocculated Suspensions

- Particles in the suspension are in form of loose agglomerates.
- Flocs are collection of particles, so rate of sedimentation is high.
- The sediment is formed rapidly.
- The sediment is loosely packed. Particles are not bounded tightly to each other. Hard cake is not formed.
- The sediment is easily redispersed by small amount of agitation.
- The flocculated suspensions exhibit plastic or pseudo plastic behaviour.
- The suspension is somewhat unsightly, due to rapid sedimentation and presence of an obvious clear supernatant region.
- The pressure distribution in this type of suspension is uniform at all places, i.e. the pressure at the top and bottom of the suspension is same.
- In this type of suspension, the viscosity is nearly same at different depth level.
- The purpose of uniform dose distribution is fulfilled by flocculated suspension.

Deflocculated System

In this type of system the solid particles exist as separate entities in dispersion medium. The sediments form hard cake. The solid drug particles settle slowly as rate of sedimentation is low. As sediments are formed eventually there is difficulty of redispersion. The suspension is more elegant as dispersed phase remain suspended for a long time giving uniform appearance. In deflocculated suspension the individual particle should remain dispersed. In some material where the quantum of surface charge is not sufficient the particle may exhibit the tendency of coming together and forming large particle. To overcome this tendency, some material carrying good charge and which can get easily absorbed on the dispersed phase particle can be added. These additives are referred as dispersants (for example darvans, daxads, marasperses). These are polymerized organic salts of alkyl/aryl substances which increase the zeta potential considerably thus encouraging particles to break energy barrier and comes together

Properties of Deflocculated Suspensions
- Particle size is less as compared to flocculated particles. Particles settle separately and hence, rate of settling is very low.
- The sediment after some period of time becomes very closely packed, due to weight of upper layers of sedimenting materials.
- After sediment becomes closely packed, the repulsive forces between particles overcome resulting in a non-dispersible cake.
- More concentrated deflocculated systems may exhibit dilatant behavior.
- This type of suspension has a pleasing appearance, since the particles are suspended for relatively longer period of time.
- The supernatant liquid is cloudy even though majority of particles have been settled.
- There is no clear-cut boundary between sediment and supernatant.

Formation of Suspension

Three precipitation methods are *organic solvent precipitation, Precipitation affected by changing the pH of the medium and double decomposition*. Water soluble drugs can be precipitated by dissolving them in water-miscible organic solvents and then adding the organic phase to distilled water under standard conditions. Examples of organic solvent include ethanol, methanol, propylene glycol, and polyethylene glycol. The important factor next to particle size control is that the correct polymorphic form or hydrates of crystals are obtained. Besides the influence of the solvent on crystals characteristics the following additional factors may need to be considered: Preparation under sterile conditions, Inherent solvent entrapment, toxicity, volume ratio of the organic to the aqueous phase, Rate and method of addition of one phase to other, temperature control, and finally, the washing of precipitate.

Precipitation affected by changing the PH of the medium and double decomposition is perhaps more readily accomplished and does not present the same difficulties associated with organic solvent precipitation. Although consideration of physical factors is needed for the production of stable suspension.

Dispersion Method

When the dispersive method is utilized for suspension precipitation, the vehicle must be formulated so that the solid phase is easily wetted and dispersed. The use of surfactant is desirable to ensure uniform wetting of hydrophobic solids. The particle size reduction may or may not result from dispersion process. If particle size reduction occur the particle obtained may have different solubility of a metastable state is involved, and this may lead to transient supersaturation of the system.

Evaluation of Suspension

Methods used for evaluation of suspension are categorized as :
- (a) Sedimentation method
- (b) Rheological method
- (c) Electrokinetic method
- (d) Micromeritic method
- (e) Stability study

Sedimentation Method

Since formation of sediment and its redispersibility are two feature related to suspension acceptability. The sediment formed should redisperse by moderate shaking to yield homogenous system. The measurement of the sedimentation volume and its ease of redispersion form two of the most common basic evaluative procedures. The sedimentation volume is the simple ratio of the height of sediment to initial height of the initial suspension. The larger the value better is the suspendability.

The simplest procedure for evaluation is to keep a measured volume of a suspension in a graduated cylinder in an undisturbed state for a certain period of time and note the volume of sediment.

Sedimentation volume is a ratio of the final or ultimate volume of sediment (V_u) to the original volume of sediment (V_O) before settling.

$$F = V_u / V_O$$

Some time 'F' is represented as 'Vs' and as expressed as percentage. Similarly when a measuring cylinder is used to measure the volume. The volume of sediment is expressed as ultimate height (Hu) and initial height of suspension (Ho).

Sedimentation volume = Hu/Ho

= ultimate height / initial height

Sedimentation volume is dependent on time and likely to vary at different period of time. Sedimentation volume can have values ranging from less than 1 to greater than1; F is normally less than 1. The products for which F = 1, such product is said to be in flocculation equilibrium, and show no clear Supernatant on standing.

Sedimentation volume (F_d) for deflocculated suspension

$$F_d = V_d / V_O$$

where, F_d = sedimentation volume of deflocculated suspension

V_d = sediment volume of completely deflocculated suspension. (Sediment volume ultimate relatively small)

V_O = original volume of suspension.

The degree of settling can be related to the amount of sediment that would be produced in the ultimate dispersed state. To obtain the completely dispersed suspension form which represent the least space for the solid phase and hence the smallest sedimentation volume, electrolytes that promotes settling may be added or the preparation may be centrifuged.

Rate of sedimentation can be estimated by the use of an oden's balance. This consists of a pan suspended in the suspension and counterbalanced against weights or attached to a painter which moves on a rotating smoking drum. As more and more particle settle on pan moves down or more weight to keep the original balance.

Redispersibility can be estimated by shaking the suspension with the help of a mechanical device.

Degree of Flocculation (β)

Degree of flocculation is an expression of the increased sediment volume resulting from flocculation. As the value of β (expressed as followed) approaches unity, the degree of flocculation decreases.

$$\beta = F / F_\infty$$
$$= \frac{V_u / V_o}{V_\infty / V_o}$$
$$= V_u / V_\infty$$
$$= \frac{\text{Ultimate sediment volume of flocculated suspension}}{\text{Ultimate sediment volume of deflocculated suspension}}$$

Rheological Methods

Rheologic methods can help in determining the settling behaviour of the suspension. In these methods low shear rates are employed and samples are evaluated undisturbed. Evaluation of thixotropy (isothermal slow reversible conversion of gel to sol) in case of parenteral suspensions is most desirable. Properly formulated suspension can prevent sedimentation, aggregation and caking by the virtue of a high yield value/ viscosity at rest which sharp agitation reduces the viscosity to permit pouring and thus dispensing of product.

This technique also indicates in which level of the suspension the structure is greater due to particles aggregates. Data obtained on aged and stored suspension reveals whether changes have taken place.

Viscosity

Various different viscometers (Fig. 5.4) are used to measure viscosity of different fluids and semisolids. Few of them are:

Ostwald Viscometer

It is a type of capillary viscometer. There is 'U' shape tube with two bulbs and two marks as shown in the Fig. 5.4a. For a liquid flowing by gravity, the time required for the liquid to pass between two marks (upper mark and lower mark) are noted; these time values are also noted with the liquid with known viscosity (like water), then the viscosity. It is used to determine the viscosity of Newtonian Liquids.

The viscosity of unknown liquid η_1 can be determined using the equation,

$$\eta_1 = \frac{\rho_1 t_1}{\rho_2 t_2} \cdot \eta_2$$

where, ρ_1 = Density of unknown liquid
ρ_2 = Density of known liquid
t_1 = Time of the unknown liquid
t_2 = Time of the known liquid
η_2 = Viscosity of known liquid

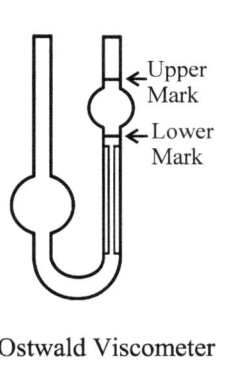

(a) Ostwald Viscometer

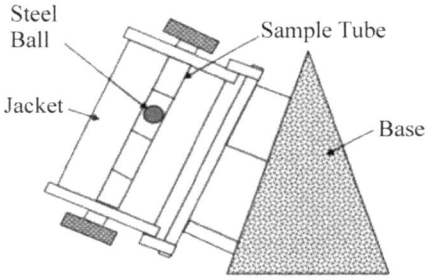

(b) Falling Sphere Viscometer

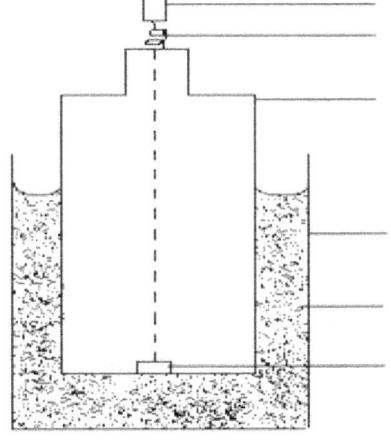

(c) Cup and Bob Viscometer

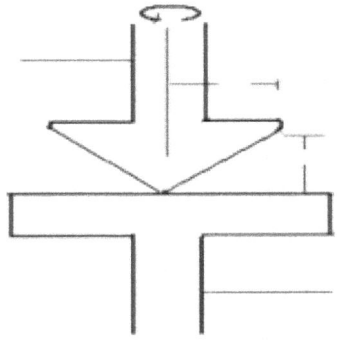

(d) Cone and plate viscometer

Fig. 5.4 Various types of viscometers.

Falling Sphere Viscometer

Falling sphere viscometer consists of cylindrical transparent tube having graduated section near the middle of its length and generally a steel ball that is allowed to fall through the tube (Fig. 5.4b). The velocity of the falling ball is measured and viscosity is calculated using stoke's law.

$$\eta = d^2 (\rho_s - \rho_l) g / 18 v$$

where, d = Diameter of the falling ball
ρ_s = Density of the sphere
ρ_l = Density of liquid
g = Gravitational acceleration
v = Terminal settling velocity

Brookfield Viscometer

By the use of Brookfield viscometer with T spindle rheological features at different depth in the sample can be studied. Brookefield viscometer with variable shear stress control can be used for evaluating viscosity of suspensions. It consist of T-bar spindle which is lowered into the suspension and the dial reading is noted which is a measure of resistance the spindle meets at various levels in the suspension.

Miscellaneous Viscometers

Cup and Bob Viscometer (Fig. 5.4c), Cone and plate viscometer (Fig. 5.4d) etc.

Electrokinetic Method

The surface electric charge or zeta potential is instrumental in deciding the stability of disperse phase system. Certain zeta potential produces more stable suspension because of controlled flocculation. The migration velocities of particles can be measured by electrophoretic method and zeta potential can be calculated from it.

Micromeritic Method

The stability of a suspension is very much dependent on to the particle size and particle size distribution of its disperse phase. A growth in the particle size is a pointer towards its instability since such an occurrence can ultimately results in the formation of lumps or cake destroying the physical structure of suspension.

Particle size analysis is performed by optical microscopy, sedimentation by using Andreasen apparatus and Coulter counter apparatus. None of these methods are direct methods. However microscopic method allows the observer to view the actual particles. The sedimentation method yields a particle size relative to the rate at which particles settle through a suspending medium

Stability Testing

It is not possible to conduct accelerated temperature studies as it can be done in solutions a rise in temperature may change the thixotropic properties of the formulations. In this physical form, the preparation would exhibit parameters that could not be extrapolated to those that would exist in the normal system. The valid temperature data could be obtained that will be useful in the estimation of the physical stability of a product at normal storage conditions. The extended aging tests must be employed under various conditions to obtain the desired information.

As per the WHO guidelines on stability testing, following physical parameters can be studied for accelerated (stress) stability testing of suspension.
- Viscosity, where appropriate
- Resuspendability
- Effects of freezing
- pH
- polymorphic conversion

Nanosuspensions

Nanosuspensions are the recently developed biphasic dosage forms which have been developed for the delivery of poorly water-soluble and poorly water- and lipid-soluble drugs (belonging to class III as classified in Biopharmaceutical Classification System or BCS).

Nanosuspensions can be defined as colloidal dispersions of nano-sized drug particles that are produced by a suitable method and stabilized by a suitable stabilizer.

Advantages of Nanosuspensions
- **Increased dissolution rate and saturation solubility of the drug**
  The dissolution rate of the nanosuspension increases due to a great increase in the surface area of the drug particles from microns to

particles of nanometer size. This effect can be explained by modified Noyes-Whitney's equation, which expresses the rate of drug dissolution at a specific time as following equation.

$$\frac{dx}{dt} = \frac{A.D.K}{h} \cdot C_s - \frac{Xd}{V}$$

where dx/dt is the dissolution rate, A is the surface area of the particle available for dissolution, D is the diffusion rate constant, K is the oil water partition coefficient, h is the thickness of the stagnant layer surrounding the particle, C_s is the saturation solubility of the drug, Xd is the amount dissolved of drug at time t and V is the volume of the dissolution media.

Due to creation of high-energy surfaces when disrupting the more or less ideal drug microcrystals to nanoparticles, saturation solubility of the drug in nanosuspension is also increased.

- **Possible diversification of products**

  As the flexibility is offered in the modification of surface properties and particle size, and ease of post-production processing of nanosuspensions, the nanosuspension can be incorporated in various dosage forms, such as tablets, pellets, suppositories and hydrogels, for various routes of administration.

- **Improved biological activity**

  Improvement in the dissolution rate and saturation solubility of a drug leads to an improvement in the *in vivo* activity of the drug.

- **Easy to manufacture and scale-up**

  Nanosuspensions are easy to manufacture. The nanosuspension's production processes (media milling and high pressure homogenization) are easily scaled up for commercial production.

- **Good stability**

  Nanosuspensions show long term physical stability due to the absence of Ostwald ripening. Ostwald ripening has been described for ultrafine dispersed systems and is responsible for crystal growth and subsequently formation of microparticles. The Ostwald ripening leads to the formation of a supersaturated solution around the large particles and consequently to drug crystallization and growth of the large particles leading to adverse effect on long term stability. The nanonsuspensions lack the Ostwald ripening due to uniform particle size, which is created by various manufacturing processes. The absence of particles with large differences in their size in nanosuspensions prevents the existence of the different saturation solubilities and concentration gradients in the vicinity of differently sized particles, which in turn prevents the Ostwald ripening effect.

Bibliography

- Attwood D. In: Aulton ME (Editor), Pharmaceutics: The science of dosage form design. 2nd Edn., 2002, Churchil Livingstone, New York, pp. 70-99.
- Billany M. In: Aulton ME (Editor), Pharmaceutics: The science of dosage form design. 2nd Edn., 2002, Churchil Livingstone, New York, pp. 334-58.
- Chingunpituk J. Walailak J *Sci & Tech* 2007; 4(2): 139-153.
- Dressman J. B., Amidon G. L., Reppas C., Shah V. P. Pharm. Res. 1998;15: 11–22.
- Emsap W, Paeratakul O, Siepmann J, In; Banker GS, Rhodes CT (Eds). Modern Pharmaceutics. 2005 (Vol. 121) Marcel Dekker, Inc. New York, Basel, US, pp 237-85.
- Martin A. and Swarbrick J., in sprowls, American Pharmacy, 6th Edition, Lippincott, Philadelphia, 1966, p.205.
- Martin A. Physical Pharmacy, 4th Edn, 1993, BI Waverly, New Delhi, pp. 393-422.
- Mu¨ller R. H., Bo¨ hm, B. H. L. (1998) Nanosuspensions. In: Mu¨ller, R. H., Benita, S., Bo¨ hm, B. H. L. (eds) Emulsions and nanosuspensions for the formulation of poorly soluble drugs. Medpharm Scientific Publishers, Stuttgart, pp 149–174.
- Müller RH and Peters K. *Int. J. Pharm.* 1998; 160, 229-37.
- Müller RH, Jacobs C and Kayer O. *Nanosuspensions for the formulation of poorly soluble drugs. In*: F Nielloud, G Marti-Mestres (ed). Pharmaceutical emulsion and suspension. New York, Marcel Dekker, 2000, p. 383-407.
- Napper DH, Polymeric Stabilization of Colloidal Dispersions, Academic Press, New York (1983).

- Nash RA. *Suspensions. In*: J Swarbrick, JC Boylan (ed). Encyclopedia of pharmaceutical technology. Second edition vol. 3. New York, Marcel dekker, 2002, p. 2045-3032.
- Patel NK, Kenon L, and Levinson RS. In; Lachman L, Lieberman HA, Kanig JL. Eds. The Theory and Practices of Industrial Pharmacy. (3rd Edition) 1986, Varghese Publishing House, Bombay, pp Pgs. 479 – 501
- Patravale V. B., Date AA and Kulkarni R.M. J Pharm Pharmacol. 2004, 56: 827–40.
- Rabinow BE. *Nat. Rev. Drug. Discov.* 2004; 3, 785-96.
- Winfield AJ, In: Winfield AJ, Richards RME (Eds). Pharmaceutical Practice, 3rd Edn, 2004, Churchill Livingstone, New York, pp. 191-97.
- World Health Organization, WHO Technical Report Series, No. 953, 2009.
- Zografi G; Schott H. and Swarbrick J., in: Remington's Pharmaceutical Sciences (18th Edition), Philadelphia College of Pharmacy and Science Pg. 257 (1990).

CHAPTER 6

Emulsions

Introduction

An emulsion is a colloidal dispersion of one liquid (disperse phase) in another (continuous phase) one. In an emulsion, however, oil and water can be forced to mix. Instead of forming two separate layers with a clear boundary between them, small droplets of one liquid (dispersed phase) are spread throughout the other liquid (continuous phase). Hence, *an emulsion can be defined as a thermodynamically unstable system consisting of at least two immiscible liquid phases, one of which is dispersed as globule (dispersed phase) in the other liquid phase (continuous phase), stabilized by the presence of an emulsifying agent (Fig. 6.1).* Typical examples of emulsion include such everyday products as milk, butter, mayonnaise and cosmetic creams.

Types of Emulsions

The most typical emulsion is one in which an oil is dispersed in water. Understandably, this is called an **oil-in-water (o/w) emulsion**. If water droplets are dispersed in oil the resulting emulsion is called **water-in-oil (w/o) emulsion**. Generally, o/w-emulsions are typically chosen for applications

142 Essentials of Pharmaceutical Technology

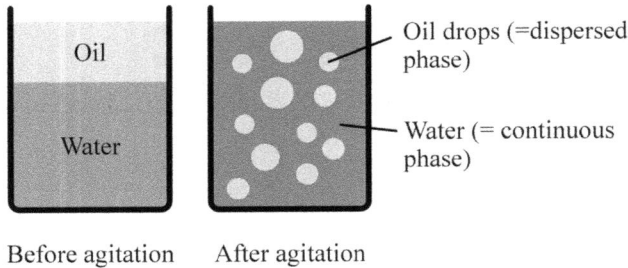

Fig. 6.1 Formation of an emulsion.

requiring a relatively small amount of fatty material as body, shaving or moisturizing creams. On the other hand w/o emulsion is preferred, when a large amount of oil is desired. This system has a greasier feel and leaves a longer-lasting residue. Typical products are emollient creams and sunscreens. In addition to the simple two-phase emulsion it is possible to make also **multiple emulsions** as w/o/w-emulsions (w/o-emulsion in water) and o/w/o-emulsions (o/w emulsion in oil) (Fig. 6.2).

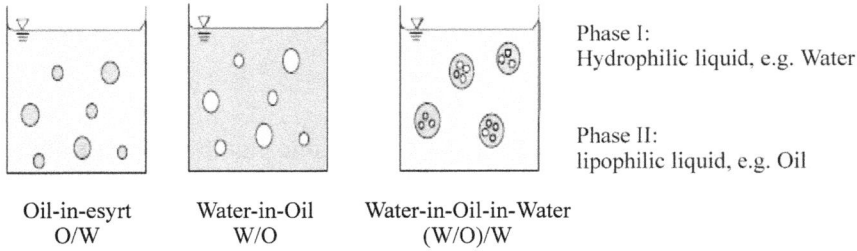

Fig. 6.2 Different types of emulsions.

When many small water droplets can be enclosed within larger oil droplets, which are themselves then dispersed in water forms water-in-oil-in-water (w/o/w) emulsions. On the other hand, when many small oil droplets can be enclosed within large water droplets, which are then themselves dispersed in oil are referred as oil-in-water-in-oil (o/w/o) emulsions. Emulsion type can be known by methods given in Table 6.1.

Table 6.1 Methods of determination of emulsion type

Test	Observation	Comments
Dilution	Emulsion can be diluted only with external phase	Useful for liquid emulsions only.
Dye test	Water soluble solid dye tints only o/w emulsions and reverse. (Microscopic observation)	May fail if ionic emulsifiers are present.
$CoCl_2$/ filter paper	Filter paper impregnated with $CoCl_2$ and dried (blue) changes to pink when o/w emulsion is added.	May fail if emulsion is unstable or breaks in presence of electrolyte.
Fluorescence	Since oils fluoresce under UV light, o/w emulsions exhibit dot pattern, w/o emulsions fluoresce throughout.	Not always applicable
Conductivity	Electric current is conducted by o/w emulsions, owing to presence of ionic species in water	Fails in nonionic o/w emulsions.

Microemulsions or Micelles Emulsions

If the dispersed globules are of colloidal dimension (1 nm to 1 micrometer) the preparations which are quite often transparent or translucent is called micro emulsions. Microemulsions are thermodynamically stable which means that they form spontaneously when the components are brought together and stay stable as long as the ingredients are intact. Microemulsions require a relatively large amount of surfactant in order to stabilize the large interfacial area created by nanodroplets. Microemulsions often require the addition of cosurfactants such as alcohols to attain appropriate fluidity or viscosity of the interface. They exhibit the properties of hydrophobic colloids.

Formulation of Emulsions

In developing the formula of an emulsion the critical decision are:
- Choice of emulsion type
- Choice of oil phase
- Choice of emulsifying agent
- Other formulation additives

Choice of Emulsion Type

The decision as to whether an o/w or a w/o emulsion is to be formulated will eliminate many unsuitable emulsifying systems. Fats or oil for oral administration, either as medicament or vehicle for oil soluble drugs, are invariably formulated as oil-in-water emulsions. In this form they are pleasant to take and inclusion of suitable flavors in the aqueous phase mask any unpleasant taste. Water in oil emulsions will have an occlusive effect by hydration of the upper layer of the stratum corneum and the inhibition of evaporation of eccrine secretions. This in turn may influence the absorption rates of drugs from these preparations.

Choice of Oil Phase

In many instance the oil phase of an emulsion is the active agent and its concentration in the product is predetermined. In many cases emulsions for external use contain oils that are present as carrier for active agent. It must be realized that the type of oil used must have an effect both on the viscosity and transport of drugs into skin e.g. liquid paraffin is the series of hydrocarbons which also include hard paraffin, soft paraffin, and light paraffin. These can be used individually or in combination with each other to control emulsion consistency (Table 6.2). Other common oils used for oil phase in emulsion are arachis oil, sesame oil, cottonseed oil etc.

Table 6.2 Emulsion consistency

The texture or feel of a product intended for external use must be also considered
For w/o emulsion:-
• Greasy texture
• High viscosity
For o/w emulsion:
• Less greasy or sticky
• Absorbed readily due to low oil content
• Easily washable

Ideally emulsion should exhibit the rheological properties of plasticity and pseudoplasticity and thixotrophy. A high apparent viscosity at very low rates of shears caused by movement of dispersed phase globules is necessary in order to retard this movement and maintains a physically stable emulsion. It is important, however, that these products should flow freely when shaken, poured from container or injected through hypodermic needles. Therefore, at these high rates of shear, a low apparent viscosity is required.

For an externally applied product a wide range of emulsion consistencies can be tolerated. Main advantage with low viscosity emulsions is their tendency to cream easily, especially if formulated with low oil concentration. Several methods by which the rheological properties of emulsion can be controlled are:

Volume Concentration of Dispersed Phase

The viscosity of the product as whole would be higher than the viscosity of the continuous phase on its own. The concentration of dispersed phase increases with the apparent viscosity of the product. If the dispersed phase concentration is increased above 60% of the total, phase inversion may occur.

Particle Size of the Dispersed Phase

It is possible under certain condition to increase the apparent viscosity of an emulsion by a reduction in mean globule diameter. This can be achieved by homogenization. The reduction in globule size may be helpful in following ways.

- A smaller mean globule size can cause increased flocculation. In a flocculated system a significant part of the continuous phase is trapped within aggregates of droplets, thus effectively increasing the apparent dispersed phase concentration. Emulsion consisting of polydispersed droplet will tends to exhibit a lower viscosity than a monodispersed system, due to differences in electrical double layer size and thus the energy of interaction curves. These variations in interaction between globules during shear may be reflected in their flow behavior.

- If a hydrophilic colloid is used to stabilize the emulsion it will form a multimolecular film round the dispersed globules. A reduction in mean globules size will increase the total surface area and therefore more colloid will adsorbed on the droplet surface. This will effectively increase the volume concentration of the dispersed phase.

Viscosity of the Continuous Phase

There is a direct relationship between the viscosity of emulsion and the viscosity of continuous phase, e.g. syrup and glycerol which is used in oral emulsion as sweetening agents will increase the viscosity of continuous phase. Their main disadvantage is in increasing the density difference between the two phases, and thus accelerating creaming.

Viscosity of Dispersed Phase

A low viscous dispersed phase would, during shear, be deformed to greater extent than a more viscous phase and thus the total interfacial area would increases slightly. This may affect double layer interaction and hence the viscosity of emulsion.

Nature and concentration of Emulsifying Agents

Hydrophilic colloids as well as colloids forming multimolecular film at the oil/water interface will also increase the viscosity of the continuous phase of an o/w emulsion. As the concentration of this type of emulgent increases, the viscosity increases. Surface active agent forming condensed monomolecular films will, by the nature of their chemical structure, influence the degree of flocculation in a similar way, by forming linkages between adjacent globules and creating a gel like structure. A flocculated system exhibits a greater apparent viscosity than deflocculated system.

Choice of Emulsifying Agent

Emulsifiers are compounds able to stabilize the dispersed droplets in the continuous phase. Emulsifiers are molecules consisting of a water loving (hydrophilic) part and water-hating but oil-loving (lipophilic) part. With their lipophilic part emulsifiers wrap around and incorporate oil drops thereby preventing them from reunite again to form a separate oily phase. In this way, the oil particles are shielded from each other resulting in a stable emulsion. The choice of emulgent to be used will depend not only on its emulsifying ability but also on its route of administration and on its toxicity (Table 6.3).

Properties of an ideal emulsifying agent

- Reduce the interfacial tension between the two immiscible liquids.
- Physically and chemically stable, inert and compatible with the other ingredients of the formulation.
- Completely non irritant and non toxic in the concentrations used.
- Organoleptically inert i.e. should not impart any colour, odour or taste to the preparation.
- Form a coherent film around the globules of the dispersed phase and should prevent the coalescence of the droplets of the dispersed phase.
- Produce and maintain the required viscosity of the preparation

Table 6.3 Factors affecting choice of emulsifying agent

- Shelf life of the product
- Type of emulsion desired
- Cost of emulsifier.
- Compatibility
- Non toxicity
- Taste
- Chemical stability.

Selection of Emulsifying Agents using HLB method: A system was developed in 1949 by William C. Griffin to assist making systematic decisions about the amounts and types of surfactants needed in stable products. The usual method for choosing an emulsifier is known as the Hydrophilic-Lipophilic Balance (HLB) system which uses a scale of 0 to 20 based on their affinity for oil and water. Emulsifiers with low HLB-values are more lipophilic, while higher HLB compounds are hydrophilic. In general, emulsifiers with HLB-values of 3-8 give w/o-emulsions, whereas those with values of above 9 are more water-soluble and result in o/w-emulsions (Table 6.4 and 6.5).

HLB numbers are experimentally determined for the different emulsifiers. An emulsifier having a low HLB number indicates that the number of hydrophilic groups present in the molecule is less and it has a lipophillic character. For example, spans generally have low HLB number and they are also oil soluble. Because of their oil soluble character, spans cause the oil phase to predominate and form a w/o emulsion.

A higher HLB number indicate that the emulsifier has a large number of hydrophilic groups on the molecule and therefore is more hydrophilic in character. Tweens have higher HLB numbers and they are also water soluble. Because of their water soluble character, tweens will cause the water phase to predominate and form an o/w emulsion. Disadvantage of the HLB system is that it does not take into account the effect of temperature, presence of additives and the concentration of emulsifier.

HLB blend = $f \times$ HLB (A) + (1-f) $\times$ HLB (B)

f = fraction of surfactant (A) in the blend of A and B

Table 6.4 HLB values for a range of oil and waxes

Oil/waxes	For w/o emulsion	For o/w emulsion
Beeswax	5	12
Cetyl alcohol	-	15
Liquid paraffin	4	12
Soft paraffin	4	12
Wool fat	8	10

Table 6.5 HLB for some pharmaceutical surfactant

Surfactant	HLB
Sorbitan triolate (span 85)	1.8
Oleic acid	4.3
Potassium oleate	20
Sorbitan mono oleate	4.3

Classification of Emulsifying Agents

Emulsifying agent are broadly classified in to three categories:
1. Surfactants
2. Hydrophilic colloids
3. Finely divided solids

Surfactants

Surface active agents (surfactants), also known as emulsifiers or emulsifying agents, are needed to provide the stability required over time. The stability of the emulsion determines its appropriate use. Surfactants are chemical compounds with a surface activity which, when dissolved in a liquid, especially water, lowers its interfacial or surface tension by preferential adsorption at the vapor/liquid surface or other interfaces. Surfactant molecules have two opposite affinities, one part is made up of a polar group yielding hydrophilic (water-loving) properties and one part is made up of a non polar radical giving it lipophilic (oil-loving) properties. There are numerous natural compounds that act as surfactants, but more commonly chemical compounds are synthesized to produce the desired characteristics. Surfactants can be grouped according to the type emulsions they yield.

Anionic surfactants: The long anion chain on dissociation imparts surface activity, while the cation is inactive. These agents are primarily used for external preparations and not for internal use as they have an unpleasant bitter taste and irritant action on the intestinal mucosa. e.g., alkali soaps, amine soaps, metallic soaps, alkyl sulphates and phosphates and alkyl sulphonates.

Cationic surfactants: The positive charge cations produced on dissociation are responsible for emulsifying properties. These are mainly used in external preparations such as lotions and creams. Quaternary ammonium compounds such as cetrimide, benzalkonium chloride and benzethonium chloride are examples of important cationic surfactants. These compounds besides having good antibacterial activity are also used in combination with secondary emulsifying agents to produce o/w emulsions for external application.

Non-ionic surfactants: These are the class of surfactants widely used as emulsifying agents. These are extensively used to produce both oil in water and water in oil emulsions for internal as well as for external use. The emulsions prepared using these surfactants remain stable over a wide range of pH changes and are not affected by the addition of acids and electrolytes. These surfactants also show low irritancy as compared to other surfactants. The examples of these surfactants include glycerol esters such as glyceryl monostearate, propylene glycol monostearate, macrogol esters such as polyoxyl stearates and polyoxyl-castor oil derivatives, sorbitan fatty acid esters such as spans and their polyoxyethylene derivatives such as tweens (polysorbates).

Hydrophilic colloids

Most of the emulsifiers form hydrated lyophilic colloids (called hydrocolloids) that form multimolecular layers around emulsion droplets. Hydrocolloid type emulsifiers (Table 6.6) have little or no effect on interfacial tension, but exert a protective colloid effect, reducing the potential for coalescence by:

- providing a protective sheath around the droplets
- imparting a charge to the dispersed droplets (so that they repel each other)
- swelling to increase the viscosity of the system (so that droplets are less likely to merge)

Table 6.6 Organic hydrocolloids used in emulsion formulation

Source	Name	Comment
Tree exudate	Gum Arabic (acacia)	Essentially neutral polysaccharide (ENP)
	Gum Ghatti	
	Karaya	ENP
	Tragacanth	ENP
Sea weeds	Agar, carrageenan	Sulfated polysaccharides
	alginates	Acidic polysaccharides
Seed extracts	Locust bean	ENP
	Guar	ENP
	Quince seed	
Synthetics cellulose	Carboxy methyl-ether	Anionic polysaccharides
Collagen synthetic	Gelatin	Amphoteric protein
	Carboxyvinyl polymer	Neutral
	Polyoxethylene poly.	Anionic

Classification of Hydrophilic Colloids
- Semisynthetic
- Natural-Plant origin and Animal origin

Semi-synthetic Polysaccharides

This class includes mainly cellulose derivatives like sodium carboxy methyl cellulose, hydroxyl propyl cellulose and methyl cellulose. They are used for formulating o/w type of emulsions. They are nontoxic, and are less subject to microbial growth. They primarily act by increasing the viscosity of the system. e.g. methyl cellulose, hydroxypropyl cellulose and sodium carboxy methyl cellulose.

Natural Emulsifying agents from Plant Origin

These consist of agents which are carbohydrates and include gums and mucilaginous substances. Since these substances are of variable chemical composition, these exhibit considerable variation in emulsifying properties. They are anionic in nature and produce o/w emulsions. They act as primary emulsifying agents as well as secondary emulsifying agents (emulsion stabilizers). Since carbohydrates acts a good medium for the growth of microorganism, therefore emulsions prepared using these emulsifying agents have to be suitably preserved in order to prevent microbial contamination. E.g. tragacanth, acacia, agar, chondrus (Irish Moss), pectin and starch.

Natural Emulsifying agents from Animal Origin

The examples include gelatin, egg yolk and wool fat (anhydrous lanolin). Type A gelatin (Cationic) is generally used for preparing o/w emulsion while type B gelatin is used for o/w emulsions of pH 8 and above. Lecithin and cholesterol present in egg yolk also act as emulsifying agent. They show surface activity and are used for formulating o/w emulsions. However they are used only for extemporaneous preparation and not for commercial preparation as it darken and degrade rapidly in unpreserved systems. Wool fat is mainly used in w/o emulsions meant for external use. They absorb large quantities of water and form stable w/o emulsions with other oils and fats. Animal derivatives are more likely to cause allergic reactions and are subject to microbial growth and rancidity. Their advantage is their ability to support formation of w/o creams.

Finely Divided Solids

Finely divided solids can be adsorbed at the oil water interface forming a coherent film that physically prevents coalescence of the dispersed phase. This group consists of finely divided solids having balanced hydrophilic lipophillic properties. They accumulate at the oil/water interface and form a coherent interfacial film around the droplets of dispersed phase globules and prevent coalescence. If the solid particles are preferentially wetted by oil, a w/o emulsion is formed; while o/w emulsion is formed when wetting is done by water. The emulsions formed using finely divided solids are stable and less prone to microbial contamination.

Other Formulation Additives

Buffers: The inclusion of buffer may be necessary to maintain chemical stability, control tonicity or ensure physiological compatibility.

Density Modifiers: From stoke's law it can be seen that if the dispersed and continuous phase both have the same density then the sedimentation and creaming will not occur. Minor modification to the aqueous phase of a emulsion by incorporation of sucrose, dextrose glycerol or propylene glycol can be achieved.

Consistency Builder: It is possible to manipulate consistency of an emulsion system to an appreciable extent by changes in surfactant concentration, phase volume ratio etc. If adjustment in these components do not serve the purpose fully hydrocolloids may be added to aqueous phase or long chain waxes to the oil phases.

Humectants: They are added to emulsion in order to reduce the evaporation of water, either from packed product when the closure is removed or from the surface of skin after application e.g. Glycerol, Polyethylene glycol and Propylene glycol.

Antioxidants: Oxidation of emulsion component leads to rancidity of oil component with resultant bad odor and bad appearance. Oxidative tendency can be countered by inclusion of 0.001% to 0.1% of antioxidants like butylated hydroxytoulene, a-tocopherol etc. Combinations of antioxidants leads to synergistic effect. Other common antioxidants are propyl, octyl and dodecyl ester of gallic acid recommended for use at concentration up to 0.001% for fixed oils and up to 0.1% for essential oils. Efficiency of antioxidants depends upon its compatibility with other ingredients, its oil/water partition coefficient, the extent of its solubilization within molecule of the emulgent and its sorption on to the container and its closure. These antioxidants are liable to discoloration by light and hence emulsions should be packed in amber color or blue color bottles.

Viscosity Enhancers: It may be difficult for aqueous based topical solution to remains in place on the skin or in the eyes for any significant time because of their low viscosity. To counteract this effect low concentration of gelling agents can be used to increase the apparent viscosity of the product. Examples include Povidone, Hydroxyethyl cellulose and Carbomer.

Preservative: When choosing a suitable preservative it must be insured that adsorption of the preservative onto the container from the product does not occur and its efficiency is not impaired by the pH of the solution or by interactions with other ingredients. Some typical preservative used in pharmaceutical and cosmetics emulsions are given in Table 6.7.

Table 6.7 Preservative used in emulsions

Type	Example	Characteristic and utility
Acids and acids derivatives	Benzoic acid sorbic acid and salt	Antifungal
Alcohol	Chlorobutanol Phenoxy-2-ethanol	Eye preparation Synergist
Aldehyde	Formaldehyde Glutaraldehyde	Broad spectrum
Formaldehyde Donors	Mono-(and-)methylodimethyl hydantoin	Broad spectrum
Phenolic	Phenol, cresol, Chlorothymol, o-phenltphenol p-Chlorometaxylenol	Broad spectrum
Quaternaries	Chlorhexidine and salt, Benzethonium chloride	Broad spectrum
Mercurials	Phenylmercuric acetate	Broad spectrum

Sweetening Agents: Low molecular weight carbohydrates and in particular sucrose, are traditionally the most widely used sweetening agents. Sucrose has the advantage of being colorless, very soluble in water, stable over a pH range of about 4 to 8 and increasing the viscosity of fluid preparation. Artificial sweeteners can be used in conjugation with sugars and alcohol to enhance the degree of sweetness, in formulations for patients who must restrict their sugar intake. They are hundred and even thousands of times sweets than sucrose and are therefore rarely required a concentration greater than about 0.2%. Polyhydric alcohols such as sorbitol, mannitol and glycerin can also be used.

Flavor and Perfumes: The simple use of sweating agents may not be sufficient to render palatable a product containing drugs with particularly unpleasant taste. In many cases, therefore, a flavoring agent can be included (Table 6.8).

Table 6.8 Suitable masking flavors for various product tastes

Type of products	Suitable Masking Flavors
Salty	Apricot, butterscotch, peach liquorice, vanilla
Bitter	Anise, chocolate, mint wild cherry.
Sweet	Vanilla. Fruits, berries
Sour	Citrous fruit, liquorice, raspberry.

Colours: The overall appearance of liquid product depends on their color and clarity. Color selection is usually made to be consistent with flavor. Green or blue for mint and Red for berry.

Theory of Emulsification

Emulsions are formed when the two phases are stabilized with the help of emulgents. The droplets can be stabilized by the following methods

A. By reducing interfacial tension

B. By preventing the coalescence of droplets.

- By formation of rigid interfacial film
- By forming electrical double layer.

Interfacial tension

The force causing each liquid to resist breaking up into smaller particle is called interfacial tension. Surfactants promote the lowering of this resistance.

Interfacial film

When water and oil are mixed in the presence of an emulsifier an interfacial film is formed at the oil water interface.

Amphiphillic molecules align themselves at a water-oil interface in the most favorable position - oleophilic portion in the oil phase and hydrophilic portion in aqueous phase. It is also well established that the surface active agents tend to concentrate at interface and that emulsifier are adsorbed at oil-water interfaces as monomolecular films. If the concentration of the emulsifier is high enough, it forms a rigid film between the immiscible phases, which acts as a mechanical barrier to both adhesion and coalescence of the emulsion droplets.

An interfacial film alters the rate of coalescence of droplets by acting as barriers. The similar film can produce repulsive electrical forces between approaching droplets. Such repulsion is due to an electrical double layer, which may arise from electrically charged groups oriented on the surface of emulsified globules. The potential produced by the double layer creates a repulsive effect between the oil droplets and thus hiders coalescence.

Manufacturing of Emulsions

These are several physical and chemical parameters are selected which favors emulsion formation. The application of energy in the form of mechanical agitation, ultrasonic vibration or electricity is required to reduce the internal phase into small droplet. The amount of worked input depends on the length of time during which energy is supplied thus timing becomes another important physical parameter. Similarly chemical parameters like chemical stability, safety, choice of lipid phase and phase ratio is important to be considered for the formulation. As also discussed in theory of emulsion, emulsification techniques (Table 6.9) involves breakup of the internal phase and stabilization and coalescence.

Table 6.9 Techniques of emulsification

Laboratory scale preparation techniques
• Continental or dry gum method
• Wet gum method
• Bottle or Forbes bottle method
• Auxiliary method
• In situ soap method
Large scale preparation techniques
• Emulsification by vaporization
• Emulsification by phase inversion
• Low energy emulsification

Laboratory Scale Preparation Techniques
Continental or Dry Gum Method

The continental method is used to prepare the initial or primary emulsion from oil, water and a hydrocolloid or "gum" type emulsifier (usually acacia). The primary emulsion or emulsion nucleus is formed from 4 parts of oil, 2 parts of water and one part of gum. The 4 parts of oil and 1 part of gum represent their total amount for the final emulsion. In a mortar the 1 part of gum (acacia) is levigated with 4 parts of oil until the powder is thoroughly wetted; then the 2 parts water is added all at once and the mixture is vigorously and continuously triturated until the primary emulsion formed is creamy white (Table 6.10).

Table 6.10 Ratio of oil: gum: water in primary emulsion

Fixed oil	= 4:1:2
Mineral oil	= 3:1:2
Volatile oil	= 2:1:2
Oleo gum resin	= 1:1:2

Additional water or aqueous solutions may be incorporated after the primary emulsion is formed. Slid substances (e.g. active ingredients, preservatives, color, flavors) are generally dissolved and added as a solution to the primary emulsion; oil soluble substances in small amounts may be incorporated directly into the primary emulsion. Any substance which might reduce the physical stability of the emulsion, such as alcohol (which may precipitate the gum) should be added as near to the end of the process as possible to avoid breaking the emulsion. When all agents have been incorporated, the emulsion should be transferred to a calibrated vessel, brought to final volume with water, then homogenized or blended to ensure uniform distribution of ingredients.

Wet Gum Method

The proportion of oil and water and emulsifier (gum) are the same as in dry gum method, but the order and technique of mixing are different. The gum is triturated with water to form mucilage; then oil is slowly added in portions, while triturating. After all the oil is added, the mixture is triturated for several minutes to form the primary emulsion. Then other ingredients are added as in continental method. Generally speaking, this method is more difficult to perform successfully, especially with more viscous oils, but may result in more stable emulsions.

Bottle Method

Bottle method is used to prepare emulsions of volatile oils, or oliogeneous substances of very low viscosities. Acacia (or other gum) is placed in a dry bottle and oil is added, the bottle is capped and thoroughly shaken. To this the required volume of water is added all at once and the mixture is shaken thoroughly until the primary emulsion is formed. It is important to minimize the initial amount of time the gum and oil are mixed. The gum will tend to imbibe the oil and will become water proof.

Auxiliary Method

An emulsion prepared by other methods can also be improved by passing it through a hand homogenizer, which forces the emulsion through a very small orifice, reducing the dispersed droplet size to about 5 microns or less.

In situ soap Method

This method involves the use of soaps as an emulsifier/ surfactants e.g. calcium soaps. Water in oil emulsions contains oils such as oleic acid, in combination with lime water (calcium hydroxide solution, USP). Emulsion is prepared by mixing equal volumes of oil and lime water.

Large Scale Preparation Techniques

Emulsification by Vaporization

Heat is important factor to be considered because vaporization is an effective way of breaking almost all the bonds between the molecules of liquids. An increase in temperature decreases the internal tension as well as viscosity. When emulsion is stored at elevated temperature for a longer period of time the kinetic energy of droplets is raised thereby facilitates their coalescence.

Changes in temperature alter the distribution coefficients of emulsifiers between the two phases and cause emulsifier migration. The distribution of the emulsifier as a function of temperature cannot be correlated directly with either emulsion formation or stability.

Emulsification by Phase Inversion

The temperature at which the inversion occurs depends upon emulsifier concentration and is called phase inversion temperature (PIT). This type of inversion can occur during emulsion formulation because they are generally prepared at high temperature and then allowed top cool at room temperature. Emulsions formed by a phase inversion technique are generally considered quite stable and are believed to contain finally dispersed internal phase. So the emulsions must have a PIT as high more possible as, always higher than the storage temperature. The phase inversion temperature is considered to be the temperature at which the hydrophilic and lipophilic properties of the emulsifier are in balance and is therefore also called the HLB temperature.

Low Energy Emulsification

The classic process of emulsification described requires considerable expenditure of energy during both the cooling and the heating cycles of emulsion formation. In this process all of internal phase, but only a portion of external phase is heated. After emulsification of heated portions, the remainder of external phase is added to the emulsion concentrate, or the preformed concentrate is blended into the continuous phase. In those emulsion in which a phase inversion temperature exists, the emulsion concentrate is preferable prepared above the phase inversion temperature, which results in emulsions having extremely small droplet size.

Equipment for Emulsification

The most important factor involved in the formation of emulsion is degree of share and turbulence required to produce a given dispersion a liquid droplets. The amount of agitation required depends on total volume of liquid to be mixed, the viscosity of the system, Interfacial tension at oil/water interface. Emulsion can be formulated using the following equipments.

- Mechanical stirrers
- Ultrasonifier
- Homogenizers
- Colloid mills

Mechanical stirrers: An emulsion may be stirred by means of various impeller mounted on shafts, which are placed directly in to system to be emulsified (Fig. 6.3). Simple top-entering propeller mixers are adequate for routine development work in the laboratory and for production purposes, if the viscosity is low. If more vigorous agitation is required or if the preparation has moderate viscosity turbine type mixers are employed both in laboratory and in production.

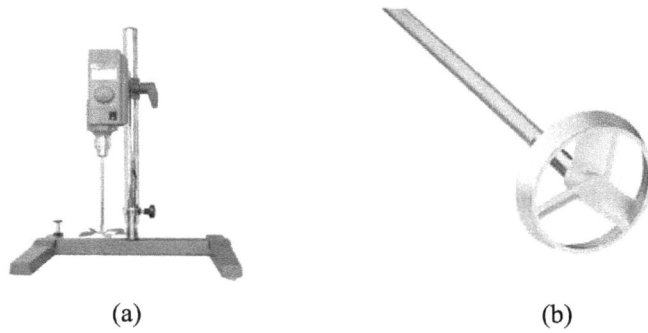

(a)　　　　　　　　　　　　(b)

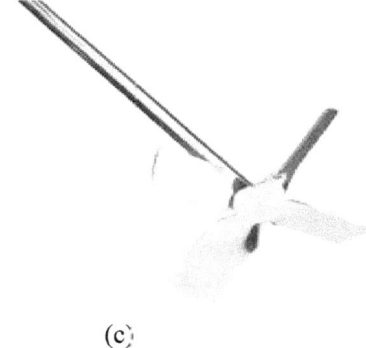

(c)

Fig. 6.3 Different types of stirrers (a) Mechanical stirrers, (b) Turbine stirrer, (c) Propeller stirrers.

Other mixers are provided with paddle blade, counter rotating blades, or planetary action blades. The degree of agitation is controlled by impeller rotation, its position in the container, the presence of baffles, and general shape of container. The pattern of liquid flow and the resultant efficiency of mixing are controlled by the time of impeller.

Ultrasonifier: These are useful for the laboratory preparation of fluid emulsions of moderate viscosity and extremely low particle size. The equipment is based upon the principle of the Pohlman liquid whistle. The dispersion is forced through an orifice at modest pressures and is allowed to impinge upon a blade (Fig. 6.4). The pressure required range from approximately 150 to 350 psi and cause the blade to vibrate rapidly to produce ultrasonic note. When the system reaches a steady state, a cavitational field is generated at the leading edge of the blade, and pressure fluctuations of approximately 60 tons psi can be achieved in commercial equipment.

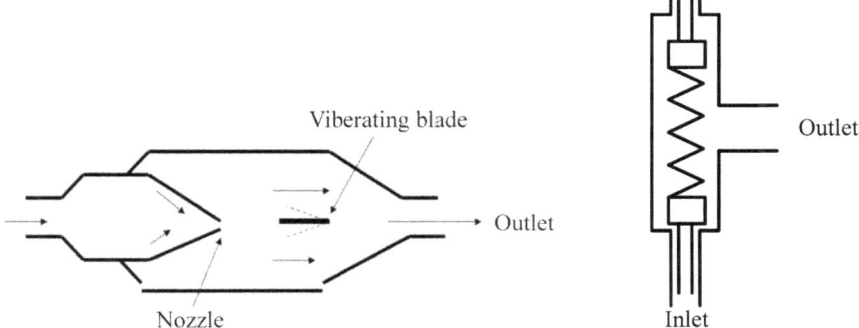

Fig. 6.4 Ultrasonifier.

Fig. 6.5 Homogenizer.

Homogenizers: In a homogenizer the dispersion of two liquids are achieved by forcing their mixture through a small inlet orifice at high pressures. A homogenizer generally consists of a pump that raises the pressure of the dispersion to a range of 500 to 5000 psi and an orifice through which this fluid impinges upon the homogenizing values held in place on the values seat by a strong spring (Fig. 6.5). As the pressure builds up, the spring is compressed, and some of the dispersion escapes between the value and the value seat. At this point the energy that has been stored in the liquid as pressure is released instantaneously and subjects the product to intense turbulence and hydraulic shear. The use of a homogenizer is warranted whenever a reasonably monodispersed emulsion of low particle size is required.

Colloid mills: Colloidal mills operate on the principle of high shear, which is normally generated between the rotor and stator of the colloidal mill. Colloidal mills are used for comminution of solids for the dispersion of suspensions containing poorly wetted solids bur are also useful for the preparation of relatively viscous emulsions (Fig. 6.6 and 6.7).

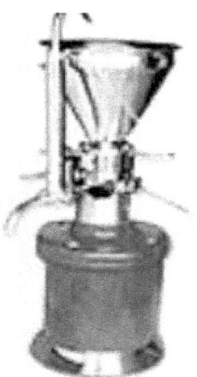
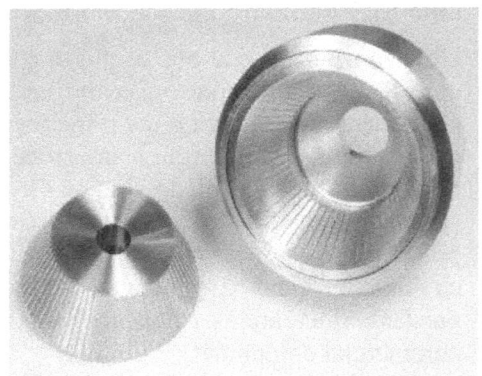

Fig. 6.6 Colloidal mill. **Fig. 6.7** Colloidal mill rotor and stator.

Stability of Emulsions

An emulsion is called physically stable if its dispersed state does not change, i.e. if its droplet size distribution remains constant regardless of time or volume element observed. For stability of emulsion droplets must not sediment, aggregate or coalesce; changes in droplet sizes.

There are different mechanisms which can cause emulsion instability. Broadly these may be of two types – physical and chemical.

Physical Stability

These may occur due to change in physical attributes of emulsion such as increase in particle size or coalescence of droplets or phase inversion (Fig. 6.8).

Creaming or Sedimentation: Creaming is the upward movement of dispersed droplets of emulsion relative to the continuous phase (due to the density difference between two phases), a fatty cream appears due to the assembly of the large drops (example: unhomogenized milk). Creaming can be reversed by agitation. Consideration of qualitative application of Stokes' law (See chapter 5: Suspension) will show that the rate of creaming can be reduced by:

- Production of an emulsion of small droplet size
- Increase in the viscosity of the continuous phase
- Reduction in the density difference between two phases
- Control of disperse phase concentration

Flocculation: It is reversible aggregation of droplet of internal phase in the form of three dimensional clusters. Flocculation of emulsion droplet can occur only when the mechanical and electrical barrier is sufficient to prevent droplet coalescence. Flocculation differs from coalescence by the fact that the interfacial films and individual droplet remains intact.

Coalescence: The oily and watery phase is completely separated due to merging droplets to form large drops. Coalescence is irreversible. An increase in the surfactant concentration or a replacement of the emulsifier being used can often improve the resistance of emulsions to coalescence. Since coalescence is a function of droplet collisions with a subsequent merger of interfacial membranes, layers with strong repulsive interactions are better suited to stabilize emulsion droplets. A strong repulsive force may prevent collisions between droplets in the first place. Repulsive interactions can be altered by modifying the charge at the droplet surface or by using a surfactant that has a different thickness of the interfacial layer. Emulsions with sufficiently small droplets, which are prevented from aggregating or coalescing by the use of suitable emulsifiers, exhibit great physical stability.

Phase inversion: Phase inversion refers to changes in the emulsion type i.e., the emulsion may spontaneously revert from oil-in-water to a water-in-oil emulsion or vice versa. This process is called phase inversion. Phase inversion occurs primarily in emulsions that have very high volume fractions. It is fairly easy to detect phase inversion, as the process generally results in sudden alterations in emulsion conductivity and viscosity.

Ostwald ripening: Ostwald ripening is the process whereby larger droplets grow at the expense of smaller ones, because of the transport of dispersed phase molecules from smaller to larger droplets through the intervening continuous phase. The driving force for this process is an increase in solubility of dispersed phase molecules in the continuous phase, which occurs when the droplet curvature increases (i.e., the droplet size decreases). Since Ostwald ripening is a function of the solubility of the dispersed phase, the addition of a second nonpolar lipid with a substantially lower solubility to the high-solubility dispersed phase can strongly reduce the growth of droplets. Another approach of minimizing the Ostwald ripening is to produce droplets as equal in size as possible (uniform size), so as to reduce the differences in capillary pressures.

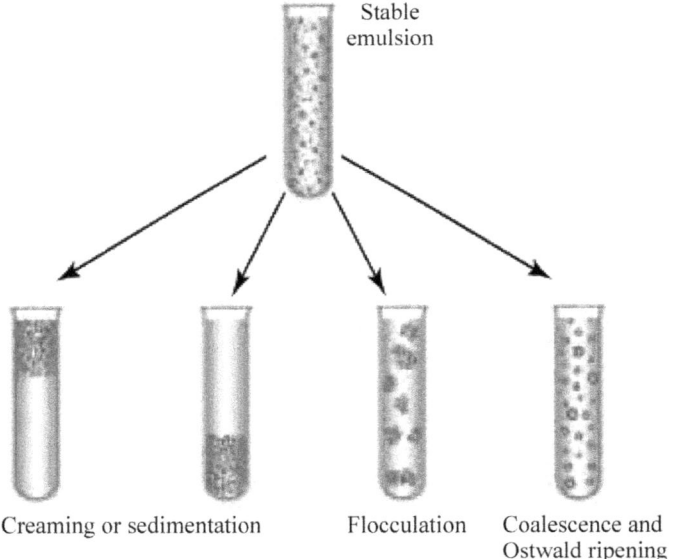

Fig. 6.8 Principal mechanisms of physical instability of emulsions.

Chemical Stability

The chemical stability of an emulsion reflects its resistance against chemical changes. Mostly oxidation of fats and oils is the critical reaction for chemical deterioration of emulsions. The addition of antioxidants and protection against external influences such as light or excessive heat, as well as suitable diffusion barriers on the surfaces between the different liquid phases, improve the chemical stability.

Emulsion Stabilization

An Emulsion can be stabilized by addition for suitable emulsifying agents. There are two stabilization mechanisms – electrostatic Stabilization and steric stabilization (Fig. 6.9).

Electrostatic Stabilization

As the name implies, this is the mechanism of stabilization involved with charged surfactants - usually anionics. On forming an aqueous solution, an ionic surfactant breaks into two components, the anionic surfactant portion and the cationic counter ion; this process is called "ionization." In the presence of a suspended oil phase, the hydrophobic tails of the anionic portion are "dissolved" in the oil droplets leaving the charged heads on the droplet surface. This molecular orientation results in a net negative charge on the surface of the droplet. This surface charge leads to the formation of a secondary shell of dissolved countering which is positively charged. The negative surface/positive secondary shell system is known as an "electrical double layer." The end result of the double layer is emulsion stabilization as two approaching oil droplets are barred from coalescing by their mutually repulsive positively charged outer shells.

Steric Stabilization

This mechanism of stabilization is prevalent with nonionic surfactants. When the hydrophobes of a nonionic are "dissolved" into a suspended oil droplet, the hydrophiles protrude a long way into the aqueous medium from the droplet surface. Much as the bristles on a hair brush preclude two brushes being pushed together head to head, the protruding hydrophiles prevent the oil droplets from coalescing. This effect is steric stabilization.

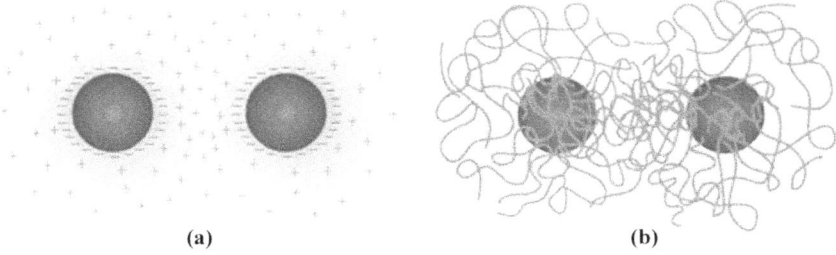

(a) (b)

Fig. 6.9 Schematic representation of electrostatic stabilization (a) and steric stabilization (b)

Evaluation of Emulsion Stability

Stability of emulsions can be done keeping the following points in focus. Final evaluation should be done in final container as:
- The ingredients may interact with the container.
- Some material may leach out from the container
- Loss of water and volatile ingredients may occur through the container or closures

Further to study emulsion stability following parameters are generally studied under stress condition (accelerated stability studies; refer Chapter 12) for:
- Thermal stress
- Aging and temperature
- Phase inversion temperature
- Gravitational stress
- Agitation

Physical Parameters of Evaluation

- **Phase separation**

  Phase separation is a phenomenon of changes in the emulsion type i.e., the emulsion may spontaneously revert from oil-in-water to a water-in-oil emulsion or vice versa. An approximate estimation may be obtained visually. Accelerating the separation by centrifugation followed by appropriate analysis of the specimen may be useful to quantitatively determine the phase separation.

- **Viscosity**

  Cone and plate viscometers are suitable for emulsions but instruments using coaxial cylinders are easy to use. Penetrometres can be used when the preparation is too viscous. Use of heliapath attachment with Brookfield viscometer helps in detection of creaming tendency and hence it is advisable to study rheological properties over extended period of time which can help in prediction of long-term behavior.

- **Globule size**

  The globule size in emulsions is measured by microscopic methods or by electronic devices such as coulter counter. In either of these two techniques the original product has to be suitably diluted before estimation. The dilution may introduce errors because of incomplete defloculation or new pattern of flocculation. Hence while making judgment about the stability of the emulsions this aspect should be kept in mind. Globule size also determines the appearance of emulsion (Table 6.11). Therefore, the appearance of an emulsion may also indicate the globule size in an emulsion.

Table 6.11 Globule size and appearance of emulsions

Globule size (mm)	Appearance
> 1	White
0.1-1.0	Blue-white
0.05-0.1	Opalescent, semitransparent
< 0.5	Transparent

- **Electrical Conductivity**

It is determined by using Platinum electrodes (diameter 0.4 mm, distance 4 mm) microamperometrically to produce a current of 15 to 50 mA. Measurements are made on emulsions stored at room temperature or at 37^0 C for short time. Stable o/w emulsions offer less resistance, but droplet aggregation increases resistance. A stable w/o emulsion doesn't conduct electricity, but with droplet coagulation conductivity increases.

- **Electrophoretic Properties**

Zeta potential (See Chapter 5; Suspension) of emulsion can be measured with the aid of moving boundary method or more quickly and directly, by observing the movement of particles under the influence of electric current. The Zeta potential is essentially useful for assessing the flocculation since electrical changes on particles influences the rate of flocculation.

Storage of Emulsions

The production rate of emulsion plants is generally greater than demand; therefore, storage facilities make it possible to have longer production runs, thus improving plant productivity. Present day emulsions may be stored for up to several months without major changes in physical properties. It is advisable to use small diameter vertical storage tanks with a minimum horizontal cross section with a dip tube filling pipe which reaches to or near the bottom of the storage tank. Emulsions of different ionic types should never be mixed and tanks should be thoroughly cleaned before refilling with a different ionic type. Provisions should also be made to ensure proper agitation of stored emulsion to prevent settling, decantation or creaming. Emulsions are sensitive to frost which can cause irreversible breaking; therefore, provisions should also be made to prevent stored emulsion from freezing.

Microemulsions

Microemulsions are recently developed advanced type of emulsions. Microemulsions can be defined as isotropic, thermodynamically stable solutions in which substantial amounts of two immiscible liquids (i.e., water and oil) are brought into a single phase by means of an appropriate surfactant or surfactant mixture. The majority of microemulsions are produced in the presence of co-surfactants of which the most commonly used are low molecular weight alcohols. Microemulsions can be sterilized by filtration and their production is relatively simple and inexpensive. Because of these properties, they have attracted a great interest as drug delivery vehicles. Some more advanced emulsions with extremely smaller globule size have also been investigated by various scientists (Table 6.12).

Major advantages of microemulsions

- Ease of preparation, clarity, stability
- Ability to be filtered
- Ability to encapsulate drugs of different HLB in the same system because the microemulsions can solubilize oil soluble, water soluble and interface soluble drugs
- Low viscosity

Preparation of Microemulsions

Microemulsions can be prepared by blending oil, water, surfactant and cosurfactants with mild agitation or mild heat. For preparing o/w microemulsions, w/o emulsion containing a lipophilic surface-active agent may be used as a base. In this process, hydrophilic surface-active agent is added by stirring which initially forms cubic structure but on further addition of hydrophilic surface-active agent forms microemulsions.

Characterization of Microemulsions

The internal structure elucidation of microemulsions can be done by Small angle X-ray scattering (SAXS), small angle neutron scattering (SANS), dynamic (or laser) light scattering (DLS), transmission electron microscopy, nuclear magnetic resonance, and time resolved fluorescence quenching methods have also been used. Other physicochemical parameters of evaluation include conductance, viscosity, dielectric permittivity, ultrasonic interferometry, ultrasonic absorption, thermal conductivity and infrared spectroscopy.

Applications of Microemulsions

Microemulsions can be applied as liquid membrane carriers to transport lipophilic substances through an aqueous medium or to carry hydrophilic substances across lipoidal medium Microemulsions have been used mainly for peroral delivery of peptides and have also been reported as drug carriers for topical, dermal, transdermal and pulmonary administrations of drugs. Microemulsions have also great potential as i.v. vehicles for sparingly soluble substances by virtue of their high solubilization capacity.

Table 6.12 Comparative features of emulsions, nanoemulsion and microemulsion

	Name	Diameter	T/D Stability	Appearance	Surfactant:Oil
R_1	Emulsion	0.1 -100 μm	No	Opaque	< 1:10
R_2	Microemulsion	10-100 nm	No	Clear Cloudy	≈ 1:1
R_3	Nanoemulsion	5-50 nm	Yes	Clear cloudy	> 1:1

Bibliography

- Aboofazeli R., Lawrence M.J. *Int. J. Pharm.* 1993; 93: 161.
- Akhtar N and Yazan Y. Formulation and characterization of a cosmetic multiple emulsion system containing Macadamia nut oil and two antiaging agents. *Turkish J. Pharm. Sciences*, 2005;2(3): 173-185.
- Attwood D. In: Aulton ME (Editor), Pharmaceutics: The science of dosage form design. 2nd Edn., 2002, Churchil Livingstone, New York, pp. 70-99.
- Becher P. Emulsions, Theory and Practice (2nd Ed.) 1965, Reinhold, New York, pp.2-149.
- Becher Paul. *Encyclopedia of Emulsion Technology.* Volume 4. Marcel Dekker, Inc.New York: 1996.

- Billany M. In: Aulton ME (Editor), Pharmaceutics: The science of dosage form design. 2nd Edn., 2002, Churchil Livingstone, New York, pp. 334-58.
- Comelles F, Pascual A. Microemulsion-based media as novel drug delivery system. *Adv.Drug Del.Rev.* 1996; 45:89-121.
- Corswant C., Thoren P., Engstrom S. Triglyceride- based microemulsion for intravenous administration of sparingly soluble substances. *J.Pharm.Sci.* 1998; 87:200-208.
- Dickinson E. 1992. An Introduction to Food Colloids. Oxford University Press, Oxford.
- Emsap W, Paeratakul O, Siepmann J, In; Banker GS, Rhodes CT (Eds). Modern Pharmaceutics. 2005 (Vol. 121) Marcel Dekker, Inc. New York, Basel, US, pp 237-85.
- Florence AT and Whitehill D. *Multiple Emulsions*, Formulation and stability. *Int. J. Pharmaceutics*, 1982;11:277-278.
- Florence AT and Whitehill D. The formulation and stability of multiple emulsions. *J. Pharm.Pharmacol.* 1982; 34: 687.
- Herbert, W. J. Multiple emulsions, a new form of mineral-oil antigen adjuvant. Lancet 1965;2: 771.
- Iliescu, Cristina-Alina. *Investigation on the thermal stability of technical and cosmetic emulsions* 2005; 30; 21-22.
- IUPAC, Brownian motion. *IUPAC Compendium of Chemical Terminology* 1990, *62*, 2177.
- Laetitia O, Monique S, Lev B, Madelein B, Thi-Nhat-Lien D and Jean-Louis G. Optimization of a thermally reversible w/o/w multiple emulsion for shear-induced drug release. *Int. J. Cont. Release*, 2003; 88:401-412.
- Latreille B. and Paquin P. Evaluation of emulsion stability by centrifugation with conductivity measurements. *J. Food Sci.* 1990;55:1666- 1672.
- Lawrance M.J., Rees G.D. Microemulsion-based media as novel drug delivery system. *Adv. Drug.Deiv Rev.* 2000; 45:89-121.
- Martin A. Physical Pharmacy, 4th Edn, 1993, BI Waverly, New Delhi, pp. 477-511.
- Olivera A.G., Scarpa M.V., Chaimovich, H. *J. Pharm. Sci.*1997; 86:616-620.

- Park K.M., Kim C.K. *Int. J. Pharm.* 1999; 181:173-179.
- Park K.M., Lee M.K., Hwang K.J., Kim C.K. *Int .J. Pharm.* 1999;183:145-154.
- Pattarino F., Marengo E., Gasco M. R., Carpignano R. *Int. J. Pharm.* 1993;91: 157.
- Rieger MM. In; Lachman L, Lieberman HA, Kanig JL. Eds. The Theory and Practices of Industrial Pharmacy. 3rd Edn, 1986, Varghese Publishing House, Bombay, pp. 502-33.
- Tenjarla S. *Ther Drug Carrier Sys* 1999;16: 461.
- Vandamme T. *Prog. Retin. Eye Res.* 2002; 21:15.
- Weiss J. Effect of Mass Transport Processes on Physicochemical Properties of Surfactant- Stabilized Emulsions. Department of Food Science, University of Massachusetts, Amherst. 1999, 280.
- Winfield AJ, In: Winfield AJ, Richards RME (Eds). Pharmaceutical Practice, 3rd Edn, 2004, Churchill Livingstone, New York, pp. 198-205.

CHAPTER 7

Oral Controlled Release Products

Introduction

Dosage forms are defined as medium of drug delivery which introduce (directly or indirectly) drug to the systemic circulation and not to a specific organ or tissue. These conventional dosage forms are also called immediate release dosage form as they do not delay or sustain the release. Conventional dosage forms have the following advantages and disadvantages.

Advantages

- Easy to manufacture or formulate.
- No chance of toxicity due to dose dumping unlike the sustained release dosage forms.
- Cost effective.

Disadvantages

- Require frequent dosing: Drugs with short biological half life ($t_{1/2}$) require frequent dosing to maintain constant therapeutic level
- Fluctuations in plasma level of drug: Inappropriate dosing interval leads to large peaks and valleys in the drug blood level.
- Drug blood level may not be within the therapeutic range at sufficient early time points.
- Patient noncompliance: Multiple-dose regimen leads to failure of therapy many a times due to patient noncompliance.
- High cost of trans-shipment due to requirement of more space for dosage forms per single therapy.

During the last two-three decades there has been remarkable increase in interest in controlled release drug delivery system. This has been due to various factor viz. the prohibitive cost of developing new drug molecules, expiration of existing international patents, discovery of new polymeric materials suitable for prolonging the drug release, and the improvement in therapeutic efficiency and safety achieved by these delivery systems.

Modified Release Dosage Forms: According to the United States Pharmacopoeia the term *'modified release dosage forms'* is used to denote the dosage forms for which the drug release characteristics of time course and/or location are chosen to accomplish therapeutic objectives not offered by the conventional dosage forms. Two types of modified release dosage forms are recognized.

- **Extended release dosage forms**

  It is defined as the one that allows at least a twofold reduction in the dosing frequency as compared to that of conventional dosage form.

- **Delayed release dosage forms**

  It is defined as one that releases the drug at a time other than "immediately" after administration.

Rationale of Controlled Drug Delivery

The basic rationale for controlled drug delivery is to alter the pharmacokinetics and pharmacodynamics of pharmacologically active moieties by using novel drug delivery system or by modifying the molecular structure and /or physiological parameters inherent in a selected route of administration.

Terminology

Different terminologies have been used for the new drug delivery system by different authors.

- **Controlled Action**

    In this type of dosage forms it provides a prolonged duration of drug release with predictability and reproducibility of drug release kinetics. In this case, the rate of drug absorption is equal to the rate of drug removal from body.

- **Sustained Action**

    In this type of dosage forms, a sufficient amount of drug is initially made available to the body to cause a desired pharmacological response. The remaining fraction is released periodically and is required to maintain the maximum initial pharmacological activity for some desirable period of time in excess of time expected from usual single dose.

- **Prolonged Action**

    These types of dosage form are designed in such a way that it release the drug over an extended period during which pharmacological response is obtained but does not necessarily maintain the constant blood level.

- **Site specific and receptor release**

    It refers to targeting of drug directly to a certain biological location.

Advantages and disadvantages of controlled release dosage forms

Advantages

Patient Compliance

Success of a drug therapy depends upon the ability of patient to comply with the regimen. But most often lack of compliance is observed with long term treatment of chronic disease. Patient compliance is affected by a combination of several factors, like awareness of disease process, patient faith in therapy, his understanding of the need to adhere to a strict treatment schedule. Moreover, the complex therapeutic regimens, the high cost of therapy and magnitude of local and or systemic side effect of the dosage form also lead to non compliance. The controlled release drug delivery system may be helpful in ensuring the patient compliance.

Reduced Fluctuation in Plasma Drug Level

Administration of a drug in a conventional dosage form (except in case of constant intravenous infusion) often results in 'see – saw' pattern of drug concentration in the systemic circulation and tissue compartments. The magnitudes of these fluctuations depend on drug kinetics such as the rate of absorption, distribution, elimination and dosing intervals. The 'see-saw' or 'peak and valley' pattern is more prominent in case of drugs with low biological half lives (less than 4 hours). A well designed controlled release drug delivery system can significantly reduce the frequency of drug dosing and also maintain a more steady drug concentration in blood circulation and target tissue cells.

Reduced dose and dosing frequency

Controlled release drug delivery systems require less amount of total drug to treat a diseased condition as compared to conventional dosage forms. Reduction in the total dose results in decreased systemic or local side effects. Moreover, the dosing frequency is also reduced. This also leads to greater cost effectiveness.

Improved Efficiency in Treatment

Optimal therapy of a disease requires an efficient delivery of active drugs to the tissues, organs that need treatment. Very often doses far in excess to those required in the cells have to be administered in order to achieve the necessary therapeutically effective concentration. This unfortunately may lead to undesirable, toxicological and immunological effects in non-target tissue. A controlled release dosage forms leads to better management of the acute or chronic disease condition by better drug utilization.

Disadvantages

Dose Dumping

Dose dumping is a phenomenon which refers to a rapid release of relatively large quantities of drug from a controlled release formulation, introducing potential toxic quantities of the drug into the systemic circulation. Dose dumping can lead to fatalities in case of potent drug, which have a narrow therapeutic index e.g. Phenobarbital.

Less flexibility in accurate dose adjustment

In conventional dosage forms, dose adjustments are much simpler e.g. tablet can be divided into two fractions. In case of controlled release dosage forms, this appears to be much more complicated. Controlled release property may get lost, if dosage form is fractured.

Poor *In Vitro-In vivo* correlation

In controlled release dosage form, the rate of drug release is deliberately reduced to achieve drug release possibly over a large region of gastrointestinal tract. Here the so called 'Absorption window' becomes important and may give rise to unsatisfactory drug absorption *in vivo* despite excellent in-vitro release characteristics.

Patient variation

The time period required for absorption of drug released from the dosage form may vary among individuals. Co-administration of other drugs, presence or absence of food and residence time in gastrointestinal tract is different among patients. This also gives rise to variation in clinical response among the patient.

Drug properties Relevant to Develop CRDF

Following criteria should be met by a drug proposed to be formulated in controlled release dosage forms (CRDF).

(a) **Short half-life**

The half life of a drug is an index of its residence time in the body. If the drug has a short half life (less than 2 hours), the dosage form may contain a prohibitively large quantity of the drug. On the other hand, drug with elimination half life of eight hours or more are sufficiently sustained in the body, when administered in conventional dosage from, and controlled release drug delivery system is generally not necessary in such cases. Ideally, the drug should have half-life of three to four hours.

(b) **Small dose**

If the dose of a drug in the conventional dosage form is high, its suitability as a candidate for controlled release is seriously undetermined. This is chiefly because the size of a unit dose controlled release formulation would become too big, to administer without difficulty.

(c) **First pass clearance**

As discussed earlier in disadvantages of controlled delivery system, delivery of the drug to the body in desired concentrations is adversely affected in case of drugs undergoing extensive hepatic first pass metabolism, when administered in controlled release forms. First pass metabolism may occur in various other sites also e.g. bacterial flora of intestine or colon, skin uptake/metabolism etc.

(d) **Desirable absorption and solubility characteristics**

Absorption of poorly water soluble drug is often dissolution rate limited. Incorporating such compounds into controlled release formulations is therefore unrealistic and may reduce overall absorption efficiency.

(e) **Desirable absorption window**

Certain drugs when administered orally are absorbed only from a specific part of gastrointestinal tract. This part is referred to as the 'absorption window'. Drugs exhibiting an absorption window like fluorouracil, thiazide diuretics, if formulated as controlled release dosage form are unsuitable.

(f) **High therapeutic index**

Drugs with low therapeutic index are unsuitable for incorporation in controlled release formulations. If the system fails in the body, dose dumping may occur, leading to fatalities e.g. Digitoxin.

Therefore, drugs with too large/too small half life, large doses, extensively first pass metabolism, low aqueous solubility, low permeability, poor absorption and low therapeutic index are not rendered suitable for modified or controlled release products.

Controlled Release Vs Sustained Release Preparations

Although this term has been interchanged widely with sustained release preparations in the past, recently it has become customary to restrict the latter term to oral formulations where the mechanism of prolonged action is dependent on one or more of the environmental factors in the gastrointestinal tract such as pH, enzymes, gastric motility etc. On the other hand, the term controlled release dosage form usually applies to preparations that are designed for all routes of administration and where the mechanism of prolonged action is inherent and determined totally by the delivery system itself. Consequently, this category offers the current state-of-the-art products where the drug release profile is controlled accurately and often can be targeted to a special body site or a particular organ.

Design and Formulation of Oral Controlled Release Drug Delivery System and the Factors Affecting

Oral drug delivery has been known for decades as the most widely utilized route of administration among all the routes that have been explored for the systemic delivery of drugs via various pharmaceutical products of different dosage forms. Indeed, for sustained-release systems, the oral route of administration has by far received the most attention with respect to research on physiological and drug constraints as well as design and testing of products. This is because there is more flexibility in dosage form design for the oral route than there is for the parenteral route. Other reasons of wide utilization of oral route are flexibility in dosage form, design and patient compliance. But here one has to take into consideration, the various pH that the dosage form would encounter during its transit, the gastrointestinal motility, the enzyme system and its influence on the drug and the dosage form. The majority of oral controlled release systems rely on dissolution, diffusion or a combination of both mechanisms, to generate slow release of drug to the gastrointestinal milieu.

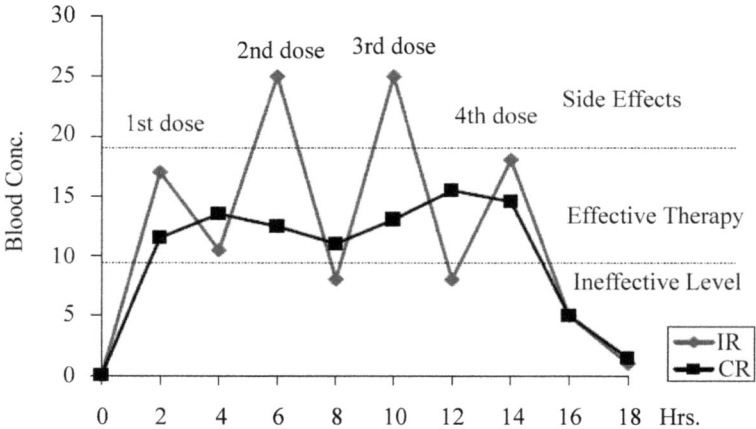

Fig. 7.1 Blood Profiles: Controlled Release (CR) vs. Immediate Release (IR).

Theoretically and desirably a controlled release delivery device, should release the drug by a zero-order process (drug release independent of time) which would result in a blood-level time profile (Fig. 7.1) similar to that after intravenous constant rate infusion.

Advantages of Sustained Release Products
1. Decreased local and systemic side effects:
   - Reduced gastrointestinal irritation.
2. Better drug utilization:
   - Reduction in total amount of drug used.
   - Minimum drug accumulation on chronic dosing.
3. Improved efficiency in treatment:
   - Optimized therapy.
   - More uniform blood concentration.
   - Reduction in fluctuation in drug level and hence more uniform pharmacological response.
   - Special effects e.g. sustained release aspirin provides sufficient drug so that on awakening the arthritic patient gets symptomatic relief.
   - Cure or control of condition more promptly.
   - Less reduction in drug activity with chronic use.
   - Method by which sustained release is achieved can improve the bioavailability of some drugs e.g. drugs susceptible to enzymatic inactivation can be protected by encapsulation in polymer systems suitable for sustained release.
4. Improved patient compliance:
   - Less frequent dosing
   - Reduced night-time dosing
   - Reduced patient care time.
5. Economy:
   Although the initial unit cost of sustained release products is usually greater than that of conventional dosage forms because of the special nature of these products, the average cost of treatment over an extended time period maybe less. Economy may also result from a decrease in nursing time and hospitalization time.

Classification of Oral Controlled Drug Delivery Systems

Controlled (zero-order) drug release has been investigated by various following classes of controlled drug delivery system.

I. Diffusion controlled system.
   (i) Reservoir type.
   (ii) Matrix type

II. Dissolution controlled system.
   (i) Reservoir type.
   (ii) Matrix type

III. Methods using Ion-exchange.

IV. Methods using osmotic pressure.

V. pH independent formulations.

VI. Altered density formulations.

I Diffusion controlled system

Basically diffusion process shows the movement of drug molecules from a region of a higher concentration to one of lower concentration (Table 7.1). The flux of the drug J (in amount / area - time), across a membrane in the direction of decreasing concentration is given by *Fick's law*.

$$J = -D \cdot \frac{dc}{dx}$$

where D = diffusion coefficient in area/ time

dc/dx = change of concentration 'c' with distance 'x'

Assuming steady state the above equation can be integrated to give,

$$J = \frac{-D \cdot \Delta c}{L}$$

In common form, when a water insoluble membrane encloses a core of drug, it must diffuse through the membrane, the drug release rate dm/dt is given by,

$$\frac{dm}{dt} = \frac{A.D.K.\Delta C}{L}$$

where A = area

K = Partition coefficient of drug between the membrane and drug core

ΔC = concentration difference across the membrane.

L = diffusion path length

(i) Reservoir type

In this system, drug core is surrounded by polymer membrane which controls release rate (Fig. 7.2). Drug partitions into the membrane and get exchanged with the fluid surrounding the particle or tablet. Additional drug will enter the polymer, diffuse to the periphery and exchange with the surrounding media. The advantages and disadvantages of this system are given in Table 7.1.

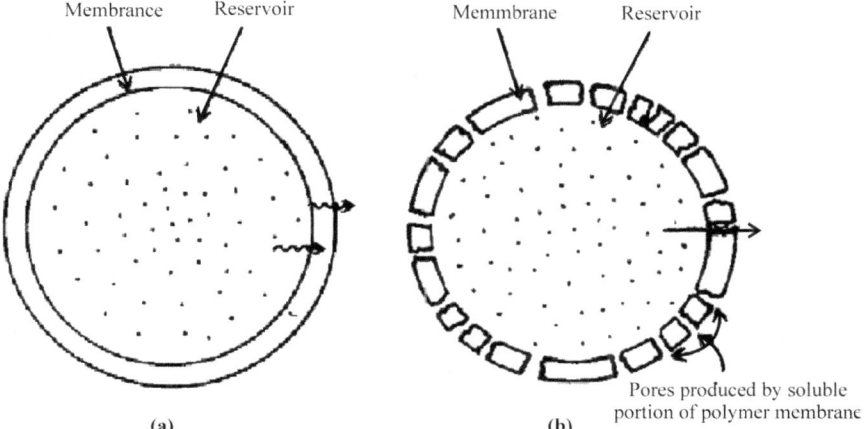

(a) Diffusion control of drug release by a water-insoluble polymer

(b) Diffusion control of drug release by a partially water-soluble polymer

Fig. 7.2 Reservoir type diffusion controlled drug release.

Table 7.1 Characteristics of oral controlled drug delivery systems

Class of CRDF	Description	Advantages	Disadvantages
Reservoir Diffusional System	Drug core surrounded by polymer membrane which controls release rate	• Zero order delivery is possible • Release rates variable with polymer type.	• System must be physically removed from implant sites • Difficult to deliver high molecular weight compound • Generally increased cost per dosage unit • Potential toxicity if system fails
Matrix Diffusional System	Homogenous dispersion of solid drug in a polymer mixture	• Easier to produce than reservoir or encapsulated devices • Can deliver high molecular weight compounds	• Cannot provide zero order release • Removal of remaining matrix is necessary for implanted system
Bioerodible Matrix System	Homogenous dispersion of drug in an erodible matrix	• Easier to produce than reservoir or encapsulated devices • Can deliver high molecular weight compounds • Removal from implant sites not necessary	• Difficult to control kinetics owing to multiple processes of release • Potential toxicity of degraded polymer must be considered.
Osmotically controlled system	Drug surrounded by semipermeable membrane and release governed by osmotic pressure	• Zero order release possible • Reformulation not required for different drugs • Release of drug independent of the environment of the system	• Much more expensive than conventional one • Quality control more extensive than most conventional tablets

(ii) **Matrix type**

A solid drug is dispersed in an insoluble matrix and the rate of release of drug is dependent on the rate of drug diffusion and not on the rate of solid dissolution.

Higuchi has derived the appropriate equation for drug release for this system,

$$M = \sqrt{Ds.Ca.\frac{p}{2Co-pCa}.t}$$

where

M = weight in gm of drug released per unit area of surface at time t

p = porosity of the matrix

T = Tortuosity of the matrix

Ds = Diffusion coefficient of drug in the release medium

Ca = solubility of drug in release medium

Co = Total amount of drug in s unit volume of the matrix

Therefore, if the drug release is directly proportional to square root of time (or the plot between amount of drug release and square root of time is linear) the drug release is said to be occur through matrix diffusion process. So, according to Higuchi Model, release of drug from a homogenous matrix system may be controlled by varying the porosity, tortuosity, polymer system forming the matrix and solubility of the drug.

A third possible diffusional mechanism is the system where a partially soluble membrane encloses a drug core. Dissolution of part of membrane allows for diffusion of the constrained drug through pores in the polymer coat.

The release rate can be given by following equation:

Release rate = $AD/L = [C_1 - C_2]$

where,

A = Area

D = diffusion coefficient

C_1 = Drug concentration in the core

C_2 = Drug concentration in the surrounding medium

L = diffusional path length

Thus diffusion controlled products are based on two approaches. The *first approach* entails placement of the drug in an insoluble matrix of some sort. The eluting medium penetrates the matrix and drug diffuses out of the matrix to the surrounding pool for ultimate absorption. The *second approach* involves enclosing the drug particle with a polymer coat. In this case the portion of the drug which has dissolved in the polymer coat diffuses through an unstirred film of liquid into the surrounding fluid.

II Dissolution Controlled Systems

A drug with a slow dissolution rate is inherently sustained and for those drugs with high water solubility, one can decrease dissolution through appropriate salt or derivative formation. These systems are most commonly employed in the production of enteric coated dosage forms. To protect the stomach from the effects of drugs such as Aspirin, a coating that dissolves in natural or alkaline media is used. This inhibits release of drug from the device until it reaches the higher pH of the intestine. In most cases, enteric coated dosage forms are not truly sustaining in nature, but serve as a useful function in directing release of the drug to a special site. The same approach can be employed for compounds that are degraded by the harsh conditions found in the gastric region.

(i) Reservoir type

Drug is coated with a given thickness coating, which is slowly dissolved in the contents of gastrointestinal tract. By alternating layers of drug with the rate controlling coats, a pulsed delivery can be achieved. If the outer layer is quickly releasing bolus dose of the drug, initial levels of the drug in the body can be quickly established with pulsed intervals. Although this is not a true controlled release system, the biological effects can be similar. An alternative method is to administer the drug as group of beads that have coating of different thickness. Since the beads have different coating thickness, their release occurs in a progressive manner.

Those with the thinnest layers will provide the initial dose. The maintenance of drug levels at late times will be achieved from those with thicker coating. This is the principle of the spansule capsule. Cellulose nitrate phthalate was synthesized and used as an enteric coating agent for acetyl salicylic acid tablets.

(ii) **Matrix type**

The more common type of dissolution controlled dosage form can be either a drug impregnated sphere or a drug impregnated tablet, which will be subjected to slow erosion.

Two types of dissolution- controlled pulsed delivery systems:

(a) Single bead – type device with alternating drug and rate- controlling layer.

(b) Beads containing drug with differing thickness of dissolving coats.

III Methods using Ion Exchange

Ion exchange resins are water-insoluble cross-linked polymers containing salt forming groups in repeating positions on the polymer chain. Drug is bound to the resin by repeated exposure of the resin to the drug in a chromatographic column, or by prolonged contact of the resin with the drug solution. Drug release from the drug-resin complex depends on the ionic environment i.e. pH and electrolyte concentration, within the GI tract as well as properties of the resin. It is based on the formation of drug resin complex formed when an ionic solution is kept in contact with ionic resins. The drug from this complex gets exchanged in gastrointestinal tract and released with excess of Na^+ and Cl^- present in gastrointestinal tract.

The rate of drug diffusion out of the resin is controlled by the area of diffusion, diffusional path length and rigidity of the resin (which is function of the amount of cross linking agent used to prepare resins). The release rate can be further controlled (Pennkinetic system by Pennwalt Coporation) by treating the drug resin complex granules with impregnating agents like polyethylene glycol 4000 (imparts plasticity and stability to complex) followed by coating with water permeable polymer membrane (e.g. ethyl cellulose) by an air suspension technique.

184 Essentials of Pharmaceutical Technology

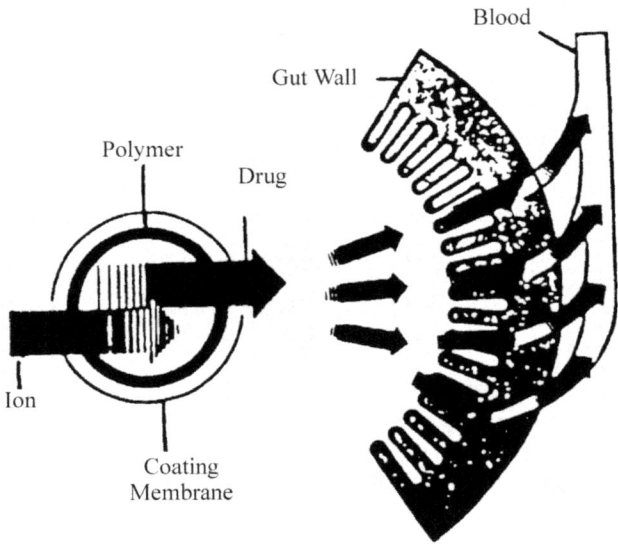

Fig. 7.3 GI absorption of ionic drugs from an advanced ion exchange controlled-gastrointestinal drug delivery system (Pennkinetic system).

The ion exchange resins prolong and sustain the drug release over 8 to 12 h into the GI tract. The resins used include Amberlite IRP-69, Indion, polysterol resins and others.

The advantages of these ion exchange-controlled gastrointestinal drug delivery systems are that (i) the rate of drug release is independent of pH conditions, enzyme activities, temperature or volume of the GI tract; (ii) the system is administered in the form of a large number of particles, which may eliminate the effect of gastric emptying; and (iii) it can be formulated as a stable liquid suspension-type pharmaceutical dosage form.

IV Methods using Osmotic Pressure

Osmotic pressure can be employed as the driving force to generate a constant release of drug provided a constant osmotic pressure is maintained and a few other features of the physical system are constrained. The advantage of the osmotic system is that it requires only osmotic pressure to be effective and is essentially independent of the environment. A semi permeable membrane (cellulose acetate) is placed around a tablet, particle or drug solution that allows transport of water into the tablet with eventual pumping of drug solution out of the tablet through a small delivery aperture or orifice in tablet coating. Characteristics of the osmotically controlled system are summarized in Table 7.1.

When an osmotically controlled system is exposed to water or any body fluid, water will flow into the core owing to the osmotic pressure difference. The rate of flow, *dV/dt,* of water into the system can be expressed as:

$$dV/dt = AK/h(\Delta\pi - \Delta P)$$

where
- K = membrane permeability
- A = area of the membrane
- h = membrane thickness
- $\Delta\pi$ = osmotic pressure difference
- ΔP = hydrostatic pressure difference

There are two types of osmotically controlled systems:

1. Type A which contains an osmotic core with drug (Fig. 7.4)
2. Type B which contains the drug in flexible bag with osmotic core surrounding (Fig. 7.5).

In the system with the bag, or if the orifice is enough in either system, the hydrostatic difference becomes negligible, and the previous equation may be expressed as:

$$\frac{dV}{dt} = \frac{Ak}{h(\Delta\pi)}$$

The equation indicates that the flow rate of the water is governed by permeability, area and thickness of the membrane. The rate of drug leaving the orifice, *dM/dt*, is equivalent to the flow rate of incoming water multiplied by the solution concentration of drug, *Cs*, within the system:

$$\frac{dM}{dt} = \left(\frac{dV}{dt}\right) \cdot Cs$$

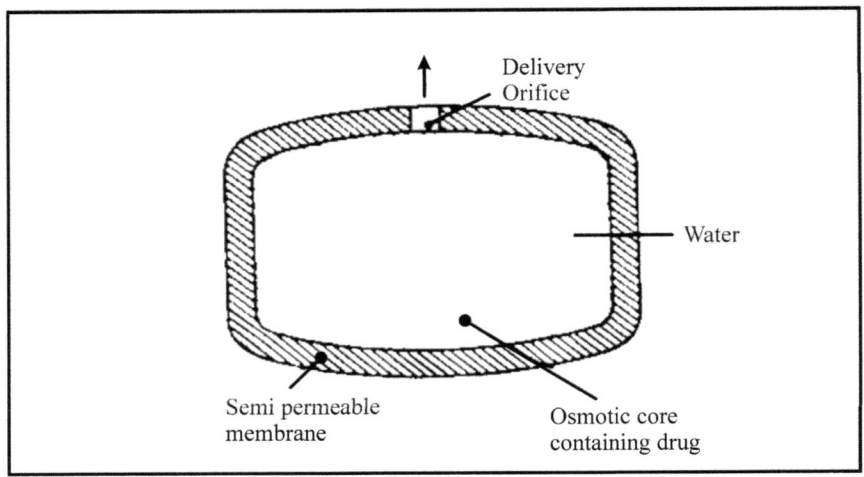

Fig. 7.4 Cross-sectional diagram of an elementary osmotic pump (OROS system Alza).

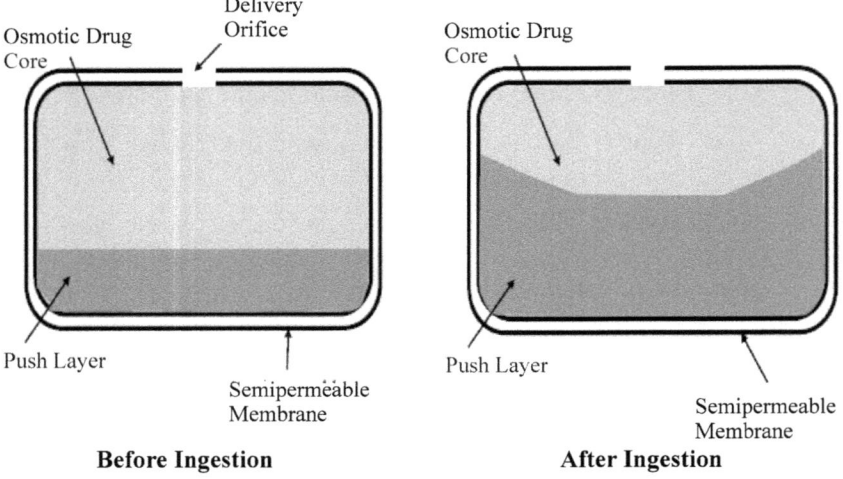

Fig. 7.5 Cross-sectional diagram of push-pull osmotic pump (After ingestion water crosses the semi permeable membrane and dissolves the osmotic agents and then expands the push layer which forces the drug release through the orifice at controlled rate).

V pH– Independent Formulations

The gastrointestinal tract present some unusual features for the oral route of drug administration with relatively brief transit time through the gastrointestinal tract, which constraint the length of prolongation, further the chemical environment throughout the length of gastrointestinal tract is constraint on dosage form design. Since most drugs are either weak acids or weak bases, the release from sustained release formulations is pH dependent. However, buffers such as salts of amino acids, citric acid, phthalic acid, phosphoric acid or tartaric acid can be added to the formulation, to help to maintain a constant pH thereby rendering pH independent drug release. A buffered controlled release formulation is prepared by mixing a basic or acidic drug with one or more buffering agent, granulating with appropriate pharmaceutical excipients and coating with gastrointestinal fluid permeable film forming polymer. When gastrointestinal fluid permeates through the membrane, the buffering agents adjust the fluid inside to suitable constant pH thereby rendering a constant rate of drug release e.g. propoxyphene in a buffered controlled release formulation, which significantly increase reproducibility.

VI Altered Density Formulations

It is reasonable to expect that unless a delivery system remains in the vicinity of the absorption site until most, if not all of its drug contents is released, it would have limited utility. To this end, several approaches have been developed to prolong the residence time of drug delivery system in the gastrointestinal tract (Table 7.2).

- **High Density Approach**

    In this approach the density of the pellets must exceed that of normal stomach content and should therefore be at least 1.4 g/cm^{-3}. Sedimentation has been employed as a retention mechanism for pellets that are small enough to be retained in the rugae or folds of the stomach body near the pyloric region, which is the part of the organ with the lowest position in an upright posture (Fig. 7.6). Dense pellets (approximately 3 g/cm^{-3}) trapped in rugae also tend to withstand the peristaltic movements of the stomach wall. With pellets, the GI transit time can be extended from an average of 5-25 hours, depending more on density than on the diameter of the pellets. Commonly used excipients are barium sulphate, zinc oxide, titanium dioxide and iron powder, etc. These materials increase density by up to 1.5-2.4 g/cm^{-3}

188 Essentials of Pharmaceutical Technology

- **Low Density Approach**

    Globular shells which have an apparent density lower than that of gastric fluid can be used as a carrier of drug for sustained release purpose. These systems float on the gastric juice for an extended period while slow releasing of drug (Fig.7.6).

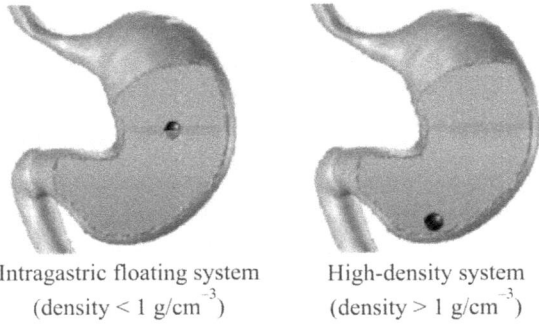

Intragastric floating system (density < 1 g/cm^{-3})   High-density system (density > 1 g/cm^{-3})

Fig. 7.6 Schematic localization of an altered density oral controlled drug delivery system in stomach

These floating drug delivery systems have bulk density lower than the gastric fluid and therefore remain floating in the stomach without affecting the gastric emptying rate for prolonged period. The drug is slowly released (by diffusion and erosion of the gel barrier) at a desired rate from the floating system and after the complete release the residual system is expelled from the stomach (Fig. 7.7).

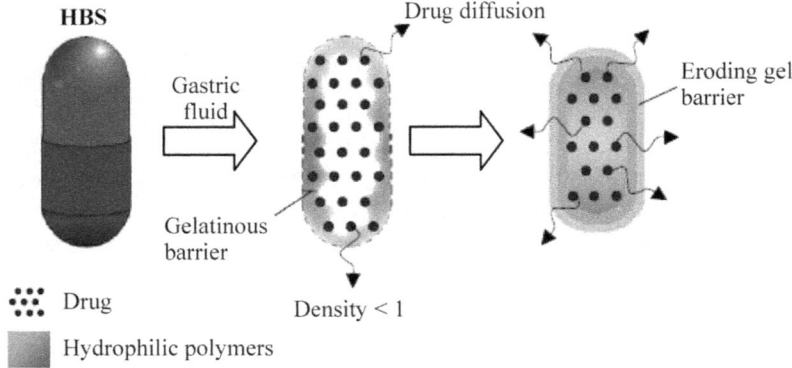

Fig. 7.7 Hydrodynamically balanced system (HBS). The gelatinous polymer barrier formation results from hydrophilic polymer swelling.

Table 7.2 Classification of altered density drug delivery system

S.No	System	Mechanism	Polymer/Ingredients
1	High-density system	Density > 1 (gastric fluid), entrapped in the folds of the antrum and withstand the peristaltic waves of the stomach.	Barium sulphate, zinc oxide, iron powder, titanium dioxide.
2	Floating system	Density < 1 (gastric fluid) and thus remain buoyant in stomach for a prolonged period. Drug released slowly at a desired rate.	Non-Biodegradable, Hydrophobic Polymers, Biodegradable polymers.
2.1	Hydrodynamically balanced system	Hydration and swelling of surface polymer.	Hydroxyproplylmethyl cellulose (HPMC), Hydroyethylcellulose (HEC), Hydroxypropyl cellulose (HPC). Sodium carboxy methylcellulose, Agar, Carrageenans or Alginic acid.
2.2	Gas-generating system	Formation of CO_2 bubbles which entrapped into polymer matrix and thus float the system.	Polyvinyl acetate and Shellac.
2.3	Raft-forming system	Formation of CO_2 bubbles which entrapped into swelled viscous cohesive gel.	Biodegradable polymers, Bioerodible polymer
2.4	Low density system	The system made up by low density material, entrapping oil or air, which make them floatable.	Polycarbonate, Eudragit S100, cellulose acetate, calcium alginate, agar and low methoxylated pectin.
3	Superporsos hydrogels system	This system is made up of pore forming polymers. When they come in contact with GI fluid due to presence pore size ≥ 100 μM fluid enter into system and thus swell within a minute and float.	Hydrophilic polymer, Croscarmellose sodium

Factors Influencing Design of Controlled Release Dosage Forms

The therapeutic efficacy of drug under clinical conditions is not simply a function of its intrinsic pharmacological activity but also depends upon the path of the drug molecule from the site of administration to the target site. Different conditions encountered by the drug molecule while traversing the path of distribution may alter either the effectiveness of the drug or affect the amount of the drug reaching the receptor site.

(a) **Formulation factors**

This refers to the development/manufacturing of an efficient delivery system in which the drug has maximum physiological stability and optimum bioavailability.

(b) **Biopharmaceutics/ pharmacokinetics**

This involves the study of absorption, distribution, metabolism and excretion of the drug, before and after reaching the target site and evaluation of the relationship between delivery system and therapeutic response.

(c) **Pharmacodynamics**

It is the study of the mechanism of action and clinical efficacy of a drug administered in dosage form in terms of onset, intensity and duration of pharmacological activity.

Drug properties influencing the design of sustained or controlled release drug delivery system are classified as:

A. Physicochemical properties of the drug

These include dose size, aqueous solubility, protein binding, molecular size, drug stability and partition coefficients.

- **Dose Size**

In general, single dose of 0.5-1.0 g is considered maximal for a conventional dosage form. This also holds true for sustained-release dosage forms. Another consideration is the margin of safety involved in administration of large amounts of drug with a narrow therapeutic range.

- **Ionization, pKa, and Aqueous Solubility**

Most drugs are weak acids or bases. Since the unchanged form of a drug preferentially permeates across lipid membranes, it is important to note the relationship between the pKa of the compound and the absorptive environment. Delivery systems that are dependent on diffusion or dissolution will likewise be dependent on the solubility of drug in the aqueous media. For dissolution or diffusion sustaining forms, much of the drug will arrive in the small intestine in solid form, meaning that the solubility of the drug may change several orders of magnitude during its release. The lower limit for the solubility of a drug to be formulated in a sustained release system has been reported to be 0.1 mg/ml.

- **Partition Coefficient**

Compounds with a relatively high partition coefficient are predominantly lipid-soluble and, consequently, have very low aqueous solubility. Furthermore these compounds can usually persist in the body for long periods, because they can localize in the lipid membranes of cells.

- **Stability**

Orally administered drugs can be subject to both acid-base hydrolysis and enzymatic degradation. For drugs that are unstable in the stomach, systems that prolong delivery over the entire course of transit in the GI tract are beneficial. Compounds that are unstable in the small intestine may demonstrate decreased bioavailability when administered from a sustaining dosage form.

B. Biological factors

These include absorption, distribution, metabolism, duration of action, margin of safety, side effects of drug, disease state and circadian rhythm.

- **Biological Half-life**

Therapeutic compounds with short half-lives are excellent candidates for sustained-release preparations, since this can reduce dosing frequency.

- **Absorption**

The absorption rate constant is an apparent rate constant, and should, in actuality, be the release rate constant of the drug from the dosage form. Compounds that demonstrate the absorption rate constants will probably be poor candidates for sustaining systems. If a drug is absorbed by active transport, or transport is limited to a specific region of the intestine, sustained-release preparations may be disadvantageous to absorptions.

- **Metabolism**

    Drugs that are significantly metabolized before absorption, either in the lumen or tissue of the intestine, can show decreased bioavailability from slower-releasing dosage forms. Most intestinal wall enzyme systems are saturable. As the drug is released at a slower rate to these regions, less total drug is presented to the enzymatic process during a specific period, allowing more complete conversion of the drug to its metabolite.

Evaluation of Controlled Release Products

Before marketing a controlled release product, it is must to assure the strength, safety, stability and reliability of a product by forming in-vitro and in-vivo analysis and correlation between the two. Various authors have discussed the evaluating parameters and procedures for controlled release formulations.

- *In-vitro Methods*

    Various official and unofficial *in-vitro* dissolution methods have been described in Chapter 2; Dissolution. These are:

    1. Official methods (USP dissolution method and IP dissolution methods)
    2. Unofficial methods: They are classified as followed (See chapter 2)
        (a) Natural convection Type: Static disc method, Sintered filter method
        (b) Forced Convection Type: Beaker method, Rotating disc method, Rotating Bottle method, Rotating Basket method, Stationary Basket Method, Oscillating tube method, Dialysis method.
        (c) Miscellaneous methods: FDA method, Tape method, Flow through dissolution cell

- *In-vivo Methods*

    Once the satisfactory in-vitro profile is achieved, it becomes necessary to conduct *in-vivo* evaluation and establish in-vitro in-vivo correlation. The various major in-vivo evaluation methods (Described in Chapter 1; Bioavailability) are:

    (a) Blood level data
    (b) Urinary excretion studies
    (c) Clinical response
    (d) Toxicity studies

- *Stability Studies*

    Adequate stability data of the drug and its dosage form is essential to ensure the strength, safety, identity, quality, purity and *in-vitro in-vivo* release rates that they claim to have at the time of use. A controlled release product should release a predetermined amount of the drug at specified time intervals, which should not change on storage. Any considerable deviation from the appropriate release would render the controlled release product useless. The *in-vitro* and *in-vivo* release rates of controlled release product may be altered by atmospheric or accelerated conditions such as temperature and humidity.

    The stability programmes of a controlled release product include storage at both nominal and accelerated conditions such as temperature & humidity to ensure that the product will withstand these conditions. The stability study protocol or methods are discussed in chapter of stability studies.

In vitro- In vivo Correlations

In-vitro studies are performed to get an idea about the expected release of drug in body (see chapter 2). Therefore, in *in-vitro* studies efforts are made to mimic the biological environment. Each parameter of dissolution is optimized to get more and more realistic result e.g. Temperature maintained to body temperature (37 ^{0}C), agitation speed to mimic gastric motility, pH of media is maintained at pH 1.2, 6.6, 6.8 or 7.4 buffer as per the required site of release etc. In spite of every effort made to mimic the biological environment, there always exists a significant difference from *in vivo* studies. So, the *in vitro* data must be correlated to *in vivo* data and their level of correlation must be studied. And these correlation are very important in the development of controlled release delivery systems. *In vitro-In vivo* Correlation is described in detail in Chapter 2; Dissolution study.

A simple *in vitro-in vitro* relationship can be established by conducting *in vitro* and *in vivo* evaluations of a potential drug delivery system simultaneously to study and compare the mechanism and rate profiles of controlled drug release. When the *in vivo* drug release mechanism is proven to be in good agreement with that observed in the *in vitro* drug release studies, then *in vitro in vivo* correlation factor is derived. For capsule type drug delivery system the factor can be represented as:

$$Q = (Q/t) \text{ in vitro} / (Q/t) \text{ in vivo}$$

where Q/t = Rate of release

'Q' values are dependent profiles of drug delivery systems upon the sites of administration and environmental conditions to which the animals are exposed during treatment (study). The above relationship can be used for optimization of controlled release Levy has classified *in-vivo – in-vitro* correlation in to:

- Pharmacological correlations based on clinical observations;
- Semi-quantitative correlations based on blood levels or urinary excretion data;
- Quantitative correlation arising from absorption kinetics. While most of the published correlations are of semi-quantitative nature, the most valuable are those based on absorption kinetics.

Bioavailability Testing

Bioavailability is generally defined as the rate and extent of absorption of unchanged drug from its site of application to the systemic circulation (see chapter 1; Bioavailability). Bioavailability is defined in terms of a specific drug moiety, usually active therapeutic entity, which may be the unchanged drug or as with prodrug, for instance, a metabolite. In contrast, the term "absorption" often refers to net transport of drug related mass from its site of application into the body. Hence, a compound may be completely absorbed but only partially bioavailable as would occur, when low bioavailability is caused by incomplete absorption. Pharmaceutical optimization of the dosage form may be warranted to improve absorption characteristics of the drug and thereby also its bioavailability.

Guidelines of bioavailability studies are given in Chapter of Bioavailability. In general, for drugs in which the exposure–response relationship has not been established or is unknown, applications for changing the formulation from immediate release to controlled release requires demonstration of the safety and efficacy of the product in the target patient population. When a new chemical entity is developed as a controlled-release dosage form, additional studies to characterize its absorption, distribution, metabolism, and excretion (ADME) characteristics are recommended.

FDA Regulation of Oral Controlled-Release Drugs

In the 1980s and subsequently in 2004, FDA introduced rigorous regulations governing bioequivalence and *in vitro–in vivo* correlations for controlled-release products. Required pharmacokinetic evaluations involve:

- relative bioavailability following single dose
- relative bioavailability following multiple doses
- effect of food
- dose proportionality
- unit dosage strength proportionality
- singe-dose bioequivalence study (experimental versus marketed formulations at various strengths)
- *in vitro–in vivo* correlation
- pharmacokinetic/pharmacodynamic (PK/PD) relationship.

Bibliography

- Collet J, Moreton C. In: Aulton ME (Editor), Pharmaceutics: The science of dosage form design. 2nd Edn., 2002, Churchill Livingstone, New York, pp. 289-306.
- Chien YW, Novel Drug Delivery System, 2nd Edn, 2005 (Vol. 50) Marcel Dekker, Inc. New York, Basel, US, pp 1-196.
- George M., Grass IV, Robinson JR. in Banker G.S., Rhodes C.T. Eds. Modern Pharmaceutics 2nd edition, Marcel Dekker, 1990: 639-658pp.
- Jantzen GM, Robinson JR. In; Banker GS, Rhodes CT (Eds). Modern Pharmaceutics. 4th Edn, 2005 (Vol. 121) Marcel Dekker, Inc. New York, Basel, US, pp 501-28.
- Longer M.A., Robinson J.R. "Sustained release drug delivery system" chapter 91 in "Remington's pharmaceutical sciences" 18th edition, Mack Publishing Company, 1990: 1675-1684pp.
- Lordi N.G. "Sustained release dosage form" In;"Theory and practice of Industrial Pharmacy" eds Lachmann et al., 3rd edition, Varghese Publishing House, 1991: 430-431pp.
- Svenson S. (Ed) Carrier Based Drug Delivery. 2004, American Chemical Society, Washington DC. ACS Symposium Series 879.
- United States Pharmacopoeia XXIV – NF XIX: 2000, USP Convention Inc.: 2059.

CHAPTER 8

Oral Drug Delivery of Proteins and Peptides

Introduction

Peptide and polypeptides are low and / or high molecular weight biopolymers, which yield two or more amino acid on hydrolysis. Peptides and polypeptides are the principle component of the protoplasm of cells and are high molecular weight compounds consisting of alpha amino acid connected together by peptide linkages. These proteins serve as enzymes, structural element, hormones or immunoglobulin and are involved in metabolic process, cell growth, immunogenic defense mechanisms and other biological activities.

Peptides and polypeptides or proteins are an important class of biological substances which are not only the essential nutrients of human body, but some of the polypeptide hormones like insulin are used in treating various diseases resulting from hormonal deficiency. As this use of peptides and polypeptides for systemic treatment of certain diseases is well accepted in medical practice, research activities are being directed towards the synthesis of large quantities by rDNA technology.

The most common route of administration for protein and peptide drug delivery has been parenteral, although many other routes have been tried with varying degree of success. Routes such as intranasal, transdermal, buccal, intraocular, rectal, vaginal and pulmonary route will deliver the drug to the systemic circulation while avoiding transit through the digestive system. A major factor that limits the usefulness of these substances for their intended therapeutic application is that they are easily metabolized by plasma proteases when they reach the peripheral circulation. In addition, adverse effects associated with applying these drugs to the pulmonary or the other mucosal surfaces, may be limiting.

Delivering therapeutically active protein and peptides by the oral route has been a challenge and a goal for many decades. Currently only two biotechnology drugs (Interferon alpha and human growth hormone) that can be given orally are known to be in clinical development in the US. For such drugs to be absorbed through the gastrointestinal tract, they must be protected from enzyme and must traverse through the luminal barriers into the blood stream in an unchanged form. This chapter reviews the problems associated with the oral delivery of proteins and peptides and presents approaches for the formulation of the delivery system for the same.

Absorption Properties of Peptides
Structure
Molecular weight and size

Molecular weight and size influence the diffusion of drugs through the epithelial layer. As a general rule very large molecules have lower diffusivities and only small molecules (< 75-100 Dalton) appear to cross the barriers rapidly. However permeability falls of markedly as the molecular size increases. Several authors have investigated the effects of the molecular weight upon oral absorption of various hydrophilic compounds.

Conformation, stereospecificity and immunogenicity

Unlike conventional drugs, peptide drugs generally have primary, secondary and tertiary structures and in solution may adopt several different conformations depending upon their size. It is the prime requisite to preserve the pharmacologically active conformation during the process of formulation and sterilization. The change in conformation can influence membrane permeability. The stereospecificity of the drug must also be preserved since the permeation systems are thought to be stereoslective.

Peptides are also recognized as often being immunogenic and the use of inert polymers like PEG, PVP and albumin for peptide delivery has been shown to increase resistance to proteolysis and simultaneously decrease peptide immunogenicity.

Electrostatic charges

Charge distribution on the peptide change may be even more important than the value of the partition coefficient in predicting permeability of peptides through oral mucosa. Terminal charges or zwitterionic peptide have a negative effect on membrane permeability even though the effective partition coefficient is relatively high. The effect of charge density can be modified to promote peptide absorption by changing the pH of the medium and thus the degree of ionization of the peptides.

Physico-Chemical Properties

Solubility and Partition Coefficient

Peptides, being amphoteric, usually have complex solubility versus pH profile. Aqueous solubility of peptide is strongly dependent upon pH, presence of metallic ion, ionic strength and temperature. At isoelectric point the aqueous solubility of peptide is minimal where the drug is neutral or has no net charge. Unless the N-and C- termini are blocked, peptides are very hydrophilic with a very low octanol -water partition coefficient (Table 8.1). Therefore, to improve the absorption of peptides by passive diffusion, their lipophilicity should be increased.

Table 8.1 Lipophilicity of selected peptides

Peptide	Partition coefficient (n-octanol/buffer, pH 7.4)
Insulin	0.0215
Thyrotropin-releasing hormone	0.0376
Luteinizing hormone-releasing hormone	0.0451
Glucagons	0.0633
Substance P	0.2750
Met-enkephalin	0.0305
Leu- enkephalin	1.1200

It is generally recognized from human buccal absorption data that the absorption of drugs from whole oral cavity obeys the pH-partition hypothesis which implies a passive diffusion mechanism. Majority of the proteins are destroyed in the very low pH of the gastric region.

Aggregation and hydrogen bonding

Self-aggregation tendency of peptides modifies their intrinsic properties. Human insulin was found to be more self-aggregating than porcine or bovine insulin. In a study it has been reported that additions of additive like non ionic surfactants (Pluronic F 68) stabilize the peptide formulation against self aggregation (Fig. 8.1).

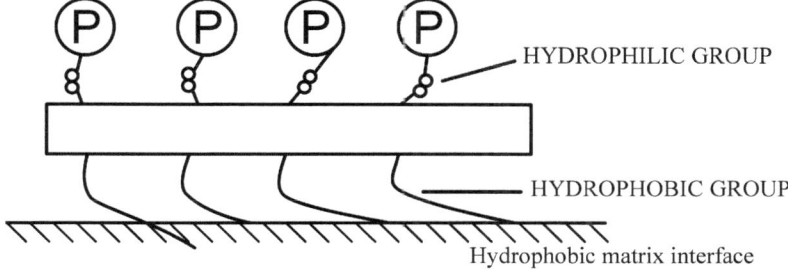

Fig. 8.1 Mechanism of action of surfactant in preventing unfolding of p protein molecule.

In aqueous solution, the three dimensional structure of a protein in its native conformation results in more hydrophobic residues being buried within the interior and more hydrophilic amino acid residues exposed to the aqueous solution. However, when the same protein comes into contact with a hydrophobic surface (like delivery matrix interface), there will be an entropic driving force for the hydrophobic residues that are normally buried within the three dimensional structure to interact with the surface and hence causing unfolding or denaturing of protein molecules. Non ionic surfactants and many other additives were found to solve the problem by preferential adsorption on hydrophobic interface (Table 8.2). Intermolecular hydrogen bonding with water decreases the permeability of protein in lipid membrane.

Basis of Oral Delivery of Proteins

It was observed that the small amount of intact protein and peptide can enter the circulation under normal circumstances. After these studies, some finding suggests that at higher peptide dosage the fraction absorbed may be expected to increase due to saturability of the degradation. These finding led the possibility of developing oral peptide delivery system.

Table 8.2 Stabilizing additives in protein delivery

S. No	Stabilizing additive	Mechanism of action	Protein stabilized
1	Sugars- trehalose, sucrose Maltose, glucose	Increase Tg thereby enhancing thermal stability of proteins	Collagan, ribonuclease, ovalbomin
2	Salts- potassium phosphate, sodium citrate, amm.sulphate	Increase Tg of proteins and self association of proteins, reduce the solubility	Collagan, ribonuclease, ovalbomin
3	Cyclodextrins- hydroxypropylcyclo dextrins	Not clear; probably by changing the properties of solvent	Porcine growth hormone
4	Heparin	Increase the unfolding temperature by 15-30^0	Acidic fibroblast growth factor
5	Metals - zinc	Complexation	hGH against urea induced denaturation Insulin
6	Chelating agent- EDTA	Complexation and decrease catalytic degradation by metal	Acidic fibroblast growth factor ribonuclease A
7	Surfactant - Non ionic- polysorbates Cationic-cetrimide Anionic - SLS	Preferential adsorption on hydrophobic interface of delivery matrix; Membrane perturbation	Nutropin^R (r-hGH) with polysorbates; hGH loaded PLG polymer matrix

Potential Problem Associated with Oral Protein Delivery

The oral administration of peptide and protein drugs faces two formidable problems. The first is protection against the metabolic barrier in GIT. The whole GIT and liver tend to metabolize protein and peptide into smaller fragments of 2-10 amino acids with the help of a variety of proteolytic enzyme (proteases). These are of four types:

1. Aspartic proteases   e.g. pepsin, rennin
2. Cystinyl proteases   e.g. papain, endopeptidase
3. Metallo proteases   e.g. carboxypeptidase – A, ACE
4. Serinyl proteases   e.g. thrombin, trypsin

The second problem is the absence of carrier system for absorption of peptides with more than three amino acids.

Approaches to circumvent metabolic barriers

The approaches to circumvent the protease action should be based entirely upon the principle sight of degradation of the peptide drug; intracellular, luminal or the brush border. The approaches may include

1. Prodrug approach
2. Co-administration of protease inhibitors
3. Use of penetration enhancers and surfactants
4. Use of carrier system
5. Formulation approaches

Prodrug Approach

Proteins are labile due to susceptibility of the peptide backbone to proteolytic cleavage, as well as their molecular size and complex secondary, tertiary and sometimes even quaternary structures. Therefore proteins can be modified chemically to give more stable prodrugs with increased plasma half-lives (Table 8.3). Some strategies for prodrug formation include olefenic substitution, d-Amino acid substitution, dehydro amino acid substitution, carboxyl reduction, retro inversion modification, polyethylene glycole (PEG) attachment to amino group and thio-methylene modification. In a recent technology known as Nobex Technology, an amphiphilic protein conjugate is prepared (Fig. 8.2). This technology reduces self-association, increases penetration and increases compatibility with formulation ingredients than parent drug. By this technology Nobex's Conjugated Insulin has also been prepared. In this technology short chain PEG and alkyl group are attached to Lys-29 of beta chain. Prepared conjugated insulin was found to be more absorbed and effective. Calcitonin oligomer prepared by this technology showed increased stability and absorption.

Table 8.3 List of prodrugs of proteins/ peptides

Parent protein/peptide	Prodrug
S-Gonadotropin Releasing Hormone	S-Gn-RH-A Nonopeptide with D-Arg-6
Growth Hormone	GHRP-6
Luteinizinghormone-releasing hormone	Buserelin, luproreline, gosereline
Vasopressin	Desmopressin
Somatostatin	Sandostatin

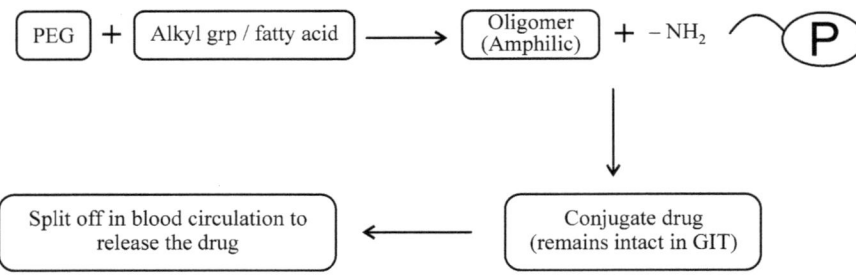

Fig. 8.2 Nobex conjugated technology for oral protein drug delivery.

(In this prodrug technology an amphiphilic protein conjugate is prepared by attaching short chain PEG and alkyl group to the amino groups of the protein molecule, which splits off in the blood circulation to release the parent protein.)

Protease Inhibitors

To alter the environment for maximum enzyme stability, protease inhibitors are co-administered with protein and peptides. Various protease inhibitors have been examined with respect to their ability to suppress proteolytic activity (Table 8.4). Positive results were observed in the oral absorption of tetragastrin, insulin, arginin, vasopressin, rennin inhibitors.

Table 8.4 Studies of protein drug delivery with protease inhibitors

Drug	Protease inhibitor	Result(s)
Insulin	Aprotinin, bactracin, bestatin, Camostat mesilate, chymotrypsin inhibitor FK – 448, sodium glycocholate, soyabean trypsin inhibitor	Significant reduction in insulin digestion and improvement in its intestinal absorption profile.
Insulin	Camostat mesilate	Plasma glucose levels decreased in a dose dependent manner.
Vasopressin and its analogues	Aprotinin	Improvement in the activity profile of the drug
Calcitonin	Camostat mesilate	Significant improvement in calcitonin delivery

Use of penetration enhancers

Penetration enhancers are compounds which, when added to a solute, increase its absorption across biological membranes. Peptide and proteins, due to their molecular size, often require penetration enhancers to achieve therapeutically significant levels of lumenal absorption.

Surfactants are one of the classes of penetration enhancers. Addition of a surfactant can stabilize a protein against denaturation during several stages from incorporation to the release at the site of delivery. Use of surfactants decreases the self-association and absorption of protein on hydrophobic interface of delivery matrix. They increase penetration and stability of protein and peptide formulations. Besides penetration enhancement, sodium glycocholate inhibits leucine amino peptidase and protect insulin from proteolysis.

Use of carrier systems

Special types of carriers are used for the poorly absorbed proteins and peptides, which are unstable in the gastro intestinal lumen for their targeting to a specific tissue or organ. A well designed carrier system protects the drug from the intestinal proteases and localizes the drug at or near the cellular membrane to maximize their driving force for passive permeation. Various novel carrier systems for protein and peptide drug delivery have been studied like lipid vesicles, particulate systems, emulsions, bioadhesive systems etc.

Formulation approaches

A variety of approaches are adopted in formulating oral peptide delivery systems as per the nature of peptide drugs and the delivery matrix. Table-8.5 shows the general formulation strategies for protein and peptide formulation.

An azo polymer, which is stable in GIT but decomposes at the ileocaecal junction have been used for insulin delivery and found to be very promising for oral insulin delivery. Chitosan-EDTA-protease inhibitor conjugates have been used for many peptide delivery. A new class of molecules-N acylated non-α, aromatic amino acid compound was found to increase the absorption of human growth hormone (hGH) by altering the conformation of molecule reversibly and facilitate transport across intestinal mucosa. Several formulations tested for the oral protein delivery include emulsions, liposomes, nanoparticles, soft gelatin coated capsules.

General method for production of protein formulations are emulsification, coacervation, extrusion, spray drying and polymerization. In all these processes it is highly emphasized that high stress, high temperature, heat and crosslinking agent must be avoided (or minimized), to ensure the stability during the formulation. Special procedures like double emulsion method and Prolease microsphere technology may also be adopted. The Prolease process is a spray method of producing microparticles containing proteins using a cryogenic process. In this method, the protein drug is incorporated as a lyophilized powder, and all manipulations involving the matrix polymer (PEG) and the proteins are performed at low temperature ($\leq -80\ ^0C$).

As proteins are more stable in solid state than in liquid, its incorporation in solid form in delivery matrix is advantageous. Spray drying and lyophillization are widely used for formulation of protein and peptide delivery system. In a study, hGH was lyophilized to get stable form with reduction in aqueous solubility. It decreased the potential for degradation during release due to decrease in protein molecule mobility and thereby ensured the stability and improved the bioavailability of orally administered peptide hormone.

Table 8.5 Approaches of formulation of oral protein drug delivery system

S. No	Protein's nature	Formulation approach
1.	Unstable in solution	Lyophilization using cryoprotectants and incorporating drug into delivery matrix as a solid powder.
2.	Adsorb to delivery matrix (PLG)	1. Incorporation of hydrophilic surfactants (Polysorbate 20/80, Pluronic F.68) 2. Addition of another protein as a competitor for adsorption surface
3.	High protein concentration required in delivery system-prone to aggregation	3. Addition of surfactant to reduce self-association 4. Use of less soluble prodrug e.g. complexation with metal (zinc-insulin)
4.	Poor stability at low pH	5. Lyophilization 6. Formulation in high pH buffer 7. Addition of soluble basic salt in delivery matrix to neutralize acid degradation products of delivery matrix 8. Formulation of microporous delivery matrix rather than monolithic device
5.	Heat sensitivity	9. Using low temperature homogenization encapsulation process.

Recent Advancements in Oral Protein Drug Delivery

Biosante Pharmaceuticals has developed a delivery system based on calcium phosphate to administer an oral form of insulin called CAPIC. Calcium phosphate particles containing insulin was synthesized in the presence of PEG-3350 and modified by aggregating the particles with caseins (the principle protein of milk) to obtain the calcium phosphate-PEG-insulin-casein (CAPIC) oral insulin delivery system. The formulation CAPIC was created through a nano-particulate technology, using microscopic particles of calcium phosphate. Studies in diabetic mice showed that oral insulin administration through the new system was effective in reduction and maintenance of normal blood glucose levels.

A group of research scientists developed mucoadhesive oral Insulin delivery systems using lectin functionalized complexation hydrogels. They developed a class of environmentally responsive complexation hydrogels composed of methacrylic acid grafted with ethylene glycol chains (P(MAA-g-EG)) functionalized with wheat germ agglutinin (WGA) to overcome the challenges of oral administration. The drug carriers were designed to (1) minimize the effects of the harsh environment of the gastrointestinal tract and (2) target delivery of the insulin to the upper small intestine by exploiting the pH shift between the stomach and the upper small intestine. Insulin entrapment in the polymer network was unaffected by the WGA functionalization and loading efficiency was determined to be 75% in both functionalized and unfunctionalized microparticles.

Recently, Pfizer Inc. got the US FDA approval for the human insulin (rDNA origin) inhalation powder (Exubera) spray. The product had been introduced in the US market in December 2006.

Bibliography

- Crommelin D, Winden EV, Mekking A. In: Aulton ME (Editor), Pharmaceutics: The science of dosage form design. 2nd Edn., 2002, Churchil Livingstone, New York, pp. 544-53.

- Chein YW, Su KSE, Chang SF. editors, Nasal Systemic Drug Delivery, New York: Marcel Dekker Inc; 1989.

- Christopher HP. Nobex Corporation: Crossing Barrier for Better Drug Delivery 2003; 3(2): 12.

- Clark AR, Shire SJ. Protein Formulation and Delivery. In: Mc Nally EJ, editors. Drugs and the Pharmaceutical Science. Vol. 99. New York: Marcel Dekker; 2000, p. 201-12.

- Cleland JL, Jones AJS. Development of stable protein formulations for microencapsulation in biodegradable polymers. Proceedings of an International Symposium on Controlled Release of Bioactive Materials. Seattle, Controlled Release society, 1995.

- Costantino HR, Langer R, Klibanov AM. Pharm Res 1994; 11 (1): 21-29.

- Dence JE. Steroids and Peptide: Selected Chemical Aspects for Biology, Biochemistry and Medicine. New York: John Willey and Sons; 1980, 89.

- Hanson MA, Roun SKE. In: Ahern, TJ, Manning MC. editors. Stability of Protein Pharmaceuticals. Part B. In Vivo Pathways of Degradation and Strategies for Protein Stabilization. New York: Plenum Press; 1992. p. 209.

- Horbett TA. In: Ahem TJ, Manning MC, editors. Stability of Protein Pharmaceuticals. Part A. Chemical and Physical Pathways of Protein Degradation. New York: Plenum Press; 1992. p. 195.

- Johnson OL. In: McNally EJ, editors. Protein Formulation and Delivery. New York: Marcel Dekker; 2000. p. 251.

- Klostermeyer H, Humble R E. Chemistry and biochemistry of insulin Angew Chem Intern 1966; 5, 807-11.

- Lewis DH. Biodegradable Polymers as Drug Delivery System. In: Chasin M, Langer R, editors. Biopolymers New York: Marcel Dekker; 1990. p. 8-24.

- Merkle HP, Wolany GJM. Intraoral peptide absorption, In: Audus K L, Raub TJ, editors. Biological Barriers to Protein Delivery. New York/London: Plenum; 1993. p. 131-60.

- Morçöl T, Nagappan P, Nerenbaum L, Mitchell A, Bell SJD. Int J Pharm 2004; 277: 91-97.

- Mumenthaler M, Hsu CC, Pearlman R. Feasibility study on spray drying protein pharmaceuticals by improved optical methods. Pharm Res 1994; 11 (1): 12-20.

- News release. New delivery system to administer insulin orally, Pharm Tech 2003; 27(7): 17.

- News Section, National Med J India 2006; 19(1): 53.

- Peppas NA. Devices based on intelligent biopolymers for oral protein delivery. Int J Pharm 2004;277: 11-17.

- Rathbone MJ, Drummond BK, Tucker IG. Oral cavity as a site for systemic drug delivery, Adv Drug Del Rev 1994; 13: 1-22.

- Tozaki H, Nishioka J, Komoike J, Okada N, Fujita T, Muranishi S, Kim SI, J Pharm Sci 2001; 90:89-97.

CHAPTER 9

Aerosols

Introduction

Pharmaceutical aerosols have been playing a crucial role in the health and well being of millions of people throughout the world for many years. These products include pressurized metered dose inhalers (MDIs), dry powder inhalers (DPIs), nebulizers, sublinguals, skin sprays (coolants, anesthetics, etc.) and dental sprays. The technology's continual advancement, the ease of use and the more desirable pulmonary-rather-than-needle delivery for systemic drugs has increased the attraction for the pharmaceutical aerosol in recent years. Moreover, the increasing incidence of asthma at an average rate of 5 % per year in developed as well as developing countries is creating a consistently high demand of inhalers or MDIs (about 50 to 60 million patients are relying on MDIs).

Definitions
- Aerosols are a suspension of small solid particles or droplets suspended in a gas or vapor.

- Aerosols are the products that depend on the power of a compressed or liquefied gas to expel the contents from the container. Aerosols are also termed as pressurized package.

Pharmaceutical aerosols: aerosol products containing therapeutically active ingredients dissolved, suspended or emulsified in a propellant or a mixture of solvent and propellant and intended for topical administration, for administration into one of the body cavities (ear, rectum and vagina) or intended for administration orally or nasally as fine solid particles or liquid mists through the pulmonary airways, nasal passages or oral cavity.

Pharmaceutical aerosols are products that are packaged under pressure and contain therapeutically active ingredients that are released upon activation of an appropriate valve system. They are intended for topical application to the skin as well as local application into the nose (nasal aerosols), mouth (lingual aerosols), or lungs (inhalation aerosols). These products may be fitted with valves enabling either continuous or metered-dose delivery; hence, the terms "[DRUG] Metered Topical Aerosols," "[DRUG] Metered Nasal Aerosols," etc. [USP definition]

Advantages

- The product is administered easily and quickly.
- Aerosols are portable and tamper-proof.
- A dose can be removed without contamination of materials.
- Stability is enhanced for these substances adversely affected by oxygen and or moisture.
- When sterility is an important factor, it can be maintained while a dose is being dispensed.
- Rapid onset of action, avoidance of degradation of the drug in the GIT and first pass effect.
- Lower dose of drug can be used and hence minimize adverse and side effects.
- The medication can be delivered directly to the affected area in a desired form, such as spray, steam, quick breaking foam or stable foam.
- Irritation produced by the mechanical application of topical medication is reduced or eliminated.
- Application of medication in thin layer

Limitations

- Costly
- Need proper use to get the effect.

There are three common types of aerosol generators for inhaled drug delivery: the small volume nebulizer (SVN), the metered-dose inhaler (MDI), and the dry powder inhaler (DPI). Because of high medication loss in the oropharynx and hand-breath coordination difficulty with MDIs, holding chambers and spacers are often used as ancillary devices with an MDI.

Uses of Pharmaceutical Aerosols

Since the mid 1950s, aerosol forms of pharmaceuticals have played an important role in treating respiratory illnesses such as asthma and chronic obstructive pulmonary disease (COPD), and MDIs and DPIs have become an important part of that treatment.

But the use of aerosol products are not limited to the pulmonary route, these can be administered by various routes of administration (ROA) for various therapeutic effects (Table 9.1). These can be administered by topical, nasal, ocular, oral, rectal and vaginal routes also.

Table 9.1 Uses of pharmaceutical aerosols

ROA	Examples	Description
Topical	Local anesthetics (e.g. Benzocaine), Wound washing, Rubiferants (e.g. Methylsalicylate), Spray on bandages, Proprietary burn applications, Antibacterials(e.g. Neomycin), Antifungal sprays (Miconazole), Anti-inflammatory steroids (e.g. Dexamethasone)	• Convenient • No need to touch skin • Minimal contamination of unused product.
Oral and Lingual	Antacids (e.g. Aluminum and magnesium silicate), Local anesthetics (e.g. Lidocaine), Antiseptics (e.g. Chloroseptic), Anti-anginals (e.g. Nitroglycerin)	• Provides access to hard-to-reach sites • Provides access to systemic circulation

Table 9.1 Contd...

ROA	Examples	Description
Vaginal	Contraceptive Foams (e.g. Noncxyenol-9)	• Provides access to hard-to-reach sites • Expands to fill available space and provide complete surface coverage
Rectal	Local anesthetics (e.g. Pramoxine), Anti-inflammatory steroids (e.g. Hydrocortisone)	• Provides access to hard-to-reach sites • Expands to fill available space and provide complete surface coverage
Nasal	Decongestants (e.g. Phenylephrine), Anti-inflammatory steroids (e.g. Beclomethasone), Antiallergics (e.g. Cromolyn sodium), Moisturizers (e.g. Normal saline), Systemic access of Antidiuretics (e.g. Desmopressin) and Antismoking (Nicotine)	• Provides access to hard-to-reach sites • Minimal dripping
Ocular	Contact lens cleaning solutions (not applied directly to eye)	• Provides access to hard-to-reach sites • Minimal dripping
Respiratory	Bronchodilators (e.g. Albuterol), Anti-inflammatory steroids (e.g. Beclomethasone), Antiallergics (e.g. Cromolyn sodium), Antivirals (e.g. Ribavirin), Smoking cessation (e.g. Nicotine), Migraine (e.g. Ergotamine tartrate)	• These act by local action • Nicotine and ergotamine act by systemic action

Components of Aerosols

An aerosol system has following major components.
- Propellant
- Container
- Valve and actuator
- Product concentrate

Propellant

Propellant is the heart of an aerosol package. It is responsible for developing the power pressure within the container and also expel the product when the valve is opened and in the atomization or form production of the product (Fig. 9.1).

Propellants provide the driving force to expel product from its container. Propellants provide dispersion medium.

Types of Propellants

I. **Liquefied gas** e.g. Hydrocarbons (HCs), Chloroflurocarbon (CFCs), Hydrofluoroalkanes (HFA)

II. **Compressed Gas Propellants**

I. **Liquefied gas:** These are materials that at room temperature and atmospheric pressure exist in the gaseous or vapor state and are capable of being liquefied at relatively low pressures or temperatures. Because the aerosol is under pressure the propellant exists mainly as a liquid, but it will also be in the head space as a vapour. As the product is used up as the valve is opened, some of the liquid propellant turns to vapour and keeps the headspace full of vapour. In this way the pressure in the can remains constant and the spray performance is maintained throughout the life of the aerosol (Fig. 9.2).

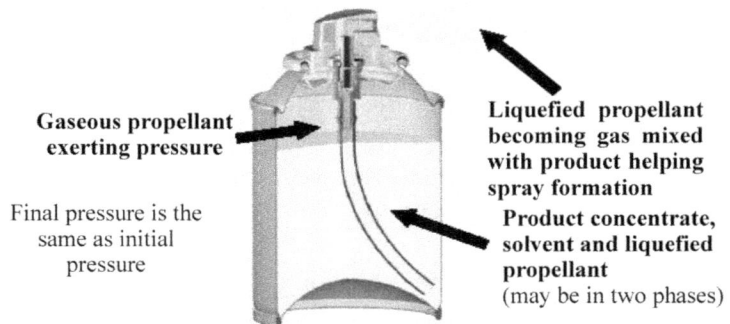

Fig. 9.1 Working of an aerosol system (with liquefied propellant).

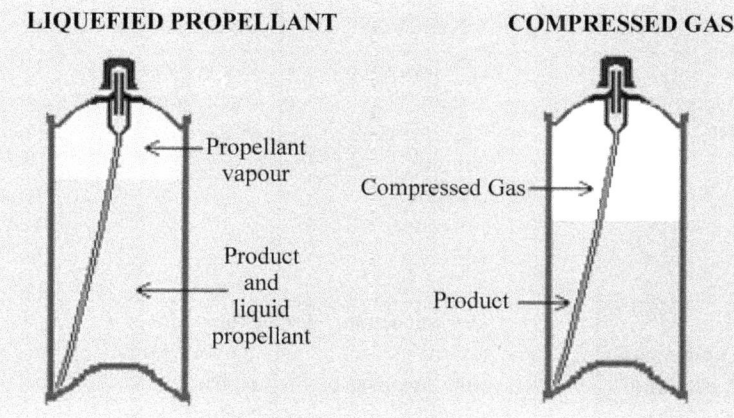

Fig. 9.2 Comparative presentation of aerosols based on two types of propellants.

These propellants have various advantages with some limitations which are listed in Table 9.2.

Table 9.2 Types, advantages and disadvantages of various propellants

Type	Advantages	Disadvantages	Examples
Ia Hydrocarbons (HCs)	• Inexpensive • Minimal ozone depletion • Negligible "greenhouse effect" • Excellent solvents • Large expansion ratio	• Flammable • Aftertaste • Unknown toxicity following inhalation • Low liquid density	n-Butane, isobutene, propane.
Ib Chlorofluorcarbons (CFCs)	• Low inhalation toxicity • High chemical stability • High purity • CFC-11 is a good solvent	• Destructive to atmospheric Ozone* • Contribute to "green house effect" • High cost	CFC-11 (CCl_3F), CFC-12 (CCl_2F_2), CFC-114 $(C_2Cl_2F_4)$**

Table 9.2 *Contd...*

Type	Advantages	Disadvantages	Examples
Ic Hydrofluoroalkanes (HFAs)	• Low inhalation toxicity • High chemical stability • High purity • Not ozone depleting	• Poor solvents • Minor "greenhouse effect" • High cost	1,1,1,2,3,3,3-Hepta-fluoropropane (HFA-227) 1,1,1,2 – Tetra-fluoroethane (HFA-134a)
II Compressed Gas Propellants	• Low inhalation toxicity • High chemical stability • High purity • Inexpensive • No environmental problems	• Require use of a nonvolatile co-solvent • Produce coarse droplet sprays (Little expansion ratio) • Pressure falls during use.	CO_2, N_2, N_2O

*CFCs have a detrimental effect on the Earth's ozone layer and the Montreal Protocol on Substances That Deplete the Ozone Layer (January 1989) set a timetable for elimination of CFC use that will take effect in January 1, 2009. HFAs are being used as alternatives and have less of an effect on the environment (Refer: Phase out of CFCs in MDIs). The use of CFCs is exempted for a very few class of aerosols- MDIs for oral/nasal steroidal drugs, bronchodilators, ergotamine tartrate, certain topical antibiotic sprays and contraceptive vaginal foams.

**CFCs are designated with 3 digits and followed by an alphabet if required. The nomenclature of a chemical structure of CFC can be given as followed.

Ist digit = No. of Carbon atoms —1; IInd digit = No. of hydrogen atoms + 1; IIIrd digit = No. of F atoms; Most symmetric structure is designated by numbers only and as the asymmetry increases a, b, c, etc follow the number (e.g. CFC-114 for dichlorotetrafluoroethane; CFC-12 (012) for dichlorodifluoromethane.

Phase-out of CFCs in MDIs

Urgent measures introduced to protect the ozone layer resulted in a ban on the production and use of fully halogenated chlorofluorocarbons (CFCs) in the developed world with effect from January 1996. The only exemption was for "essential" uses. However, these "essential" CFCs are no longer deemed essential because there are now many alternatives/substitutes to CFC containing MDIs available. As a result, Germany has already banned CFC-MDIs containing drugs of the following classes:

- short-acting beta-sympathomimetic bronchodilators (salbutamol, terbutaline, fenoterol, bitolterol, and procaterol) as of January 2001,
- inhaled steroids (beclomethasone, dexamethasone, flunisolide, fluticasone, budesonide and triamcinolone) as of January 2003,
- and intends to ban CFC-MDIs containing anticholinergic bronchodilators comprising ipratropium bromide and oxitropium bromide.

Various other national transition strategies for the phase-out of CFCs in MDIs are published, among others in Australia, Europe, New Zealand, Japan, USA and Canada. The Canadian Transition Strategy is as follows:

- as of January 2003: CFC-MDIs containing salbutamol prohibited
- as of January 2004: CFC-MDIs containing corticosteroids forbidden
- as of January 2005: Prohibition of all MDIs containing CFCs (production and import).

Furthermore, Austria, Belgium, Denmark, Finland, France, Germany, The Netherlands, Portugal and the United Kingdom formally determined that most of the short-acting beta-agonist CFC-MDIs are no longer essential.

In Europe, this has already resulted in a more than 50 % reduction in the total CFC quantities used in MDIs; from 5,600 tonnes required in 1997 to approx. 2,500 tonnes in 2002.

In total, approx. 500 million MDIs are manufactured, corresponding to approx. 8,500 tonnes of propellant, traditionally consisting of CFCs. When substituted by HFAs, the global warming potential is reduced by more than 75 %. The total global warming contribution of HFA-MDIs is less than 0.5 % of the total greenhouse gas emissions.

II. Compressed Gas Propellants

Compressed gas (e.g. nitrogen, nitrous oxide, carbon dioxide) propellants only occupy the head space above the liquid in the can. When the aerosol valve is opened the gas 'pushes' the liquid out of the can (Fig. 9.2). The amount of gas in the headspace remains the same but it has more space, and as a result the pressure will drop during the life of the can. Moreover, use of compressed gas propellants is typically restricted to applications where spray characteristics are not critical e.g. dental creams, hair spray, germicide etc.

Container

Aerosol's container must withstand pressure as high as 140 to 180 psig (pounds per sq. inch gauge) at 130 ^{0}F (Table 9.3). Containers may be made of followings:

A. Metals
  1. Tinplated steel
  2. Tin free steel
  3. Aluminum
  4. Stainless steel
B. Glass
  1. Uncoated glass
  2. Plastic coated glass

Table 9.3 Maximum tolerable pressure by different aerosol containers

Container	Maximum pressure (psig)	Temperature ^{0}F
Tinplated steel	140 to 180	130
Aluminum	Up to 180	130
Stainless steel	Up to 180	130
Plastic	Less than 25	70
Uncoated glass	Less than 18	70
Coated glass	Less than 25	70

- **Tinplated steel:** It is light and inexpensive. Prior to fabrication, this may be further coated with organic coating, e.g. oleoresin, phenolic, vinyl or epoxy coating for additional protection against corrosion. The coating also decreases the compatibility problems. These are used in topical pharmaceutical aerosols

- **Aluminum:** It is less reactive, light weight, seamless, easy to fill and crimp and shows greater resistance from corrosions. Aluminum containers can be screen printed, therefore visually appealing. But these are incompatible with some propellants and solvents. So, this may be coated with organic coating, e.g. oleoresin, phenolic, vinyl or epoxy coating for additional protection. These are used in oral, topical and most MDIs.

- **Stainless steel:** It is extremely strong, resistant to most materials. There is no need of any extra protection with coatings. It is limited to the smaller sizes (due to cost and production problems). It is used for inhalation aerosols.
- **Glass:** These have characteristics of aesthetic value and compatibility with most formulations. They allow level of contents to be seen. But its use is limited for products having lower pressure (upto 25 psig) and lower percentage (about only upto 15%) of propellant. Uncoated glasses are costing low but show high clarity. On the other hand, plastic coated glass has the characteristics to prevent the glass from shattering in the event of breakage. Plastic coating absorbs "neckshock" during crimping and provides barrier to broken glass. The glass containers are used for some topical and MDI aerosols.

Valves

It is the vital component of an aerosol package. It helps to deliver the drug in desired form. It determines the performance of a pressurized package. Major functions of valves are as followed:
- To regulate the flow of product from the container
- To provide a means of discharging desired amount when needed and prevent loss at other times.
- To exert a major effect on the characteristics of dispensed product.

Types

- *Continuous spray valve*

    These valves release the product as long as pressure is maintained on the actuator. These are employed in high speed production technique.

- *Metering valves*

    A finite volume (25 -150 µml for inhalation aerosols, up to 5 ml for topical aerosols) of product is released when the actuator is pressed. No more product is released unless the actuator is returned to its rest position and repressed. Dispersing of potent medication at proper dispersion can be done by these valves.

Components of Valves

In general a pharmaceutical aerosol valve comprises of following components (Fig. 9.3).

Valve Cup (Mounting Cup/ferulae)

It is used to attach the valve properly to the container. It is typically constructed from tinplated steel or aluminum.

Outer Gasket

This is the seal between the valve cup and the aerosol can.

Valve Housing (Valve body)

It is manufactured from nylon or delrin. It contains an opening at the point of the attachment of the dip tube (0.013 inch to 0.08 inch). Sometimes it may contain another opening called vapor tap. Vapor tap prevents clogging, helps in satisfactory dispensing, decreases the chilling effect (of propellant on skin) and flame extension. It contains the valve stem, spring and inner gasket.

Valve Stem

It is the tap through which the product flows. It is made of nylon or delrin.

Inner Gasket

It covers the hole in the valve stem. It is made of BUNA-N and neoprene rubber.

Valve Spring

It holds the gasket in place and closes or opens the gasket. It is usually made of stainless steel.

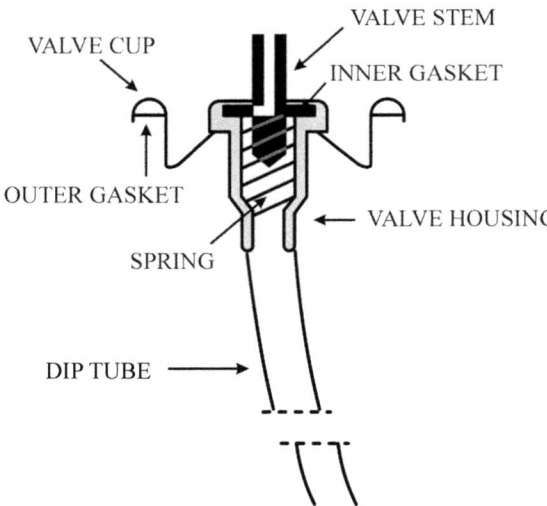

Fig. 9.3 Components of valves.

Dip Tube

It allows the liquid to enter the valve. It prevents propellants from escape without dispensing the contents. Its inner diameter is 0.120 inch to 0.125 inch, while it may be slightly large (upto 0.195 inch) for viscous products.

Actuator

It provides rapid and convenient means for releasing the contents from a pressurized container. An actuator fits onto the valve stem (Fig. 9.4). It ensures that aerosol product is delivered in the proper and desired form i.e. fine mist, wet spray or semisolid stream etc. Different types of actuators are available for different type of dispensing like Spray actuators, Foam actuators, Solid steam actuators, Special actuators etc. Mechanical breakup actuators are used for systems with low percentage of propellant.

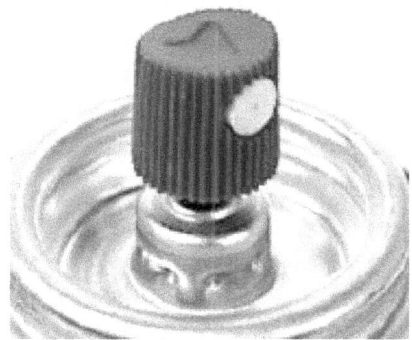

Fig. 9.4 A typical actuator of aerosol package.

Types of Aerosol Preparations

An aerosol system consist of product concentrate (mixture of active ingredients and other such as solvents, antioxidants and surfactants) and propellant (single or blend of various propellants). The aerosol systems can be classified as followed.

A. On the basis of propellant or container

    I. Liquefied gas system

        (i) Two phase system (space spray, surface coating spray)

        (ii) Three phase system (aquasol, foam system)

II. Compressed gas system (semisolid, foam or spray dispensing)

III Barrier type systems

(i) Piston type

(ii) Plastic Bag type

(iii) Can in Can type

B. Dosage form based

I. Solution system

II. Suspension or Dispersion systems

III. Emulsion systems

I. Liquefied gas system

These systems employ liquefied gas propellants. The liquefied gas propellants generally have boiling point below 21 °C. They generally exert a vapor pressure of 13.4 to 135 psia at 21 °C.

In the system pressure on liquid phase push product concentrate and propellants up in dip tube and dispensed due to large expansion in atmospheric pressure. Initially there is just a temporary fall in pressure, which is restored when pressure is released and sufficient molecules change from liquid to vapor state.

Two Phase system

- **Solution system**

    Drug may be dissolved in the propellant system. It consists of a solution of active ingredients in pure propellant or a mixture of propellant and solvents. It is easy to formulate, provided that the ingredients are soluble in the propellant. Smaller spray particle size can be achieved after complete propellant evaporation. Chemical degradation may occur faster in solution systems. A general formula of solution system is as followed.

Ingredients	wt%
Drug/active ingredient	10-15
Propellants 12/11 (50:50) to	100

- **Suspension/dispersion system**

    These systems can be used to deliver insoluble drugs. Higher doses can be delivered by suspension systems. Constant agitation during manufacturing and use is required for these systems. But these systems may be associated with physical instability (due to agglomeration, caking, particle-size growth and valve clogging or closing). A general formula of suspension system is as followed.

Ingredients	wt%
Drug/active ingredient	0.5 to 1
Sorbiton trioleate (STO)	0.5
Propellants 12/114 (49.5:49.5) to	100

Following methods can be adopted for improving the stability of aerosol dispersion

- Moisture content < 300 ppm
- Use of derivative of active ingredient
- Reduction of particle size < 5 µ (50-100 µ for topical aerosols)
- Adjust density of propellants and /or suspenoid
- Use of dispersing agent like surfactant with HLB < 10 *e.g.* Sorbiton trioleate (STO), Sorbiton mono-oleate (SMO), Isopropyl myristate (IPM), Minerol oil

Three Phase/water based system

It allows greater use of liquid components not miscible with the propellants. These include formation of three phases consisting of liquid propellant, vaporized propellant and aqueous solution of active ingredient. As low percentage of propellants is used in these systems, special types of actuators (Mechanical breakup actuators) are needed. A general formula of water based systems or aquasol is as followed.

Ingredients	wt%
Drug/active ingredient	40-85
Surfactant	0.5-2
Propellants to	5-10

Mechanism of working of Aquasol

Vapor phase of propellants + Product → Mixing chamber in actuator through special ducts. Vaporized propellant enters moving at tremendous speed and product is forced to actuator by the pressure of propellants. So the product and vaporized propellants get mixed and dispensed in spray form.

Foam or Emulsion Systems

In these systems propellants are emulsified. These are suitable for topical aerosols. Propellants are used at 40-50 psig at 21 ^0C with 4-7 % concentration. Two types of emulsions can be formulated-o/w or w/o.

- If the product concentrate is dispersed throughout the propellant→ W/O emulsion→ the product is dispensed as wet stream
- If the propellant is in the internal phase →O/W emulsion→foam is emitted.

II. **Compressed gas system**

These are used to dispense semisolid, foam or spray discharge. An initial high pressure of 90-100 psig at 21 ^0C is required for these systems.

III. **Barrier type systems**

These systems are equipped with the provision of separation of propellants from the product with some physical barrier. The pressure outside the barrier pushes the contents from the container. On the basis of type of barrier these aerosol systems are classified as followed.

(i) **Piston type:** For semisolid dispensing, e.g. Ointment, cake decorating creams

(ii) **Plastic Bag type:** Provides stream, fine mist dispensing, e.g. Creams, ointment, gels.

(iii) **Can in Can type:** Nasal aerosols with aqueous solution of Insulin

Manufacturing of Aerosols

Aerosols are generally manufactured by following methods:
- Pressure filling
- Cold filling apparatus

Pressure filling

The concentrate may be chilled slightly (15-20°C) to reduce vaporization of any volatile solvent or propellant→ The concentrate is added to an open container → The valve is crimped in place → The propellant is added under pressure through the valve → The filled container is passed through the water path (for leak test).

Cold filling apparatus

Lowering the temperature of the concentrate (solution or suspension) below room temperature (– 30°C to – 60°C)→ The cold concentrate is added to chilled (cooled) container → The propellant is added → The valve is crimped in place → The container is passed into a water path (55°C) to ensure there is no leakage or distortion in the container.

Selection of Drug Particle Size with Reference to Pulmonary Delivery

Administration of drugs by the pulmonary route is technically challenging because oral deposition can be high, and variations in inhalation technique can affect the quantity of drug delivered to the lungs. Therefore, there have been considerable efforts to provide more efficient and reproducible aerosol systems through improved drug delivery devices and through better formulations that disperse more readily during inhalation.

The size of the suspended drug particles depends on the intended use of the product. Particle size plays an important role in lung deposition, along with particle velocity and settling time. As particle size increases above 3 µm, there is a shift in aerosol deposition from the periphery to the conducting airways. Oropharyngeal deposition also increases as particle sizes increase above 6 µm. Exhaled loss is high with very small particles of 1 µm or less. These data support the view that particle sizes of 1-5 µm are best for reaching the lung periphery, while 5-10 µm particles deposit preferentially in the conducting airways (Fig. 9.5).

Aerosol devices in clinical use produce *heterodisperse* (also termed *polydisperse)* particle sizes, meaning that there is a mix of sizes in the aerosol.

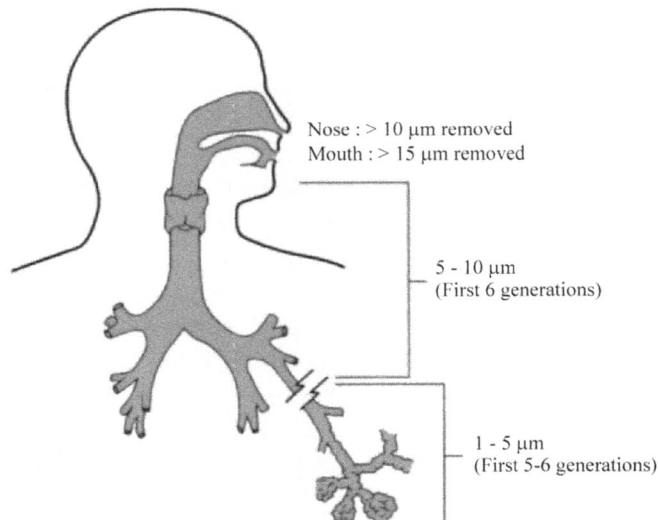

Fig. 9.5 A simplified view of the effect of aerosol particle size on the site of preferential deposition in the airways.

This is contrasted with *monodisperse* aerosols, which consist of a single particle size. A measure that can be useful in describing a polydisperse aerosol is the *mass median diameter* (MMD), which is defined as the particle size (in μm) above and below which 50% of the mass of the particles is contained. This is the particle size that evenly divides the *mass*, or amount of the drug in the particle size distribution. This is usually given as the mass median aerodynamic diameter, or MMAD, due to the way sizes are measured. The higher the MMAD, the more particle sizes are of larger diameters and lesser is their respirable fraction (Table 9.4).

Table 9.4 Respirable fractions as designated by the American Conference of Government and Industrial Hygienist (ACGIH) and the U.S. Atomic Energy Commission (USAEC)

Mass median aerodynamic diameter (MMAD) in μm	Respirable fraction (%)*	Respirable fraction (%)**
10	1	0
8	5	-
5	30	25
4	50	-
2	91	100
1	97	-

* ACGIH; ** USAEC

So for pulmonary delivery, the dry particles of drug in product concentrate of aerosol device must be prepared in respirable sizes. The production of respirable aerosol particles has traditionally been achieved by micronization of the drug. This involves the introduction of bulk particles on a gas stream under high pressure. Particles impact on each other and are thereby ground into small particles, which ultimately pass through a cyclone separator and are collected in a vessel or a bag filter. These particles can be produced in size ranges less than 5 µm, which is suitable for lung deposition. Nowadays spray drying is more popular for the production of more spherical particles. Spray drying is also more suitable method than jet milling for the production of thermolabile substances. The recently developed and more successful method for the production is the supercritical fluid technology. This technology involves controlled crystallization of drugs from dispersion in supercritical fluid, notably carbon dioxide.

Types of Aerosol Inhalors

There are three common types of aerosol generators for inhaled drug delivery of drugs in treating pulmonary diseases (Table 9.5).

- Metered dose inhalers (MDIs)
- Dry powder inhalers (DPIs)
- Small volume nebulizers (SVN)

Because of high medication loss in the oropharynx and hand-breath coordination difficulty with MDIs, holding chambers and spacers are often used as ancillary devices with an MDI.

Advantages and disadvantages of the inhalation route of administration with aerosolized drugs in treating pulmonary diseases.

Advantages

- Aerosol doses are generally smaller than systemic doses; e.g. oral albuterol is 2 to 4 mg; inhaled albuterol is 0.2 mg (MDI) to 2.5 mg (SVN).
- Onset of effect with inhaled drugs is faster than with oral dosing; e.g. oral albuterol is $\leq$ 30 min; inhaled albuterol is ~ 5 min.
- Drug is delivered directly to the target organ (lung), with minimal systemic exposure.
- Systemic side effects are less frequent and severe with inhalation compared to systemic delivery (injection, oral); e.g. less muscle

tremor, tachycardia with ß2-agonists; lower hypothalamic-pituitary-adrenal (HPA) suppression with corticosteroids.

- Inhaled drug therapy is less painful and relatively comfortable.

Disadvantages

- Lung deposition is a relatively low fraction of the total aerosol dose.
- A number of variables (correct breathing pattern, use of device) can affect lung deposition and dose reproducibility.
- Difficulty coordinating hand action and inhalation with MDIs.
- Lack of knowledge of correct or optimal use of aerosol devices by patients and clinicians.
- The number and variability of device types confuses patients and clinicians.
- Lack of standardized technical information on inhalers for clinicians.

Metered Dose Inhalers (MDIs)

MDIs dispense each dose from a metering chamber fed by a formulation reservoir, contained within a glass or metal container (Figure 9.6a). Drug is either homogeneously dissolved (in solution) or micronized and suspended in the formulation. On actuation of the MDI, the MDI's metering chamber becomes closed to the formulation reservoir and opens to the atmosphere, resulting in the expansion of the propellant-based formulation and atomization through the actuator orifice. The MDI has seen significant developments during recent years as the original chlorofluorocarbon (CFC) propellants are replaced by the non-ozone-depleting hydrofluoroalkane (HFAs) propellants HFA 134a and HFA 227ea in accordance with the Montreal Protocol (1989).

Metering valves are the most critical component of MDIs. The metering valve crimped onto the container is the most critical component of the pMDI (pressurized metered-dose inhaler), and has a volume ranging from 25 µL to 100 µL. While there are many designs of metering valve, they all operate on the same basic principle. Before firing, a channel between the body of the container and the metering chamber is open, but as the pMDI is fired, this channel closes, and another channel connecting the metering chamber to the atmosphere opens. The pressurized formulation is expelled rapidly into the valve stem, which, together with the actuator seating, forms an expansion chamber in which the propellant begins to boil (Fig. 9.6b). The canister is used in the inverted position, with the valve below the container so that the valve will refill under gravity. Some valves are surrounded by a retaining cup that contains the next few doses of drug. Several other valve designs aimed at improving the precision of dosing have also been reported.

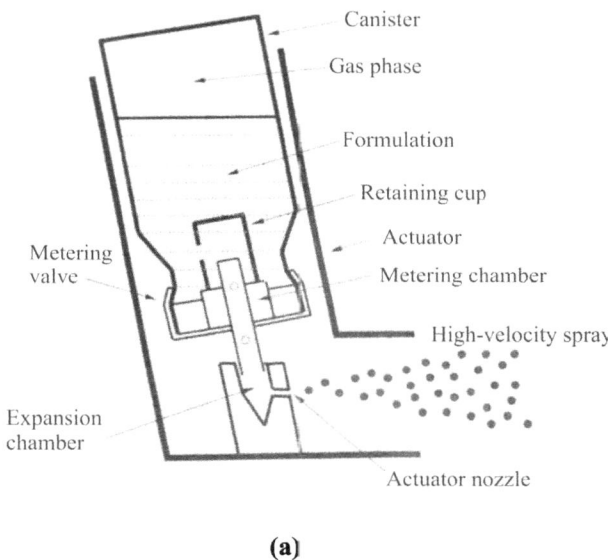

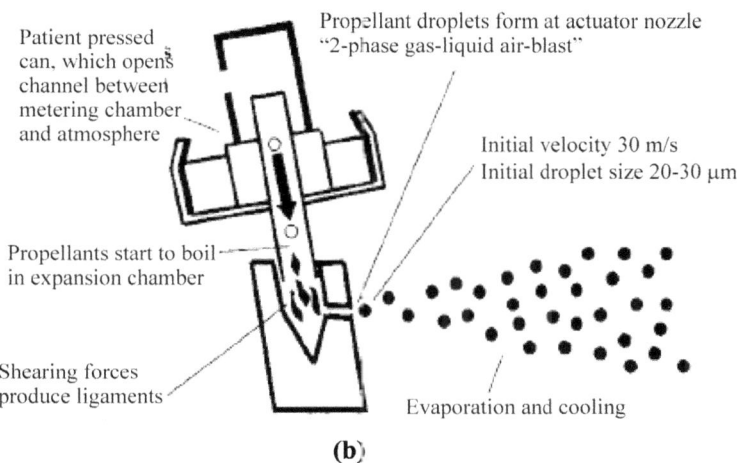

Fig. 9.6 Metered-dose inhaler (a) Standard components (b) Dispensing of spray from a MDI.

Small Volume Nebulizers (SVN)

Nebulizers convert solutions or suspensions into aerosols of a size that can be inhaled into the lower respiratory tract.

Pneumatic jet nebulizers are the oldest form of aerosol generator, and their basic design and performance have changed little in the past 30 years (Fig. 9.7a). A pneumatic nebulizer delivers compressed gas through a jet, causing a region of negative pressure. The solution to be aerosolized is entrained into the gas stream and is sheared into a liquid film. This film is unstable and breaks into droplets due to surface tension forces. A baffle in the aerosol stream produces smaller particles.

Ultrasonic nebulizers, which have been available for many years but are not commonly used for inhaled drug delivery, use electricity to convert a liquid into respirable droplets. The ultrasonic nebulizer converts electrical energy to high frequency ultrasonic waves. The transducer vibrates at the frequency of the ultrasonic waves applied to it (piezoelectric effect). Ultrasonic waves are transmitted to the surface of the solution to create an aerosol (Fig. 9.7b). Small volume ultrasonic nebulizers are commercially available for delivery of inhaled bronchodilators. A potential issue with the use of ultrasonic nebulizers is the possibility for drug inactivation by the ultrasonic waves, although this has not been shown to occur with common aerosol medications. Use of these devices has been hampered by their tendency for mechanical malfunction.

The newest generation of nebulizers uses mesh technology (use of a mesh or plate with multiple apertures to produce a liquid aerosol). This operating principle uses an aperture plate attached to a piezoelectric material that vibrates at high frequency. The rapid vibration of the aperture plate creates a pumping action to produce the aerosol from a liquid solution (Fig. 9.7c). Alternatively, the solution can be forced through the mesh to create the aerosol. These devices are able to generate aerosols with a high fine-particle fraction, which results in more efficient drug delivery compared to conventional nebulizers. The aerosol is generated as a fine mist, and no internal baffling system is required. They have a high rate of aerosol production and they are portable and battery-operated. They have minimal residual dead volume and some are breath-actuated.

The General advantages and disadvantages with use of small volume nebulizers are listed in Table 9.5.

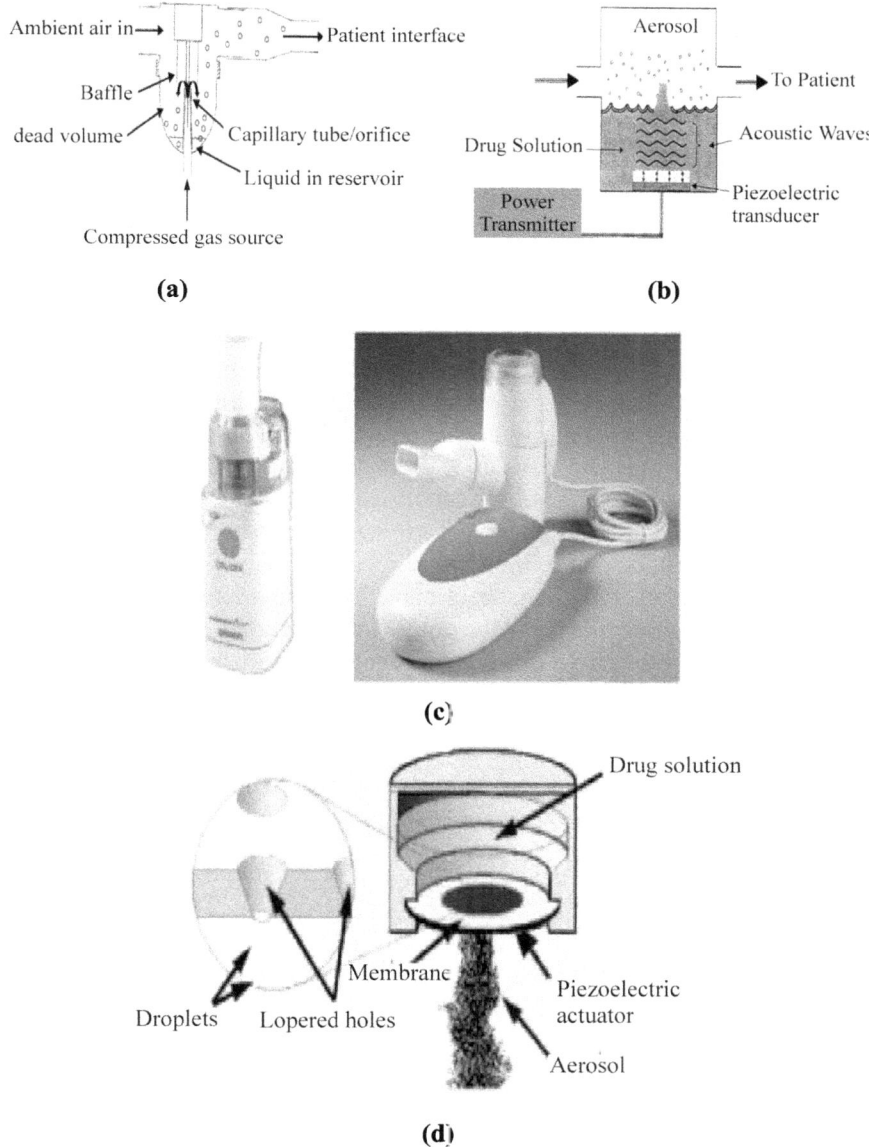

Fig. 9.7 Types and functions of nebulizers (SVN): (a) pneumatic jet nebulizer, (b) Ultrasonic nebulizers; (c) Principle of operation of mesh nebulizer and (d) Some commercial mesh nebulizer

(In Fig. 9.7a, Dead volume refers to the solution that is trapped inside the nebulizer and is thus not made available for inhalation. Dead volume is typically

230 Essentials of Pharmaceutical Technology

in the range of 0.5-1 mL. In an attempt to reduce medication loss due to dead volume, clinicians and patients tap the nebulizer periodically during therapy in an effort to increase nebulizer output.)

Dry Powder Inhalers (DPIs)

DPIs are small portable, propellant free, breath-actuated (thereby ensuring coordination between release of drug and inhalation) inhalers (Fig. 9.8). Further impetus to the development of aerosol formulations as powders came with the Montreal Protocol and the phase-out of ozone-destroying CFC propellants in MDIs. Advantages and disadvantages of DPIs are listed in Table 9.5.

DPIs do not contain propellants, and all current devices are breath-actuated. The patient's inspiratory effort, both inspiratory flow and volume, provide the energy to disperse and deliver the drug powder. All DPIs have an intrinsic resistance to airflow that differs among devices. The resistance determines how much inspiratory flow occurs through the device for a given inspiratory effort. As airflow occurs, a pressure drop between the intake and exiting mouthpiece occurs, thus lifting the powder from the drug reservoir, blister or capsule. The patient's inspiratory effort also deaggregates the powder into finer particles. Higher inspiratory flows generally improve drug deaggregation, fine particle production, and lung delivery. Excessive inspiratory flow, however, can increase impaction on the oral cavity and theoretically decrease lung deposition, although for current DPIs this is higher than the patient's capability.

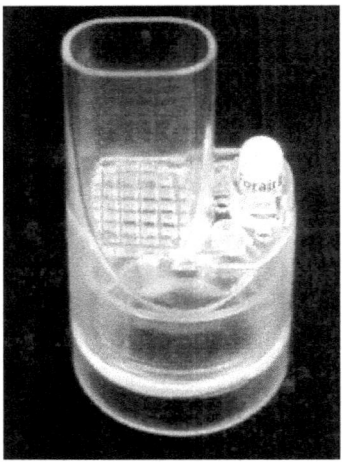

Fig. 9.8 Commonly used dry powder inhaler.

Recently, EXUBERA® [human insulin (rDNA origin); Pfizer], a dry powder, that is an inhaled form of fast-acting insulin developed by Pfizer and the sanofi-aventis group in conjunction with Nektar Therapeutics, has been approved by the FDA as the first inhaled insulin system (Table 9.7). Peak activity of inhaled insulin occurs about 60 min after inhalation making it satisfactory for prandial use. Approximately 30% of the inhaled dose is absorbed into the alveolar capillary circulation, 20% is deposited in the throat and bronchial tree. Between 20 and 40% of the insulin that reaches the alveoli is actually taken up into the bloodstream.

Table 9.5 Types, advantages and disadvantages of inhalation aerosols

Type of Inhalation aerosols	Advantages	Disadvantages
Small Volume Nebulizers (SVNs)	• Ability to aerosolize many drug solutions • Ability to aerosolize drug mixtures (>1 drug), if drugs are compatible • Normal breathing patterns can be used • Useful in very young, very old, debilitated, or distressed patients • An inspiratory pause (breath-hold) is not required for efficacy • Drug concentrations can be modified	• Treatment times are lengthy for pneumatically-powered nebulizers • Equipment required may be large and cumbersome • Need for power source (electricity, battery, compressed gas) • Variability in performance characteristics among different brands • Possible contamination with inadequate cleaning Wet, cold spray with facemask delivery Potential for drug delivery into the eyes with facemask delivery
Metered-dose inhalers (MDIs)	• Portable and compact • Short treatment time • Reproducibile dose emitted	• Hand–breathing coordination is difficult for many patients • Proper inhalation pattern (slow inspiration to total lung capacity) and breath-hold can be difficult • Canister depletion is difficult to determine (no dose counter) • High oropharyngeal impaction unless a holding chamber or spacer is used

Table 9.5 *Contd...*

			• Failure to shake can alter drug dose • Fixed drug concentrations • Reaction to propellants or excipients have occurred in some patients • Foreign body aspiration from debris-filled mouthpiece • Limited range of drugs
Dry powder inhalers (DPIs)	• Small and portable • Built-in dose counter • Propellant-free • Breath-actuated • Short preparation and administration time		• Dependence on patient's inspiratory flow • Patients less aware of delivered dose • Relatively high oropharyngeal impaction can occur • Vulnerable to ambient humidity or exhaled humidity into mouthpiece • Limited range of drugs

Table 9.6 Recently developed inhaled insulin formulations and their description

Insulin	Onset (min)	Peak (min)	Duration (h)	Formulation	Advantages/ Disadvantages
EXUBERA®	30	30 – 90	6	Dry powder	• Available only as 1- or 3-mg blister packs • Slight ↓ FEV1 and DLCO levels
AERx® iDMS	10	50 – 60	5 – 8	Liquid	• Microprocessor in delivery device that minimizes inhalation variability • Device durability is a concern • Duration of action is dose dependent • Similar lung cautions as EXUBERA

Table 9.6 *contd…*

Insulin	Onset (min)	Peak (min)	Duration (h)	Formulation	Advantages/ Disadvantages
AIR®	15	45	6 – 8	Dry powder	• Device is simple to use • Dosing limited to 2- and 6-unit capsules • Similar lung cautions as EXUBERA
Technosphere/ Insulin®	Minutes	13	2 – 3	Dry powder	• Microencapsulation delivery most likely gives insulin unique kinetics • No PFT changes in published reports
Alveair™	–	–	–	Liquid	• Unmodified human insulin; most likely to have the same kinetics/concerns as other inhaled insulins, but no kinetic/ PFT data in humans as yet
Kos	15 – 30	90	6 – 8	Liquid	• Meter-dose style inhalation device

PFT: Pulmonary function test.

FEV: forced expiratory volume

DLCO: carbon monoxide diffusion capacity

Evaluation of Aerosols

A. Flammability and combustibility

- Flame Projection
- Flash point

B. Physiochemical characteristics
- Vapor pressure
- Density
- Moisture content
- Identification of propellants

C. Performance
- Aerosol valve discharge rate
- Dose uniformity
- Net contents
- Leakage
- Particle size distribution

D. Therapeutic activity

A. Flammability and combustibility

- Flame Projection

This test indicates the effect of an aerosol formulation on the extension of an open flame. In this test the product is sprayed for 4 sec into flame. Depending on the nature of formulation, the flame is extended, and exact length is measured with ruler.

- Flash point

Flash point is determined by using standard ***Tag Open Cap Apparatus***. Steps are as followed.

Aerosol product is chilled to temperature of $-25°$ F and transferred to the test apparatus. →Temperature of test liquid increased slowly, and the temperature at which the vapors ignite is taken a flash point. → Calculated for flammable component, e.g. topical hydrocarbons.

B. Physiochemical characteristics

Physiochemical characteristics are evaluated as followed.

- Vapor pressure - Determined by pressure gauge.
- Density - Determined by hydrometer or a pycnometer.
- Moisture content - By Karl Fischer method
- Identification of propellants - By I.R spectrophotometry

C. Performance (methods prescribed by USP)

- *Aerosol valve discharge rate/Delivery Rate:*

  Select not fewer than four aerosol containers, shake, if the label includes this directive, remove the caps and covers, and actuate each valve for 2 to 3 seconds. Weigh each container accurately, and immerse in a constant-temperature bath until the internal pressure is equilibrated at a temperature of 25 as determined by constancy of internal pressure, as directed under the Pressure Test below. Remove the containers from the bath, remove excess moisture by blotting with a paper towel, shake, if the label includes this directive, actuate each valve for 5.0 seconds (accurately timed by use of a stopwatch), and weigh each container again. Return the containers to the constant-temperature bath, and repeat the foregoing procedure three times for each container. Calculate the average Delivery Rate, in g per second, for each container.

- *Delivered-Dose uniformity:*

  The test for Delivered-Dose Uniformity is required for topical aerosols fitted with dose-metering valves. For collection of the minimum dose, proceed as directed in the test for Delivered-Dose Uniformity under Metered-Dose Inhalers and Dry Powder Inhalers, as described below, except to modify the dose sampling apparatus so that it is capable of quantitatively capturing the delivered dose from the preparation being tested. Unless otherwise stated in the individual monograph, apply the acceptance criteria for Metered-Dose Inhalers (MDIs) and Dry Powder Inhalers (DPIs) as mentioned below.

  ### *Delivered-Dose Uniformity for nasal spray*

  Unless otherwise directed in the individual monograph, the drug content of the minimum delivered doses (minimum number of sprays per nostril as described on the label, or instructions for use) collected at the beginning of unit life (after priming as described on the label, or instructions for use) and at the label claim number of metered sprays, from each of 10 separate containers, must meet the following acceptance criteria: not more than 2 of the 20 doses are outside the range of 80% to 120% of label claim, and none are outside the range of 75% to 125% of label claim, while the mean for each of the beginning and end doses falls within the range of 85% to 115% of label claim. If 3–6 doses of the 20 doses collected are outside of 80% to 120% of the label claim, but none are outside of 75% to 125% of label claim, and the means for each of the beginning and end doses fall within 85% to 115% of label claim, select 20 additional containers for second-tier testing. For second-tier testing, the requirements are met if not more than 6 of the 60 doses collected are outside the range of 80% to 120% of label claim, none are outside the range of 75% to 125% of label claim, and the means for each of the beginning and end doses fall within the range of 85% to 115% of label claim.

General Sampling Procedure

To ensure reproducible in-vitro dose collection, it is recommended that a mechanical means of actuating the pump assembly be employed to deliver doses for collection. The mechanical actuation procedure should have adequate controls for the critical mechanical actuation parameters (e.g., actuation force, actuation speed, stroke length, rest periods, etc.). The test must be performed on units that have been primed according to the patient-use instructions. The test unit should be actuated in a vertical or near vertical, valve-up, position. The two doses collected at the beginning and end of the container life should be the dose immediately following priming and the dose corresponding to the last label claim number of doses from the container.

For suspension products, the delivered dose should be delivered into a suitable container (e.g., scintillation vial) in which quantitative transfer from the container under test can be accomplished. A validated analytical method is employed to determine the amount of drug in each delivered dose, and data are reported as a percent of label claim. For solution products, the delivered dose can be determined gravimetrically from the weight of the delivered dose, and the concentration and density of the fill solution of the product under test.

Delivered-Dose Uniformity for MDIs and DPIs

Unless otherwise directed in the individual monograph, the drug content of the minimum delivered dose from each of 10 separate containers is determined in accordance with the procedure described below.

Unless otherwise specified in the individual monograph, the requirements for dosage uniformity are met if not less than 9 of the 10 doses are between 75% and 125% of the specified target-delivered dose and none is outside the range of 65% to 135% of the specified target-delivered dose. If the contents of not more than 3 doses are outside the range of 75% to 125% of the specified target-delivered dose, but within the range of 65% to 135% of the specified target-delivered dose, select 20 additional containers, and follow the prescribed procedure for analyzing 1 minimum dose from each. The requirements are met if not more than 3 results, out of the 30 values, lie outside the range of 75% to 125% of the specified target-delivered dose, and none is outside the range of 65% to 135% of the specified target-delivered dose.

Delivered-Dose Uniformity over the Entire Contents

The test for Delivered-Dose Uniformity over the Entire Contents is required for inhalers (e.g., metered-dose inhalers or dry powder inhalers) containing multiple doses of drug formulation (e.g., solution, suspension, or dry powder) either in reservoirs or in premetered dosage units (e.g., blisters), and for drug formulations packaged in reservoirs or in multiple-dose assemblies of premetered dosage units that have a predetermined dose sequence, where these multiple-dose assemblies are labeled for use with a named inhalation device. The test for Delivered-Dose Uniformity over the Entire Contents also ensures that multidose products supply the total number of discharges stated on the label. Unless otherwise directed in the individual monograph, the drug content of at least 9 of the 10 doses collected from one inhaler, in accordance with the procedure below, are between 75% and 125% of the target-delivered dose, and none is outside the range of 65% to 135% of the target-delivered dose. If the contents of not more than 3 doses are outside the range of 75% to 125%, but within the range of 65% to 135% of the target-delivered dose, select 2 additional inhalers, and follow the prescribed procedure for analyzing 10 doses from each. The requirements are met if not more than 3 results, out of the 30 values, lie outside the range of 75% to 125% of the target-delivered dose, and none is outside the range of 65% to 135% of the target-delivered dose.

Note: The sampling apparatus and sampling procedures prescribed specifically in USP should be followed for sampling in all the above.

- *Net contents/ Minimum fill:*

    Select a sample of 10 filled containers, and remove any labeling that might be altered in weight during the removal of the container contents. Thoroughly cleanse and dry the outsides of the containers by suitable means, and weigh individually. Remove the contents from each container by employing any safe technique (e.g., chill to reduce the internal pressure, remove the valve, and pour). Remove any residual contents with suitable solvents, then rinse with a few portions of methanol. Retain as a unit the container, the valve, and all associated parts, and heat them at 100 for 5 minutes. Cool, and again weigh each of the containers together with its corresponding parts. The difference between the original weight and the weight of the empty aerosol container is the net fill weight. Determine the net fill weight for each container tested. The requirements are met if the net weight of the contents of each of the 10 containers is not less than the labeled amount.

- *Leakage:*

    The test is used to estimate the weight loss over a 1-year period. Perform this test only on topical aerosols fitted with continuous valves. Select 12 aerosol containers, and record the date and time to the nearest half hour. Weigh each container to the nearest mg, and record the weight, in mg, of each as $W1$. Allow the containers to stand in an upright position at a temperature of 25.0 ± 2.0 for not less than 3 days, and again weigh each container, recording the weight, in mg, of each as $W2$, and recording the date and time to the nearest half hour. Determine the time, T, in hours, during which the containers were under test. Calculate the leakage rate, in mg per year, of each container taken by the formula:

    $$(365)(24/T)(W1 - W2).$$

    Where plastic-coated glass aerosol containers are tested, dry the containers in a desiccator for 12 to 18 hours, and allow them to stand in a constant-humidity environment for 24 hours prior to determining the initial weight as indicated above. Conduct the test under the same constant-humidity conditions. Empty the contents of each container tested by employing any safe technique (e.g., chill to reduce the internal pressure, remove the valve, and pour).

Remove any residual contents by rinsing with suitable solvents, then rinse with a few portions of methanol. Retain as a unit the container, the valve, and all associated parts, and heat them at 100 for 5 minutes. Cool, weigh, record the weight as W3, and determine the net fill weight (W1 − W3) for each container tested. [note—If the average net fill weight has been determined previously, that value may be used in place of the value (W1 − W3) above.] The requirements are met if the average leakage rate per year for the 12 containers is not more than 3.5% of the net fill weight, and none of the containers leaks more than 5.0% of the net fill weight per year. If 1 container leaks more than 5.0% per year, and if none of the containers leaks more than 7.0% per year, determine the leakage rate of an additional 24 containers as directed herein. Not more than 2 of the 36 containers leak more than 5.0% of the net fill weight per year, and none of the 36 containers leaks more than 7.0% of the net fill weight per year. Where the net fill weight is less than 15 g and the label bears an expiration date, the requirements are met if the average leakage rate of the 12 containers is not more than 525 mg per year and none of the containers leaks more than 750 mg per year. If 1 container leaks more than 750 mg per year, but not more than 1.1 g per year, determine the leakage rate of an additional 24 containers as directed herein. Not more than 2 of the 36 containers leak more than 750 mg per year, and none of the 36 containers leaks more than 1.1 g per year. This test is in addition to the customary in-line leak testing of each container.

- *Particle size distribution:*

  The particle or droplet size distribution in the spray discharged from metered-dose inhalers, and the particle size distribution in the cloud discharged from dry powder inhalers, are important characteristics used in judging inhaler performance. While particle size measurement by microscopy can be used to evaluate the number of large particles, agglomerates, and foreign particulates in the emissions of metered-dose inhalers (e.g., Epinephrine Bitartrate Inhalation Aerosol), whenever possible this test should be replaced with a method to determine the aerodynamic size distribution of the drug aerosol leaving the inhaler. The aerodynamic size distribution defines the manner in which an aerosol deposits during inhalation. When there is a log-normal distribution, the aerodynamic size distribution may be characterized by the mass median aerodynamic diameter (MMAD) and geometric standard deviation (GSD). The aerodynamic size distribution of the drug leaving metered-dose and dry powder inhalers is determined using Apparatus 1, 2, 3, 4, 5, or 6 as specified in USP. A fine particle dose or fine particle fraction can also be determined as that portion of the inhaler output having an aerodynamic diameter less than the size defined in the individual monograph. This may be expected to correlate with the drug dose or that fraction of the drug dose that penetrates the lung during inhalation. Individual monographs may also define the emitted fractions of the delivered dose in more than one aerodynamic size range.

Particle size are generally evaluated by using Cascade Impactor,

In this apparatus particles are carried in a stream of air through a series of consecutively smaller jet openings → The heavier and larger diameter particles are impacted on a slide under the larger opening → As the openings get smaller, the velocity of the stream increases and the next larger particles are deposited on the next slides.

D. Therapeutic activity

It is done by standard *in vivo* tests and pharmacological models. Specially designed insufflators are used to deliver powders or solutions to rats, mice or guinea pigs. The dosage of the product has to be determined for inhalation aerosols, and this must be related to particle size distribution. Methods like Gamma scintigraphic and single positron emission computer aided tomography imaging are used to evaluate the site of deposition of drugs administered as aerosols.

Topical preparations are applied to the test areas in the usual manner, and absorption of therapeutic ingredients can be determined.

Bibliography

- American Association for Respiratory Care. AARC Clinical Practice Guideline: Selection of a device for delivery of aerosol to the lung parenchyma. *Respir Care* 1996; 41:647-653.
- Byron PR. Respiratory Drug Delivery, CRC Press, Boca Raton, FL, 1990.
- Dalby R, Suman J. *Adv Drug Deliv Revs* 2003; 55:779–791
- Dean R, Timothy R, Joseph L. A Guide to Aerosol Delivery Devices. American Association for Respiratory Care, www.AARC.org.

- Gennaro R., Remington's Pharmaceutical Sciences.
- Hausmann M, Dellweg S, Heinemann L, Buchwald A, Heise T. *Diabetes* 2005; 54(Suppl. 1):A102.
- Hickey AJ, In: Banker GS, Rhodes CT (Eds). Modern Pharmaceutics, 4th Edn., Marcel Dekker Inc., New York, 2005, pp. 479-96.
- Jani R, Triplitt C, Reasner C & DeFronzo RA, *Expert Opin. Drug Deliv. 2007; 4(1):63-76.*
- Lachman L, Lieberman HA, Kanig JL. The Theory and Practices of Industrial Pharmacy. 3rd Edn, 1986, Varghese Publishing House, Bombay, pp. 589-618.
- Leung FK, Wong S, Li J, Leung E, Liu N: *Diabetes* 2004; **53** (Suppl. 1):A467-A468.
- Lewis D. *Expert Opin. Drug Deliv.* 2007; **4**(3):235-245.
- McDonald KJ, Martin GP. *Int J Pharm* 2000; 201(1):89–107.
- Newman SP, Hollingworth A, Clark AR. *Int J Pharm* 1994; 102:127-132.
- Newman SP. *Respir Care*, 2005; 50(9): 1177-90.
- Partridge MR, Woodcock AA. Propellants. In: Bisgaard H, O'Callaghan C, Smaldone GC, editors. Drug delivery to the lung. New York: Marcel Dekker; 2002:371–388.
- Patton Js, Baker J, Nagarajan S: Inhaled insulin. *Adv. Drug Deliv. Rev.* 1999; 35:235-247.
- Patton JS, Platz RM: *Adv. Drug Deliv. Rev.* 1992; 8:179-228.
- Patton JS. *Adv. Drug Deliv. Rev* 1996; 19:3-36.
- Patton JS. *Chemtech* 1997;27:34-48.
- Pfutzer A, Mann AE, Steiner SS. *Diabetes Technol. Ther.* 2002; 4:589-594.
- Rau JL. *Respir Care* 2005;50(3):367-382.
- Rau JL. *Respir Care* 2006;51(2):158-172.
- Schuster JA, Farr SJ, Cipolla D *et al*: In: Resp. Drug. Deliv. V. Dalby RN, Bryon PR, Farr SJ (Eds.) Interpharm Press, Buffalo Grove, IL 1998; 83-90.
- Smyth HD. *Adv Drug Deliv Revs* 2003;55(7):807–828.

- Taylor K, In: Aulton ME (Editor), Pharmaceutics: The science of dosage form design. 2nd Edn., 2002, Churchil Livingstone, New York, pp. 473-84.
- Taylor K. In: Aulton ME (Editor), Pharmaceutics: The science of dosage form design. 2nd Edn., 2002, Churchil Livingstone, New York, pp. 473-88.
- USP24, 601. Aerosols, metered dose inhalers, and dry powder inhalers, (2000) 1895–1912.
- Vervaet C, Byron PR. *Int J Pharm* 1999;186(1):13-20.

CHAPTER 10

Parenteral Products

Introduction

The parenteral or injectables are the most popular dosage forms which have always been proven to be vital in emergency treatments, protein or hormonal delivery and the delivery of drugs which can not be given by oral route. An Injection is a preparation intended for parenteral administration and/or for constituting or diluting a parenteral preparation prior to administration. Parenteral administration is injection or infusion by means of a needle or catheter inserted into the body. The term *parenteral* comes from Greek words "para" meaning outside; "enteron", meaning the intestine. These are the preparations which are given by other than oral routes.

Parenteral articles are preparations intended for injection through the skin or other external boundary tissue, rather than through the alimentary canal, so that the active substances they contain are administered using gravity or force, directly into a blood vessel, organ, tissue, or lesion.

United States Pharmacopoeia

All parenteral products are designed to bypass the body's natural defenses against microorganisms' invasions associated with skin and mucosal tissues. Parenteral products are prepared meticulously by methods designed to ensure that they meet Pharmacopoeial requirements for sterility, pyrogens, particulate matter, and other contaminants, and, where appropriate, contain inhibitors of the growth of microorganisms. Not only the sophisticated process but also a well designed and maintained manufacturing plant layout is the utmost requirement for formulation of parenterals. The parenteral formulations have various advantages.

Advantages of Parenterals
- Rapid onset of action
- Predictable effect, predictable and nearly complete bioavailability,
- Avoidance of the gastrointestinal (GI) tract and hence, the problems of variable absorption, drug inactivation and GI distress.
- Reliable drug administration in very ill or comatose patients.
- Suitable for nutritive like glucose & electrolyte.
- Suitable for the drugs which are inactivated in GIT

Disadvantages of Parenterals
- Frequent pain and discomfort of injections, with all the psychological fears associated with the needle.
- An incorrect drug or dose is often harder or impossible to counteract when it has been given parenterally, particularly intravenous.
- Termination of therapy is not possible after administration, if adverse reaction occurs
- Only trained person is required.
- Correct syringe, needle, and technique must be used
- If given by wrong route, difficult to control adverse effect
- Difficult to save patient in case of overdosing.
- Sensitivity or allergic reaction at the site of injection
- Requires strict control of sterility.

Table 10.1 Necessities of parenteral preparations

- Sterility (must)
- Pyrogen free(must)
- Free from particulate matter (must)
- Clarity (must)
- Stability (must)
- Isotonicity (should)
- Solvents or vehicles used must meet special purity and other standards.
- Restrictions on buffers, stabilizers, antimicrobial preservative. Do not use coloring agents.
- Must be prepared under aseptic conditions.
- Specific and high quality packaging.

A parenteral dosage form must have certain characteristics/properties which are shown in the table 10.1. Parenterals can be administered by various routes which can be classified as primary and secondary parenteral routes (Table 10.2).

Subcutaneous (s.c.), Intravenous (i.v.) and Intramuscular (i. m.) routes constitutes primary, while Intra-arterial, Intrathecal, Intraarticular, Intrapleural, Intracardial and Intradermal constitutes other routes of parenteral administration.

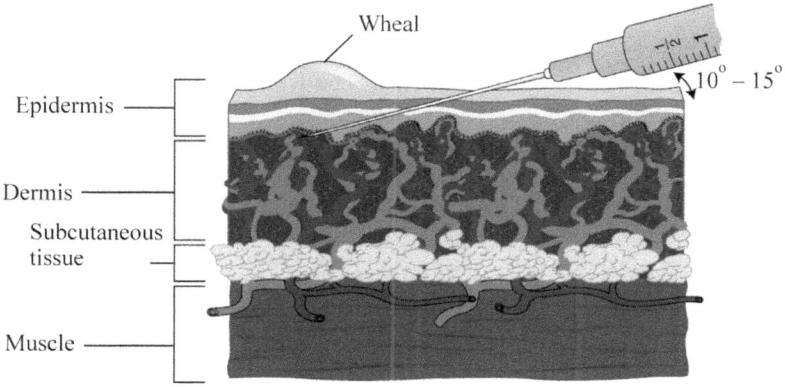

(a) s.c.

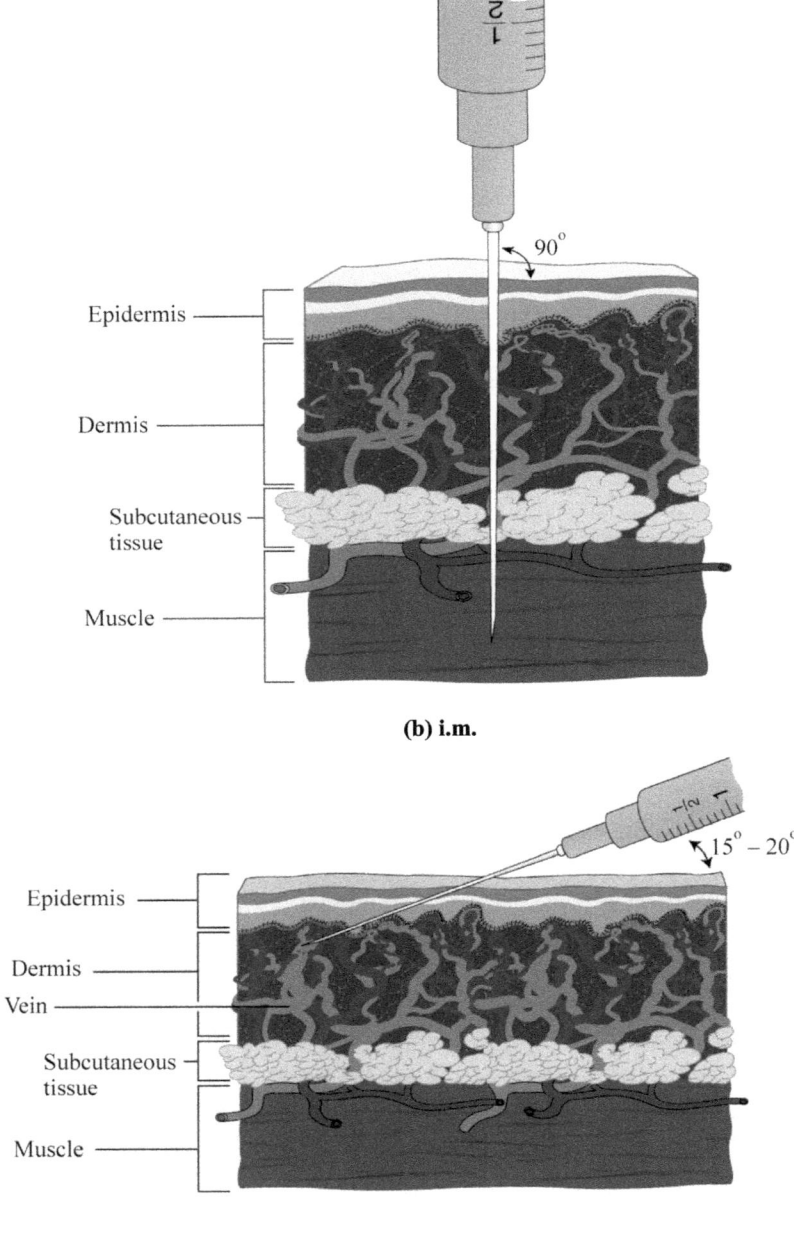

Fig. 10.1 Parenteral routes of dug administration

Table 10.2 Parenteral routes of drug administration

Routes	Usual volume (ml)	Needle commonly used	Types of medication administered
Primary parenteral routes			
Small volume parenterals			
Subcutaneous	0.5-2	5/8 in., 23 gauge	Insulin, vaccines
Intramuscular	0.5-2	1½ in., 22 gauge	Nearly all drug classes
Intravenous	1-1000	Veinpuncture 1½-in., 20-22 gauge	Nearly all drug classes
Large volume parenterals	101 and larger (infusion units)	Venoclysis 1½ in., 18-19 gauge	Nearly all drug classes like electrolytes and nutrients to restore blood volume & to prevent tissue dehydration.
Other parenteral routes			
Intra-arterial: directly into an artery (immediate action sought in peripheral area)	2-20	20-22 gauge	Radiopaque media, antineoplastics, antibiotics
Intrathecal (intraspinal)	1-4	24-28 gauge	Local anesthetics, analgesics; neurolytic agents
Intraepidural (into epidural space near spinal column)	6-30	5 in., 16-18 gauge	Local anesthetics, narcotics, steroids
Intra-articular: directly into the joint, usually for a local effect there, as for steroid anti-inflammatory action in arthritis	2-20	1.5-2 in., 18-22 gauge	Morphine, local anesthetics, steroids, NSAIDs, antibiotics
Intracardial: directly into the heart when life is threatened	0.2-1	5 in., 22 gauge	Cardiotonic drugs, calcium
Intrapeural: directly into the pleural cavity or a lung (also used for fluid withdrawal)	2-30	2-5 in., 16-22 gauge	Local anesthetics, narcotics, chemotherapeutic agents

Preformulation

Prior to the development of dosage forms with a new drug, it is essential to determine some fundamental physical and chemical properties of the drug molecule and other derivative properties of drug powder. These sets of information govern the possible approaches in formulation development. This stage of product development is known as preformulation. Therefore, preformulation may be described as a stage of development during which the physicochemical properties of the drug in question are characterized so as to provide all the necessary information for the formulation of a stable, safe and effective dosage form.

With respect to the preformulation studies of drugs intended to be developed as parenteral dosage forms, the physical, chemical and biological properties of the drug need to be assessed in order to make rational decisions on the selection of a suitable vehicle (aqueous or non-aqueous), selection of added substances or excipients (antioxidants, antimicrobials, preservatives, buffers, solubilising agents and tonicity adjusters), and selection of containers and closures.

For the preformulation studies of drugs formulated as parenteral dosage form, solubility and dissolution are the important properties. The most important factor affecting dissolution is the aqueous solubility of the drug itself, but other factors that can be important are the physical state of the drug (crystallinity, polymorphism etc.), particle size, and formulation pH. In general, it has been suggested that unless a compound has an aqueous solubility in excess of 1% (10 mg/ml) over the pH range of 1-7 at 37 ^{0}C then potential bioabsorption problems may occur. The water solubility may be improved by various means (Refer Chapter 1) like use of suitable crystalline state (amorphous/crystalline, hydrates/solvates), salt form, polymorph type, formulation's pH, complexation (lipid or metal).

Crystal Characteristics

Crystalline characteristics are analyzed by microscopy and X-ray powder diffratctometry (XRPD). Crystal habit or the external shape (cubic, tetragonal, hexagonal etc.) of a crystal may be determined by microscopy. In XRPD the sharp peaks in diffractograms generally indicate the crystalline nature of the drug. While on the other hand the diffused peaks indicate the amorphous form. Many dry solid parenteral products, such as cephalosporins, are prepared by sterile crystallization techniques. Control of the crystallization process to obtain a consistent and uniform crystal form, habit, density, and size distribution is particularly critical for drug substances to be utilized in sterile suspensions. For example, when the crystallization process for sterile ceftazidime pentahydrate was modified to increase the density and decrease volume of the fill dose, the rate of dissolution increased significantly.

Each crystallization procedure has to be designed to ensure sterility and minimize particulate contamination. The use of unsuitable solvent during the washing procedure can destroy the crystalline structure. Drugs that associate with water to produce crystalline forms are called Hydrates. A particular hydrate with the best stability (even in extreme humidity conditions) should be selected for parenteral dosage form.

Amorphous form of the drug is generally rapidly absorbed but show a short duration of action (e.g. amorphous or semilente insulin). On the other hand crystalline form is slowly absorbed but show a prolonged duration of action (e.g. crystalline or ultralente insulin). So the combination of crystalline and amorphous form of a same drug may provide a dosage form with combined benefits of rapid onset and prolonged duration of action (e,g. lente insulin, a physical mixture of 70% crystalline ultralente and 30% amorphous semilente insulin). Moreover, the crystalline form of the drug can withstand the high thermal stress (dry heat for several hours) as compared to amorphous form (e.g. Pencillin G).

Chemical Modification of the Drug

Chemical modification of the parent drug can be done for improvement of the properties of a drug. The properties like stability, solubility and depot action can be improved; while formulation difficulties and pain on injection can be minimized by the preparation of an ester, salt, or other modification of the parent structure of parenteral drugs. These modified drugs that convert back to the active parent structure are known as a prodrugs. Benzathine penicillin, procaine penicillin, metronidazole phosphate and chloramphenicol sodium succinate are some examples of Antibiotic Prodrugs; while methylprednisolone sodium succinate, hydrocortisone sodium succinate are some steroidal Injectable prodrugs

The preparation of salts of parenteral drugs is one of the most important and popular tools for improvement of stability and modulating solubility. IV and IM Injectable solutions may require high solubility for loading or incorporating more quantity of drug into acceptable volumes for bolus administration. Sodium and potassium salts of weak acids and hydrochloride and sulfate salts of weak bases are widely used in parenterals requiring highly soluble compounds, based on their overall safety and history of clinical acceptance.

If the solubility of a drug is to be reduced to enhance stability or to prepare a suspension, the formulator may prepare water insoluble salts. Ex: Procaine Penicillin G: decrease solubility (7 mg/ml) of which, when compared with the very soluble penicillin G potassium, is utilized to prepare stable parenteral suspensions. Another alternative to prepare an insoluble drug is to use the parent acidic or basic drug and to buffer the pH of the suspension in the range of minimum solubility.

Polymorphism

Several crystal forms of a given chemical exhibits different physical properties, this phenomenon is called polymorphism. Polymorphs have different relative intermolecular and/or inter-atomic distances and unit cells, resulting in different physical and chemical properties, such as density, solubility, dissolution rate, bioavailability, and so on.

The conversion of one polymorph to another may cause a significant change in the physical properties of the drug and in critical quality attributes of drug products. In parenteral formulations the most stable polymorphic form (generally the one with the lowest melting point; or with lower free energy at a given temperature) of the drug should only be used. Physical stresses that occur during suspension manufacture may also give rise to changes in crystal form.

pH and pKa

Profiles of pH (and acid dissociation constant or pKa) versus stability and solubility are needed for solution and suspension formulations to assure physicochemical stability as well as to maximize or minimize solubility. This information is also valuable for predicting the compatibility of drugs with various infusion fluids.

Parenteral products with pH value above pH 9 causes tissue necrosis, while if it is below pH 3, it causes extreme pain at site of injection.

In a nut shell, the physical and chemical data that should be obtained on the drug substance include the following:
- Melting point
- Thermal profile
- Particle size and shape
- Hygroscopicity potential
- Ionization constant
- Light stability
- Optical activity
- pH solubility profile
- pH stability profile
- Polymorphism potential
- Solvate formation

Formulation of Parenterals

General steps of parenteral formulations are given in Fig. 10.2 and the components are listed in Table 10.3.

Vehicles

Aqueous Vehicles:

Water for injection (WFI) is the most widely used solvent for parenteral preparations.

Preparation: The source water usually must be pretreated by one or combination of the following treatments: Chemical softening, filtration, deionization, carbon absorption, or reverse osmosis purification. Preparation techniques of water for injection are shown Table 10.4 and the preparation assemblies are shown in Fig. 10.3.

252 Essentials of Pharmaceutical Technology

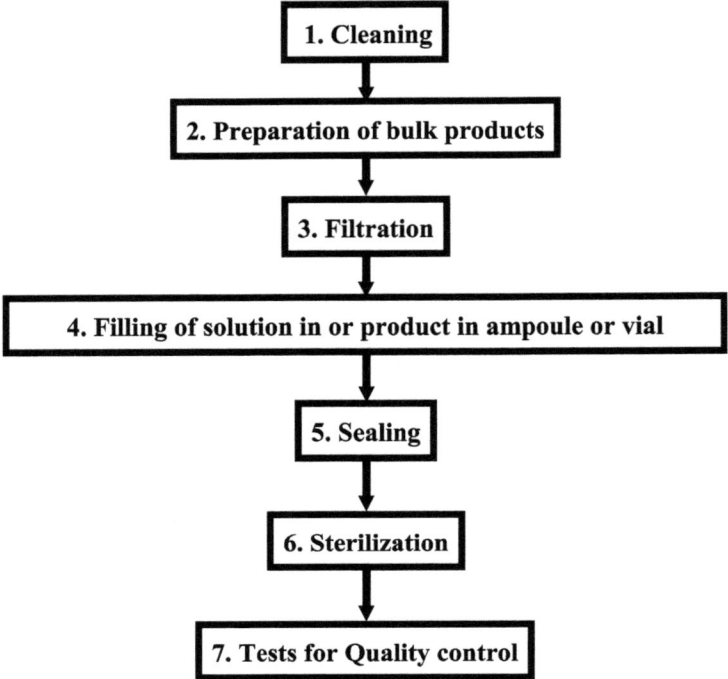

Fig. 10.2 Steps involved in formulation of parenterals.

Table 10.3 Formulation of parenteral

- Therapeutic agents
- Vehicles
  - Water
  - Water miscible vehicles
  - Non- aqueous vehicles
- Added substances (Additives)
  - Antimicrobials
  - Antioxidants
  - Buffers
  - Bulking agents
  - Chelating agents
  - Protectants
  - Solubilizing agents
  - Surfactants
  - Tonicity adjusting agents

WFI can be prepared by distillation or by membrane technologies (reverse osmosis or ultra filtration). USP: "distillation or a purification process that is equivalent of superior to distillation".

Permissible limits for WFI as per USP are

- Conductivity ≤ 1.3 μS/cm @ 25° C
- Total Organic Carbon (TOC) ≤ 500 ppb
- Microbial ≤ 10 cfu / 100 ml
- Endotoxin requirement < 0.25 EU/ml

Table 10.4 Preparation techniques of water for injection

- Multi-Effect Still (MES)
  - Uses Plant Steam to convert feedwater to pure steam
  - Separators allow impurities to drop out of the pure steam
  - Pure steam from first effect used to convert feedwater to pure steam in subsequent effects
- Vapor Compression (VC)
  - Uses plant steam to convert initial feedwater to vapor (pure steam)
  - Pure steam is compressed, elevating temperature
  - Compressed vapor is used to evaporate new feedwater, giving up latent heat and condensing as WFI
  - Higher electrical demand, but lower steam demand

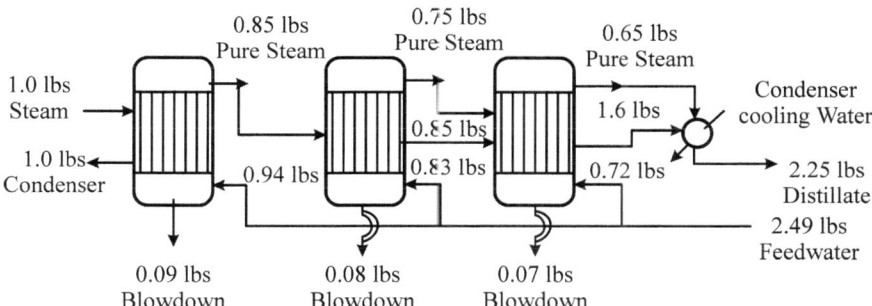

(a) Multi-Effect Still (MES)

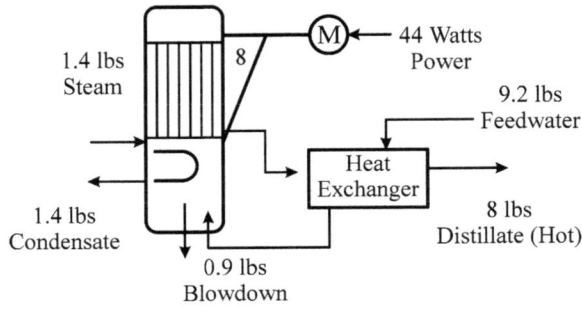

(b) **Vapor Compression (VC)**

Fig. 10.3 Preparation assemblies of water for injection

Storage and Distribution

The rate of production of WFI usually is not sufficient to meet processing demands; therefore, it is collected in a holding tank for subsequent use. The USP requires that the WFI be held at a temperature too high for microbial growth. Normally this temperature is a constant 80 ^{0}C.

The USP also permits the WFI to be stored at room temperature but for a maximum of 24 hrs and requires frequent sanitization to minimize the risk of viable microorganisms being present. The stainless steel storage tanks in such systems usually are connected to a welded stainless steel distribution loop supplying the various use sites with a continuously circulating water supply. The tank is provided with a hydrophobic membrane vent filter capable of excluding bacteria and non-viable particulate matter. Such a vent filter is necessary to permit changes in pressure during filling and emptying. Such systems are carefully designed and constructed and often constitute the most costly installation within the plant.

When the water cannot be used at 80 ^{0}C, heat exchangers must be installed to reduce the temperature at the point of use. Bacterial retentive filters should not be installed in such systems because of the risk of bacterial buildup on the filters and the consequent release of pyrogenic substances.

The Sterile Water for injection (SWFI) requirements differ in that since it is a final product, it must pass USP sterility test. WFI and SWFI may not contain added substances. Bacteriostatic Water for Injection (BWFI) contains one or more suitable antimicrobial agents in containers 30 ml or less. This restriction is designed to prevent the administration of large quantity of a bacteriostatic agent that probably would be toxic in the accumulated amount of large volume of solution, even though the concentration was low.

Other aqueous vehicles that may be used in place of SWFI and BWFI for reconstitution or administering drugs include dextrose (5%), sodium chloride (0.9%), and a variety of other electrolyte and nutrient solution.

Non-aqueous vehicles

Fixed oils are used as vehicles for non-aqueous injections are of vegetable origin, are odorless and have no odor suggesting rancidity. They meet the requirements of the test for solid paraffin under mineral oil, have a saponification value of between 185 and 200, have an iodine value of between 79 and 128 and meet the requirements of free fatty acids tests. They must be ensured that they exhibit no pharmacological action, non-toxic and none irritating, and are compatible and stable with all ingredients of the formulation. A non-aqueous solvent or a mixed aqueous solvent system may be necessary to stabilize drugs, (such as the barbiturates that are readily hydrolyzed by water) or to improve solubility (e.g. Digitoxin).

Commonly used oils are corn oil, cottonseed oil, peanut oil and sesame oil. Because fixed oils can be quite irritating when injected may cause sensitivity reactions in some patients, the oil used in the product must be stated on the label. Fixed oils must never be administered intravenously and are, in fact, restrict to intramuscular use.

The main use of such oils is with steroids, with which they yield products that produce a sustained-release effect. Ex: sesame oil has also been used to obtain slow release of fluphenazine esters given IM. Benzyl benzoate may be used to enhance steroid solubility in oils if desired. Example of injectable products formulated with nonaqueous solvents are – Diazepam Injection USP and Phenytoin Sodium USP.

Water miscible vehicles are used primarily to solubilize certain drugs in an aqueous vehicle and to reduce hydrolysis. They are widely used in parenterals to enhance drug solubility and to serve as stabilizers.

The more common solvents include glycerin, ethyl alcohol, propylene glycol, and polyethylene glycol 300.The most important solvents in this group are ethyl alcohol, liquid polyethylene glycol and propylene glycol. Ethyl alcohol is used particularly in the preparation of solution of cardiac glycosides, certain alkaloids.

Methods of Adjusting Tonicity

Based on the theoretical background provided earlier, individual methods to adjust the tonicity of solution can be devised, based on the principles of colligate properties. However, in the practice of pharmacy, a number of simple methods to adjust the tonicity of a formulation in a prescription order were developed on an extemporaneous basis to help the pharmacist. These methods can be classified into two types.

In Class 1 methods, an inert substance such as sodium chloride or dextrose is added to the solution to lower its freezing point to match that of blood, $-0.52°$ C, that is the solution is made isotonic by the addition of an inert excipient.

In Class II methods, a calculated quantity of water is added to the total solute content (drug) of the prescription to make it isotonic and then diluted with sufficient isotonic diluting solution to bring it to the final volume. These methods are explained below followed by a simple example illustrating the method. However, the assumption inherent in all these methods needs to be considered carefully. The first assumption is that colligative properties are additive for mixtures of solutes, and that they are linearly related to their concentration expressed in molarity, molality, or in percentages. This assumption is true in dilute solution of nonelectrolytes and electrolytes. However, for concentrated solutions, this assumption may not be valid. In case if chemical interaction, association, or complextion or micellar interaction between solutes in solution, the colligative properties of solutes may not be additive. The second assumption is that all solutes present in solution contribute to its tonicity. But all biological membranes are not truly semipermeable and hence some solutes do not contribute to the tonicity of the solution across a membrane, for example, boric acid across an erythrocyte membrane. Nevertheless, the errors introduced are small and slight deviations from isotonicity on either side do not result ininsignificant adverse effect. In the literature, the L-value method or the L_{iso} method can also be found. It is identical to the theoretical method described above for solutes for which the freezing point depression can be calculated based on their molecular weight and ionic *nature*. Knowing the freezing point depression, any of the Class 1 or Class II methods can then be used to adjust their solution to isotonicity.

Class 1 Methods

Freezing Point Depression (Cryscopic Method)

The freezing point depression of a number of drug and excipients, either experimentally determined by the method described earlier or a calculated theoretically using the L_{iso} method, are available in the literature. Basically the freezing point of the solution is calculated from the percentage of drug present in solution. This number is subtracted from the freezing point of blood (-0.52 °C) to obtain the freezing point depression to be achieved by the addition of sodium chloride. Knowing that 0.9% sodium chloride is isotonic and freezes at -0.52°C, the amount to be added s calculated as shown by Example 1.

Example 1: Calculation of the amount of sodium chloride needed to prepare 100 mL of 2% isotonic physostigmine salicylate solution:

Freezing point depression of 2% physostigmine salicylate

$$= 2 \times 0.09 \,°C = 0.18 \,°C$$

Tonicity Adjustment

Therefore, the freezing point depression to be achieved by adding sodium chloride

$$= 0.52° - 0.18 \,°C = 0.34 \,°C$$

Since 0.9% sodium chloride products a freezing point depression of $-0.52°$, the percentage of sodium chloride needed

$$= \{0.34°C/0.52°C\} \times 0.9\% = 0.59 \,\% \text{ g/100 mL}$$

Sodium Chloride Equivalent (E) Method

The sodium chloride equivalent (E) is the amount of sodium chloride that is equivalent to 1 g of the drug in exerting the same osmotic effect. The E value for a new drug can be calculated from its L_{iso} value or the freezing point depression as shown below.

The freezing point depression of a 1 g/L of solution of a new drug can be expressed as in Eq. (1)

$$\Delta T1 = Liso \cdot 1g/ MW \qquad \ldots(1)$$

By definition E g of sodium chloride (MW = 58.45, L_{iso} = 3.4) in 1 L has a similar freezing point depression, as shown in Eq. (2).

$$\Delta T_1 = 3.4 \cdot E \text{ g}/ 58.45 \qquad \ldots(2)$$

Therefore, combining Eqs (1) and (2) gives Eq. (3).

$$E = 17. L_{iso}/ MW \quad \ldots(3)$$

Wells developed a monogram based on Eq. (3) to readily calculate E values from the MW and L_{iso} value of the drug. Thus, the E value for physostigmine salicylate (MW 413.46) calculated by using $L_{iso} = 3.4$ for a uni-univalent electrolyte is equal to 0.14 which is close to the E value of 0.16. This small deviation is due to the difference between the experimentally determined L_{iso} (3.9) of physostigmine salicylate and the theoretical value of 3.4 for a uni-univalent electrolyte. Knowing the E value, the solution can be adjusted to isotonicity as shown by Example 2.

Example 2: Calculate of the amount of sodium chloride needed to prepare 100 mL of 2% isotonic physostigmine salicylate solution.

2 g/100 mL of physostigmine salicylate is equivalent to

$2 \times 0.16 (E) = 0.32$ g/100 mL of sodium chloride

Therefore, Amount of sodium chloride to be added to 100 mL of this solution to make it isotonic shall be

$= (0.9 - 0.32)g = 0.58$ g

Note that the answers by the two methods are not identical but very close.

Class II Methods

The Class II method involve the calculating of the quantity of water needed to make an isotonic solution for a given amount of a drug, followed by dilution with an isotonic solution to make up the volume. These methods were developed to enable pharmacists to prepare parenteral and ophthalmic formulation with simplicity and case.

The White-Vincent Method (USP Method)

In this method, the weight of the drug (w) is first multiplied by sodium chloride equivalent (E) to obtain the quantity of sodium chloride osmotically equivalent to the weight of drug. Since 0.9 g sodium chloride dissolved in 100 mL, results in an isotonic solution, the volume of isotonic solution that can be prepared from w g of drug is given by Eq. (4)

$$V = w . E .100 / 0.9 = 111.1 \; w . E \quad \ldots(4)$$

Thus, dissolving w g of drug in V mL of water results in an isotonic solution which can be further diluted with isotonic solutions such as 0.9% sodium chloride or isotonic dextrose solution to make up the volume. The method can be illustrated by Example 3.

Example 3: Prepare 100 mL of 2% physostigmine salicylate solution isotonic with blood (E of physostigmine salicylate = 0.16).

Using Eq. (4) the volume of water needed to prepare an isotonic solution

$$V = 2 \text{ g} \times 0.16 \times 111.1 \text{ mL/g} = 35.55 \text{mL}$$

This solution can be diluted with 64.45 mL of any isotonic diluting to obtain 100 mL of 2% isotonic physostigmine salicylate solution.

To verify the results, it is assumed that the above solution is diluted with 64.45 mL isotonic sodium chloride solution; the equivalent amount of sodium chloride added is 0.58 g, which matches with results obtained by the Class 1 methods.

The Sprowls Methods

In the early days of practice of pharmacy, many prescriptions were written to prepare one fluid ounce of a 1% drug solution; thus, the amount of drug (w = 0.3 g) and the final volume were fixed (1 fluid ounce or 30 mL). Sprowls recognizing this fact suggested a modification of the White-Vincent method to further simplify the calculations for the practicing pharmacist.

In this method, the amount of drug is fixed at 0.3 g (30 mL of 1% solution), and the volume of water required to prepare this isotonic solution is calculated using Eq. (4) for all drugs which are commonly used in parental and ophthalmic formulation and for which the sodium chloride equivalents are known. The pharmacist then proceeds to make up the volume of the preparation to 30 mL with an isotonic diluting solution to fill the prescription. For example, if one fluid ounce of 1% physostigmine salicylate solution is to be prepared, 5.3 mL of water is required for 0.3 g of physostigmine salicylate to prepare an isotonic solution. Following its preparation, this 5.3 mL solution can be diluted with any isotonic diluting solution to make up the volume to one fluid ounce.

If 100 mL of a 1% solution are needed, the volume of water (V) should be multiplied by 3.33 to obtain the amount of water necessary to make it isotonic.

Summary of Methods of Adjusting Tonicity

A. Freezing Point Depression

- freezing point depressions of 1 w/v% drug solutions ($DT_f^{1\%}$)
- choose appropriate solute for adjusting tonicity
    - using $DT_{f,ref}^{1\%}$ determine required amount (w_{ref}) to cover remaining DT_f

$$w_{ref} = \left[\frac{0.52 - C\Delta T_f^{1\%}}{\Delta T_{f,ref}^{1\%}}\right] V_{req}$$

V_{req} = volume of water required

C = drug concentration (w/v%)

B. Sodium Chloride Equivalent (E) Method

$NaCl\ (w/v\%) = 0.90 - E \times [drug]\ (w/v\%)$

$E = NaCl$ equivalent

C. White-Vincent Method (USP Method)

calculates volume (V) in ml of isotonic solution that can be prepared by mixing drug with water/isotonic buffered solution

$V = w \times E \times 111.1$

w = wt. of drug (g)

Table 10.5 Classes and examples of parenteral additives

Additives	Examples	Usual concentration (%)
Antimicrobials	Benzalkonium chloride	0.01
	Benzyl alcohol	1-2
	Chlorobutanol	0.25-0.5
	Metacresol	0.1-0.3
	Butyl p-hydroxybenzoate	0.015
	Methyl p-hydroxybenzoate	0.1-0.2
	Propyl p-hydroxybenzoate	0.2
	Phenol	0.25-0.5
	Thimerosal	0.01

Table 10.5 Contd...

Antioxidants	Ascorbic acid	0.01-0.05
	Cysteine	0.1-0.5
	Monothioglycerol	0.1-1.0
	Sodium bisulfite	0.1-1.0
	Sodium metabisulphite	0.1-1.0
	Tocopherols	0.05-0.5
Buffers	Acetates	1-2
	Citrates	1-5
	Phosphates	0.8-2.0
Bulking agents	Lactose	1-8
	Mannitol	1-10
	Sorbitol	1-10
	Glycine	1-2
Chelating agents	Salts of ethylenediaminetetraacetic acid	0.01-0.05
Protectants	Sucrose	2-5
	Glucose	2-5
	Lactose	2-5
	Maltose	2-5
	Trehalose	2-5
	Human serum albumin	0.1-1.0
Solubilising agents	Ethyl alcohol	1-50
	Glycerine	1-50
	Polyeyhylene glyccl	1-50
	Propylene glycol	1-50
	Lecithin	0.2.0
Surfactants	Polyoxyethylene	0.1-0.5
	Sorbitan monooleate	0.05-0.25
Tonicity-adjusting agent	Dextrose	4-5
	Sodium chloride	0.5-0.9

Types of Parenteral preparation

Solutions of drugs suitable for parenteral administration are referred as injection. According to USP injections are separated into

- [Drug] Injection: Liquid preparations that are drug substances or solutions thereof, e. g. Insulin.
- [Drug] *for* Injection: Dry solids that, upon addition of suitable vehicles, yield solutions conforming in all respects to the requirements for injections, e.g. Cefamandole Sodium
- [Drug] injectable emulsion: Liquid preparations of drug substances dissolved or dispersed in a suitable emulsion medium, e.g. Propofol

- [Drug] injectable suspension: Liquid preparations of solids suspended in a suitable liquid medium, e.g. Methyl Prednisolone Acetate.
- [Drug] *for* Injectable suspension: Dry solids that, upon the addition of suitable vehicles, yield preparations conforming in all respects to the requirements for injectable suspensions, e.g. Sterile Ampicillin for Suspension

Boylan and Nail has discussed the formulation of major types of parenteral products as solutions, suspensions, emulsions and dry powders.

Solutions

Aqueous (hydroalcoholic/ mixtures of water with glycols) injectables are relatively less painful on injection (Table 10.6). However other nonaqueous solvents are also used in solutions. The injectable solutions are manufactured by dissolving the drug and any excipients, adjusting the pH, sterile filtering the resultant solution through a 0.22 µm membrane filter and, when possible, autoclaving the final product. Sterile filtration is used for thermolabile substances followed by filling. Thermostable drugs should be terminally autoclave sterilized after filling. This is the best way to ensure the product sterility. Large volume parenterals (LVPs) and small volume parenterals (SVPs) which do not have antimicrobial agent should be terminally sterilized. Only multiple dose-SVPs commonly include an antimicrobial agent.

Parenteral solutions are generally filtered through 0.22 µm membrane filters to achieve sterility and remove particulate matter. Talc or carbon filtration aid (or other filter aids) may also be necessary. If talc is used it should be pretreated with a dilute acid solution to remove surface alkali and metals.

In filtering protein solutions the chances of adsorption of protein onto membrane filters must be avoided. To avoid the loss of very expensive (mostly) protein materials, a membrane (such as hydrophilic polyvinylidene difluoride and hydroxyl-modified hydrophilic polyamide membranes) with minimum protein adsorbing properties should be used.

The total fluid volume that must be filled into a unit parenteral container is typically greater than the volume that would contain the exact labeled dose. The fill volume is dependent on the viscosity of the solution and the retention of the solution by the container and stopper. The USP provides a procedure for calculating the fill dose that is necessary to ensure the delivery of the stated dose. It also provides a table of excess volumes that are usually sufficient to permit withdrawal and administration of the labeled volume (refer USP).

Suspension

Suspension parenteral dosage forms are one of the most difficult formulations due to the requirement of easy resuspendability and syringeability or injectability (so that it can be ejected through an 18 to 21 gauge needle). Table 10.6 provides the comparison between solution and suspension parenteral dosage forms.

To achieve these properties it is necessary to select and carefully maintain particle size distribution, zeta potential, and rheological properties, as well as the manufacturing steps that control wettability and surface tension. Suspensions Solid content ranges from 0.5 to 5% (but may go as high as 30% in some antibiotic preparation).

Cake formation by solid granules is a major problem associated with the suspension. This cake formation may be prevented by the use of surface active agent which may reduce the interfacial tension between particle and vehicle e.g. Polysorbate 80, lecithin. Hydrocolloids like sodium CMC increase the effect of surfactant. Stability of the suspension sometime increases on increasing the viscosity (by adding some amount of protective colloid or compounds such as sorbitol).

Two basic methods are used to prepare parenteral suspensions.

Sterile vehicle and powder are combined aseptically: e.g. Penicillin G Procaine Injectable Suspension USP.

(a) Sterile solutions are combined and crystals formed in situ: e.g. Sterile Testosterone Injectable Suspension USP.

In the first method (of preparation of Procaine penicillin injectable suspension) an aqueous vehicle containing the soluble components (such as sodium citrate, povidone, lecithin) is filtered through a 0.22 µm membrane filter, heat sterilized, and transferred into a pre sterilized mixing-filling tank. The sterile antibiotic powder, which has previously been produced by freeze drying, sterile crystallization, or spray drying, is aseptically added to the sterile solution while mixing. After all tests have been completed on the bulk formulation, it is aseptically filled.

In the second method (of preparation of Testosterone suspension) the vehicle is prepared and sterile-filtered. The testosterone is dissolved separately in acetone and sterile filtered. The testosterone-acetone solution is aseptically added to the sterile vehicle, causing the testosterone to crystallize. The resulting suspension is then diluted with sterile vehicle, mixed, crystals allowed to settle and the supernatant solution siphoned off. This procedure is repeated several times until all the acetone is removed. The suspension is then brought to the volume and filled in the normal manner.

The critical nature of the flow properties of parenteral suspensions becomes apparent as these products are frequently administered through 1 in. or longer needles having internal diameters in the range of only 300-600 µm. The flow properties of parenteral suspensions are usually characterized on the basis of syringeability or injectability. The syringeability and injectability characteristics of a suspension are closely related to viscosity and to particle characteristics.

***Syringeability* refers to the handling characteristics of a suspension while drawing it into and manipulating it in syringe. It includes characteristics such as case of withdrawal from the container into the syringe, clogging and foaming tendencies, and accuracy of dose measurement.**

The term *injectability* refers to the properties of the suspension during injection; it includes factors as pressure or force required for injection, evenness of flow, aspiration qualities, and freedom from clogging.

Table 10.6 Solutions and suspension injectables

Solutions	Suspensions
• The simplest and thus preferred form	• Particles suspended in a solution
• Risk of low stability of the active compound	• Not thermodynamically stable
• Normally rapid uptake	• Used for substances of low solubility or for controlled released formulations

• Important quality parameters
  • pH
  • Osmolality (ionic strength)
  • Sterility
  • Content and impurities
	• Critical parameter the same as for solutions plus particle size

Emulsion

In emulsions type parenterals maintenance of uniform oil droplets of 1-5 μ size (as internal phase) is the main problem. The selection of emulgent is a vital part. The emulsion must be able to withstand sterilization. The condition of dry heat sterilization may produce coalescence of dispersed phase. The high mechanical stress (excessive shaking) may cause acceleration of rate of creaming. Small amount of some stabilizers like gelatin, dextran & microcrystalline cellulose are added to stabilize the emulsion. Most often emulgents and stabilizer are needed in formulation of parenteral emulsion with the aim of controlling particle size, preventing emboli in blood vessel and preventing the rancidity of oil phase. But due to availability of very limited choice of emulsifier and stabilizer (of low toxicity) for preparation of parenteral emulsion, it becomes very typical to develop the same.

Various emulsion based novel formulation are used to prepare sustained and control release formulation. These include carrier system like microsphere parenteral emulsions, used for several purposes including w/o emulsions of allergenic extracts (s.c.) and o/w sustained release depot preparation (i.m.). An increasingly popular class of i.v emulsions is lipid emulsions. Fat is transported in the bloodstream as small droplets known as chylomicra. Intravenous fat emulsions yield triglycerides that provides essential fatty acids and calories during total parenteral nutrition of patients who are unable to absorb nutrients through the GIT. Intravenous lipid emulsions are usually administered in combination with dextrose and amino acids. Drugs are not added to these admixtures, with common exceptions being heparin, insulin and ranitidine.

Dry Powders

Many drugs are too unstable, either physically or chemically, in an aqueous medium to allow formulation as a solution, suspension or emulsion. Instead the drug is formulated as dry powder that is reconstituted by addition of water before administration. The reconstituted product is usually aqueous solution; occasionally it may be an aqueous suspension (e.g. Ampicillin trihydrate). Dry powders for reconstitution as an injectable product may be produced by following methods:

A. Aseptic Crystallization and Dry Powder Filling

This method is primarily used for manufacturing of sterile aqueous suspension. In aseptic crystallization the drug is dissolved in a suitable solvent and sterile filtered through an appropriate membrane filter. A second solvent, a sterility filtered nonsolvent for the drug, is then added at a controlled rate causing crystallization and precipitation of the drug. The crystals are collected on a funnel, washed if necessary, and dried by vacuum dryer. After drying it may be necessary to mill or blend the drug crystals. The powder is then transferred to dry powder filling equipment and filled into vials.

Disadvantages

- Batch to batch variability in crystal habit and crystal size results in variability in physical properties troublesome consistent product quality.
- Maintenance of asepsis between sterile crystallization and filling of the powder during material handling.
- Maintenance of fill weight uniformity.

B. Spray Drying

A solution of drug is sterile filtered and metered into the drying chamber, where it passes through an atomizer that creates an aerosol of small droplets of liquid. The aerosol comes in contact with a stream of hot sterile gas, usually air. The solvent evaporates quickly, allowing drug to be collected as a powder in the form of uniform hollow spheres. The powder is then filled into vials using conventional powder filling equipment. Limitations of spray drying include: sterile filtration of very large volumes of air; constructing and maintaining a spray dryer that can be readily sterilized; aseptic transfer of powder from the spray dryer to the powder filling line; and precise control of the drying conditions to prevent overheating of the product while providing adequate drying.

C. Freeze Drying

The most common form of sterilized powder is a freeze dried or lyophilized powder.

Advantages

- Water can be removed at low temperature, avoiding damage to heat sensitive materials.
- Proper freeze drying provides dried product with high specific surface area, which facilitates rapid, complete reconstitution of the solid.

- From operation point of view, freeze dried dosage forms allow drug to be filled into vials as a solution which makes control of the quantity filled into each vial more precise than filling drug into vial as a powder. In addition, there is minimal concern with dust contaminant, cross contamination and potential work exposure to hazardous drugs.

Limitations

- Some drugs, particularly biological systems such as proteins, liposomal systems, and vaccines are damaged by freezing, freeze drying or both. Although the damage can be often minimized by using protective agents in the formulation.
- The stability of a drug in a solid state depends on its physical state. If freeze drying produces an amorphous solid and the amorphous form is not stable, then freeze drying will not provide acceptable product.
- Freeze drying is a relatively extensive drying process; it can be an issue for more cost-sensitive products.

Procedure: a solution is filled into vials, a special slotted stopper is partially inserted into the neck of the vial, and trays of filled vials are transferred to the freeze dryer. The solution is frozen by circulation of a fluid, such as silicone oil, at a temperature ranging between $-35°c$ to $-45°c$ through internal channels in the shelf assembly. When the product has solidified sufficiently, the pressure in the freeze dryer chamber is reduced to a pressure less than the vapor pressure of ice at the temperature of the product, and heat is applied to the product by increasing the temperature of the circulating fluid. Under these conditions, water is removed by sublimation of ice.

Freeze drying takes below the triple point of water, at which solid, liquid and vapor all coexist in equilibrium. The most important objective in freeze dried product is to assure that critical quality attributes are met initially and throughout its shelf life. Critical quality attributes include recovery of original chemical or biological activity after reconstitution, rapid and complete dissolution, appropriate residual moisture level and acceptable cake appearance. In addition, process conditions should be those conditions that minimize drying time without adversely affecting product quality. Freeze drying should be carried out at the highest allowable product temperature that maintains the appropriate attributes of a freeze dried product.

While crystallinity of a drug is generally desirable for freeze drying, it is often important for excipients to remain amorphous. In particular, disaccharides (sucrose etc.) are important as formulation additives to stabilize proteins against damage caused by freezing, freeze drying or both. However, in order to be effective stabilizers, it is essential for these compounds to remain amorphous both during freeze drying and subsequent storage.

Lay out and Production facilities of parenterals

The manufacturing of sterile products is subjected to special requirements in order to minimize risks of microbial contamination and of particulate and pyrogen contamination (Fig.10. 4 and Table 10.7)

- Clean- up area
- Preparation area
- Aseptic area
- Quarantine area
- Finishing and packaging area

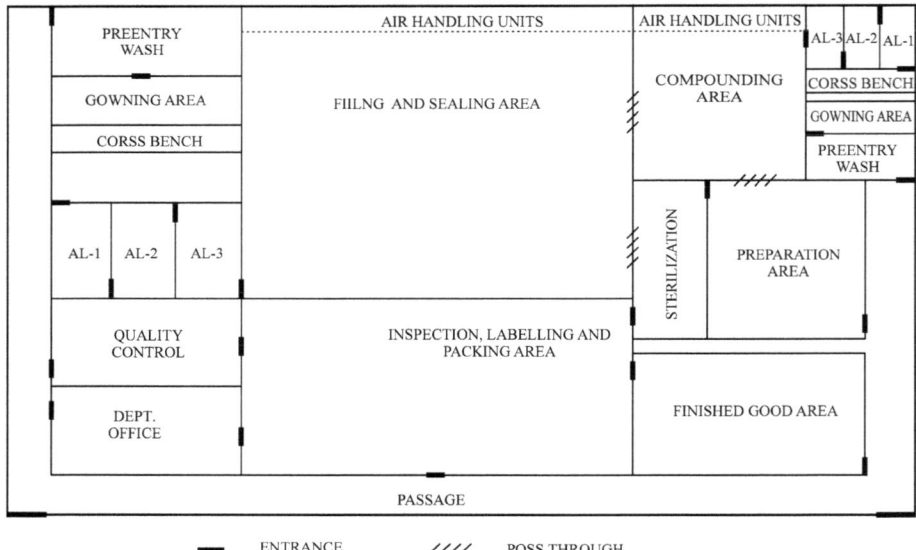

Fig. 10.4 Layout of sterile product manufacturing

Table 10.7 Layout of sterile product manufacturing

Clean- up area:
- Non aseptic area
- Free from dust, fibers & micro-organisms
- Constructed in such a way that should withstand moisture, steam & detergent
- Ceiling & walls are coated with material to prevent accumulation of dust & micro-organisms
- Exhaust fans are fitted to remove heat & humidity
- The area should be kept clean so that to avoid contamination to aseptic area
- The containers & closures are washed

Preparation area:
- The ingredients are mixed & preparation is prepared for filling
- Not essential that the area is aseptic
- Strict precaution is taken to prevent contamination from outside
- Cabinets & counters: SS
- Ceiling & walls : sealed & painted

Aseptic area:
- Filtration & filling into final containers & sealing is done
- The entry of outside person is strictly prohibited
- To maintain sterility, special trained persons are only allowed to enter & work
- Person who worked should wear sterile cloths
- Should be subjected for physical examination to ensure the fitness
- Minimum movement should be there in this area
- Ceiling & walls & floors : sealed & painted or treated with aseptic solution and there should not be any toxic effect of this treatment
- Cabinets & counters
- Mechanical equipments
- Air
    - Free from fibers, dust & micro organisms
    - HEPA filters are used which removes particles upto 0.3 micron
    - Fitted in laminar air flow system, in which air is free from dust & micro organisms flows with uniform velocity
    - Air supplied is under positive pressure which prevents particulate contamination from sweeping
    - UV lamps are fitted to maintain sterility

Table 10.7 Contd...

> **Quarantine area:**
> - After filling, sealing & sterilization the products or batch is kept in this area
> - The random samples are chosen and given for analysis to QC dept.
> - The batch is send to packing after issuing satisfactory reports of analysis from QC
> - If any problem is observed in above analysis the decision is to be taken for reprocessing or others.

Production Facilities for Parenterals

Principle

The manufacture of sterile products is subject to special requirements in order to minimize risks of microbiological contamination, and pyrogen contamination. Much depends on the skill, training and attitudes of the personnel involved. Quality Assurance is particularly important, and this type of manufacture must strictly follow carefully established and validated methods of preparation and procedure. Sole reliance for sterility or other quality aspects must not be placed on any terminal process or finished product test.

Note:

This guidance does not lay down detailed methods for determining the microbiological and particulate cleanliness of air, surfaces etc. Reference should be made to other documents such as the EN/ISO standards.

General

1. The manufacture of sterile products should be carried out in clean areas entry to which should be through airlocks for personnel and/or for equipment and materials. Clean areas should be maintained to an appropriate cleanliness standard and supplied with air which has passed through filters of an appropriate efficiency.

2. The various operations of component preparation, product preparation and filing should be carried out in separate areas within the clean area.

Manufacturing operations are divided in two categories; firstly those where the product is terminally sterilized, and secondly those which are conducted aseptically at some or all stages.

3. Clean areas for the manufacture of sterile products are classified according to the required characteristics of the environment. Each manufacturing operation requires an appropriate environmental cleanliness level in the operational state in order to minimize the risk of particulate or microbial contamination of product or materials being handled.

In order to meet "in operation" condition these areas should be designed to reach certain specified air –cleanliness levels in the at least occupancy state. The at-rest state is condition where the installation is installed and operating, complete with production equipment but with no operating personnel present. The in operation state is the condition where the installation is functioning in the defined operating mode with the specified number of personnel working.

The in operation and at rest states should be defined for each clean room or suite of clean rooms.

For the manufacture of sterile medicinal products 4 grades can be distinguished.

Grade A: The local zone for high risk operations, e.g. filling zone, stopper bowls, open ampoules and vials, making aspects connections. Normally such conditions are provided by a laminar air flow work station. Laminar air flow systems should provide a homogeneous air speed in range of 0.36-0.54 m/s (guidance value) at the working position in open clean room applications.

The maintenance of laminarity should be demonstrated and validated.

A uni-directional air flow and lower velocities may be used in closed isolators and glove boxes.

Grade B: For aseptic preparation and filling, this is the background environment for grade A zone.

Grade C and D: Clean areas for carrying out les critical stages in the manufacture of sterile products.

Personnel

- Only the minimum number of personnel required should be present in clean areas; this is particularly important during aseptic processes.

Inspections and controls should be conducted from outside such areas as far as possible.

- All personnel (including those concerned with cleaning and maintenance) employed in such areas should receive initial and regular training in disciplines relevant to the correct manufacture of sterile products, including hygiene and the basic elements of microbiology. When outside staff who have not received such training (e.g. building or maintenance contractors) need to be brought in, particular care should be taken over their instruction and supervision.

- Staff who have been engaged in the processing of animal-tissue materials or of cultures of microorganisms other than those used in the current manufacturing process should not enter sterile-product areas unless rigorous and clearly defined decontamination procedures have been followed.

- High standards of personal hygiene and cleanliness are essential, and personnel involved in the manufacture of sterile preparations should be instructed to report any conditions that may cause the shedding of abnormal numbers or types of contaminants; periodic health checks for such conditions are desirable. The action to be taken in respect of personnel who might be introducing undue microbiological hazards should be decided by a designated competent person.

- Outdoor clothing should not be brought into clean areas, and personnel entering changing rooms should already be clad in standard factory protective garments. Changing and washing should follow a written procedure designed to minimize the contamination of clean area clothing or the carry-through of contaminants to clean areas.

- Wrist-watches and jewellery should not be worn in clean areas, and cosmetics that can shed particles should not be used.

- The clothing worn and its quality should be appropriate for the process and the grade of the working area (workplace). It should be worn in such a way as to protect the product from contamination. The clothing required for each grade is as follows:
    - *Grade D.* The hair and, where relevant, beard and moustache should be covered. Protective clothing and appropriate shoes or overshoes should be worn. Appropriate measures should be taken to avoid any contamination from outside the clean area.

- *Grade C.* The hair and, where relevant, beard and moustache should be covered. A single or two-piece trouser suit, gathered at the wrists and with a high neck, and appropriate shoes or overshoes should be worn. The clothing should shed virtually no fibers or particulate matter.

- *Grades A/B.* Headgear should totally enclose the hair and, where relevant, beard and moustache. A single or two-piece trouser suit, gathered at the wrists and with a high neck, should be worn. The headgear should be tucked into the neck of the suit. A face mask should be worn to prevent the shedding of droplets. Appropriate, sterilized, non-powdered rubber or plastic gloves and sterilized or disinfected footwear should be worn. Trouser-bottoms should be tucked inside the footwear and garment sleeves into the gloves. The protective clothing should shed virtually no fibers or particulate matter and should retain particles shed by the body.

- Outdoor clothing should not be brought into changing rooms leading to grade B and C rooms. For every worker in a grade A/B room, clean sterilized or adequately sanitized protective garments should be provided at each work session, or at least once a day if monitoring results justify this. Gloves should be regularly disinfected during operations. Masks and gloves should be changed at least at every working session. The use of disposable clothing may be necessary.

- Clothing used in clean areas should be laundered or cleaned in such a way that it does not gather additional particulate contaminants that can later be shed. Separate laundry facilities for such clothing are desirable. If fibers are damaged by inappropriate cleaning or sterilization, there may be an increased risk of shedding particles. Washing and sterilization operations should follow standard operating procedures.

Premises

- All premises should, as far as possible, be designed to avoid the unnecessary entry of supervisory or control personnel. Grade B areas should be designed so that all operations can be observed from outside.

- In clean areas, all exposed surfaces should be smooth, impervious and unbroken in order to minimize the shedding or accumulation of particles or microorganisms and to permit the repeated application of cleaning agents and disinfectants, where used.
- To reduce the accumulation of dust and to facilitate cleaning, there should be no uncleanable recesses and a minimum of projecting ledges, shelves, cupboards and equipment. Doors should be carefully designed to avoid uncleanable recesses; sliding doors are undesirable for this reason.
- False ceilings should be sealed to prevent contamination from the space above them.
- Pipes and ducts and other utilities should be installed so that they do not create recesses, unsealed openings and surfaces that are difficult to clean.
- Sinks and drains should be avoided wherever possible and should be excluded from grade A/B areas where aseptic operations are carried out. Where installed, they should be designed, located and maintained so as to minimize the risks of microbiological contamination; they should be fitted with effective, easily cleanable traps and with air breaks to prevent back-flow. Any floor channels should be open and easily cleanable and be connected to drains outside the area in a manner that prevents the ingress of microbiological contaminants.
- Changing rooms should be designed as airlocks and used to separate the different stages of changing, thus minimizing particulate and microbiological contamination of protective clothing. They should be effectively flushed with filtered air. The use of separate changing rooms for entering and leaving clean areas is sometimes necessary. Hand-washing facilities should be provided only in the changing rooms, not in areas where aseptic work is done.
- Airlock doors should not be opened simultaneously. An interlocking system and a visual and/or audible warning system can be installed to prevent the opening of more than one door at a time.
- A filtered air supply should be used to maintain a positive pressure and airflow relative to surrounding areas of a lower grade under all operational conditions; it should flush the area effectively. Adjacent rooms of different grades should have a pressure differential of approximately 10–15 pascals. Particular attention should be paid to the protection of the zone of greatest risk, i.e. the immediate

environment to which the product and the cleaned components in contact with it are exposed. The various recommendations regarding air supplies and pressure differentials may need to be modified where it becomes necessary to contain certain materials, e.g. pathogenic, highly toxic, radioactive or live viral or bacterial materials or products. The decontamination of the facilities and the treatment of air leaving a clean area may be necessary for some operations.

- It should be demonstrated that airflow patterns do not present a contamination risk; for example, care should be taken to ensure that particles from a particle-generating person, operation or machine are not conveyed to a zone of higher product risk.

- A warning system should be included to indicate failure in the air supply. An indicator of pressure difference should be fitted between areas where this difference is important, and the pressure difference should be regularly recorded.

- Consideration should be given to restricting unnecessary access to critical filling areas, e.g. grade A filling zones, by means of a physical barrier.

Equipment
- A conveyor belt should not pass through a partition between a grade A or B clean area and a processing area of lower air cleanliness, unless the belt itself is continuously sterilized (e.g. in a sterilizing tunnel).

- Whenever possible, equipment used for processing sterile products should be chosen so that it can be effectively sterilized by steam or dry heat or other methods.

- As far as possible, equipment fittings and services should be designed and installed so that operations, maintenance and repairs can be carried out outside the clean area. Equipment that has to be taken apart for maintenance should be re-sterilized after complete reassembly, wherever possible.

- When equipment maintenance is carried out within a clean area, clean instruments and tools should be used, and the area should be cleaned and disinfected again, where appropriate, before processing recommences if the required standards of cleanliness and/or asepsis have not been maintained during the maintenance work.

- All equipment, including sterilizers, air-filtration systems, and water treatment systems, including stills, should be subject to planned maintenance, validation and monitoring; its approved use following maintenance work should be documented.
- Water-treatment plants and distribution systems should be designed, constructed and maintained so as to ensure a reliable source of water of an appropriate quality. They should not be operated beyond their designed capacity.

Consideration should be given to including a testing programme in the maintenance of a water system. Water for injection should be produced, stored and distributed in a manner which prevents the growth of microorganisms, e.g. by constant circulation at a temperature above 70 °C or not more than 4 °C.

Environment Control/Air Control

The air quality/movement, care and maintenance of the area and personnel movement are the main elements of environment control. The air quality in manufacturing area can be the greatest source of contamination. This problem can be minimized using special bacterial and particulate filters. Depth type filters, electrostatic filters and dehumidification systems are used to remove the major portion of airborne contaminants. Air for aseptic area is then passed through high efficiency particulate air (HEPA) filters. HEPA filters remove 99.7% of all particles 0.3 μm or larger. A positive pressure is maintained relative to corridors, to prevent outside air from entering aseptic areas.

A Laminar air flow system provides a means for environment control of an aseptic area. Laminar air flow system contains three basic elements- a blower, a high efficiency air filter, and a plenum. The flow is called laminar because the turbulent air upstream is changed by the filter into a straight-line flow off the downstream face of the filter. Many blowers, many filters, and very large plenums but all have the same basics. The necessity of laminar air flow is to remove most of the particulate matter, as a matter of fact 99.99% of everything air-borne down to 0.3 microns should be screened out to have an environment whose air supply is free of bacteria, fungi, pollen, and practically all air-borne dirt. The HEPA filters are validated by DOP-dioctylphthalate-method.

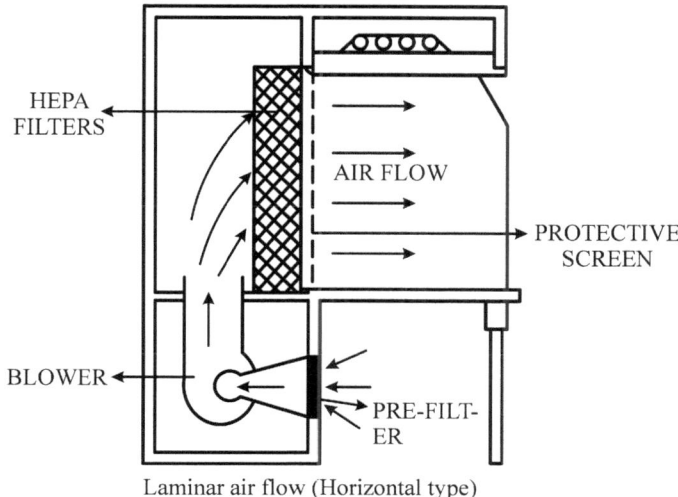

Laminar air flow (Horizontal type)

Fig. 10.5 Horizontal laminar air flow system

Validation of HEPA filter, by the DOP (dioctyl phthalate) method

when manufactured, DOP liquid plasticiser, heated to the point of vaporisation and reconstituted into 0.3 micron particles to form a monodisperse aerosol. These single size particles are diluted with air until a conc. of 100 µg per litre is reached and aerosol mixture allow to passed through the filter. The amount of penetration is measured on the downstream side with a forward light scattering photometer, giving the familiar reading of 0.03% or better studies were made of the effect of different size leaks on typical types of work such as photoresist, microweld, sterile transfers, and the like where it was shown that a leak of 0.01% was the border at which reject rates began to increase and excessive contamination was detected for in-situ DOP test this also represents the linear mass photometer threshold accuracy

Salient Features of Laminar Air Flow
- The underlying principle of a laminar air flow hood is that a constant flow of HEPA filtered air at a rate of approximately 90 linear feet per minute physically sweeps the work area and prevents the entry of contaminated air.

- The hood workspace is used to prevent the contamination of compounded sterile products and parenteral preparations.
- The space between the HEPA filter and sterile product being prepared is referred to as the critical work surface.
- HEPA filter – (High Efficiency Particulate Air filter) removes 99.97% of all air particles 0.3 μm or larger.
- Horizontal Flow (Laminar Flow Hood)
  - Air blows towards worker
  - Used for non-chemotherapy preparations
- Vertical Flow (Biological Safety Cabinet or Chemotherapy Hood)
  - Air blows from top down to maintain sterility and protect the worker
  - Used to make chemotherapy

Air Classification Technique of Environmental Control

Electronic air borne particle-monitoring instruments determine number and size of particulate matter in the sampled air irrespective of viability or non-viability of the particles. Air Classification is defined as the number of particles per cubic foot of air that are larger than 0.5 μm in diameter. e.g. Class 100, Class 1000, Class 10000.

Pyrogens and pyrogenisity

A pyrogen substance gives rise to an elevated body temperature when injected. Endotoxin produced by Gram-negative bacteria is of increasing concern in biotechnology. Highly toxic to mammalian cells, endotoxin is one of the most potent modulators of the immune system. Endotoxin, also referred as lipopolysaccharide (LPS), is composed of hydrophobic fatty acid and hydrophilic carbohydrate domains (Fig. 10.6). The primary hydrophobic domain, known as lipid A, carries many of the biological activities associated with LPS. Lipid A contains fatty acid chains attached to a phosphorylated disaccharide. The lipid composition of lipid A exhibits strain-specific variations. The core is made of carbohydrates, some of which are phosphorylated and ethanolaminylated. The repeat units are trisaccharides, the number of which varies among the different strains.

Pyrogens (The key points)

- Pyrogens cause fever, leucopenia and alteration in blood coagulation
    - Exogenous pyrogens are chemically lipopolysaccharides of bacterial origin, but not necessarily produced mostly by gram-negative bacteria
- Endotoxin - complex of pyrogenic **lipopolysaccharide**, a protein and inert lipid;
- lipid part of the lipopolysaccharide is the main pyrogenic agent;
- polysaccharide part increases solubility

Most properties of endotoxins are accounted for by the active but insoluble "Lipid A" fraction being solubilized by the various sugar moieties. Although the general structure is similar, individual endotoxins vary according to their source and are characterized by the O-specific antigenic chain.

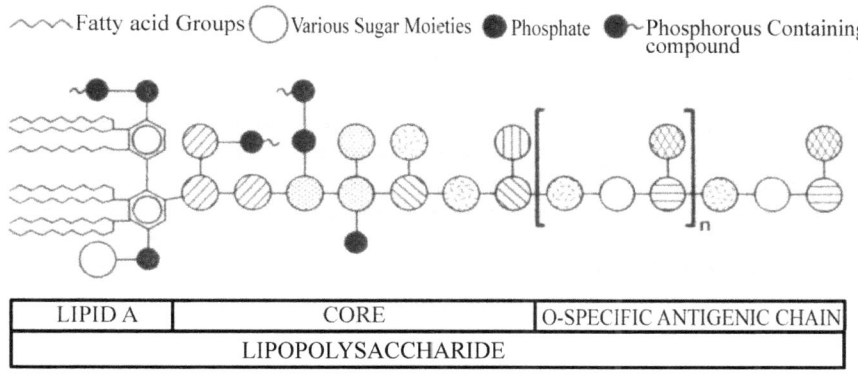

Fig. 10.6 Generalized structure of endotoxin

Sources of pyrogen contamination

- Solvent - possibly the most important source
- The medicament
- The apparatus
- The method of storage between preparation and sterilization

Pyrogen detection

This heterogeneity of pyrogenic bacterial products raises a question about the effectiveness of pyrogen detection in parenteral pharmaceuticals. Both the United States Pharmacopeia and the European Pharmacopoeia specify the rabbit pyrogen test and the *Limulus* amebocyte lysate (LAL) test. However, the LAL test detects only LPS and results in false negatives with certain products. Technically, the rabbit test is an acute toxicity test with an arbitrarily selected end point. There are reports that some parenteral products (e.g., human serum albunin) have caused pyrogenic reactions in patients even after passing the rabbit and LAL tests. Therefore, it is possible that even the rabbit test cannot detect all pyrogenic bacterial products.

An alternative pyrogen test is the monocyte activation cytokine assay. In this assay, monocytes isolated from human peripheral blood are incubated with test samples and their supernatant assayed for pyrogenic cytokines such as IL-1 or TNF-α. A variation of this test is the whole blood-IL-6 assay. A monocytic cell based assay also has been developed. The disadvantage of the monocyte activation-cytokine assay is that the sensitivity of freshly isolated monocytes can vary depending on the immunological responsiveness of the donors. To make this assay suitable for quality control purposes, a well-defined monocytic cell line, which retains its ability to synthesize and secrete cytokines, is needed. This could lead to the development of a quantitative pyrogen test with a broader range of applicability. The Mono-Mac-6 and THP-1 cell lines have been characterized for their suitability in a cell-based pyrogen assay and were found to have the ability to detect bacterial pyrogens.

Elimination of pyrogens

Pyrogens can be eliminated by adsorption on the surface of selective adsorbants, but the often concurrent phenomenon of the adsorption of solute ions or molecules may prevent the use of such method. Solvent extraction methods are useful in the production of antibiotics where heavy pyrogen contamination results from the fermentation process. Ultrafilteration is also sometimes used to eliminate pyrogens.

Quality control of parenterals

Quality control of parenteral includes:
- Test for pyrogens: Rabbit test and Bacterial endotoxins test (BET).
- Particulate evaluation
- Leakers Test
- Sterility test

Test for pyrogens (Rabbit test)

Preliminary test (Sham Test)

Intravenous injection of sterile pyrogen-free saline solution is given to the animal to exclude any animal showing an unusual response to the trauma (shock) of injection any animal showing a temperature variation greater than 0.6°C is not used in the main test.

Main test:

- Group of 3 rabbits
- Preparation and injection of the product:
    - Warming the product
    - Dissolving or dilution
    - Duration of injection: not more than 4 min
    - The injected volume: not less than 0.5 ml per 1 kg and not more than 10 ml per kg of body mass
- Determination of the initial and maximum temperature
- All rabbits should have initial T: from 38.0 to 39.8°C
- The differences in initial T should not differ from one another by more than 1°C

Interpretation of the results If the sum of the responses of the group of three rabbits does not exceed 1.4° and if the response of any individual rabbit is less than 0.6°, the preparation under examination passes the test. If the response of any rabbit is 0.6° or more, or if the sum of the response of the three rabbits exceeds 1.4°, continue the test using five other rabbits. If not more than three of the eight rabbits show individual responses of 0.6° or more, and if the sum of responses of the group of eight rabbits does not exceed 3.7°, the preparation under examination passes the test. (Table 10.8)

Table 10.8 Interpretation of the results

No. of Rabbits	Individual Tempt. Rise (°c)	Tempt. Rise in group (°c)	Test
3 rabbits	< 0.6	≤ 1.4	Passes
If above not passes take additional 5 rabbits (for 3+5 = 8 rabbits)	< 0.6 (not more than 3 should show ≥ 0.6)	≤ 3.7	Passes
If above test not passes the sample is said to be pyrogenic perform the test again			

Limulus Amebocyte Lysate (LAL) test or Bacterial Endotoxins Test
(Official in I.P. and B.P.)

The test is used to detect or quantify endotoxins of gram-negative bacterial origin. LAL test is based on the primitive blood-clotting mechanism of the horseshoe crab (Fig. 10.7). The presence of pyrogen is indicated by the formation of a proteinaceous gel, upon incubation of the mixture of LAL reagent and test solution (Fig. 10.8).

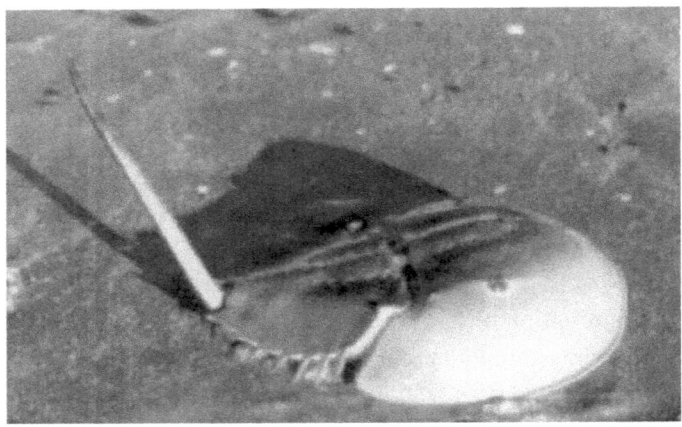

Fig. 10.7 *Limulus polyphemus* or horseshoe crab

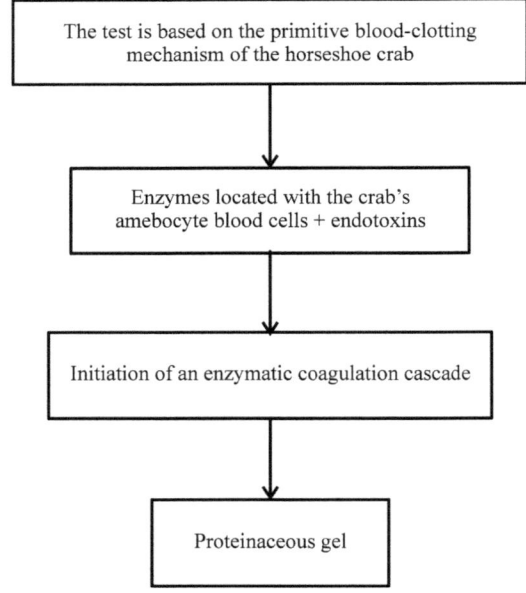

Fig. 10.8 Mechanism of LAL Test

LAL Test performance (The key points)
- Avoid endotoxin contamination
- Before the test:
  - interfering factors should not be present
  - equipment should be depyrogenated
  - the sensitivity of the lysate should be known
- Test:
  - equal volume of LAL reagent and test solution (usually 0.1 ml of each) are mixed in a depyrogenated test-tube
  - incubation at 37°C, 1 hour
  - remove the tube, invert in one smooth motion (180°), read (observe) the result
  - pass-fail test
    - If a firm gel is formed- Pyrogen present.
    - If an intact gel is not formed – Pyrogen absent.

Note:

1. A lysate of amoebocytes from either of the species of the horseshoe crab, Limulus polyphemus, Tachypleusgigas, Tachypleus tridentatus or Carcinoscorpius rotundicauda may be used for the LAL test. The species from which the lysate is obtained is mentioned on the label and reconstituted as stated on the label.
2. The LAL test or BET may be used as qualitative as well as quantitative (and also semi-quantitaive) measure of detecting the presence of pyrogens. IP and BP may be referred for further studies about the same.

Particulate evaluation

The entire product should be inspected by human inspectors under good light baffled against reflection into the eye and against black and white background (Fig. 10.9). Any container with visible particle if seen is discarded.

Limitations
- Size of the particles that can be seen (Visible in unaided eye: 50 μm) only be observed
- Variations of visual acuity from inspector
- Emotional stress
- Eye Strain
- Fatigue

284 Essentials of Pharmaceutical Technology

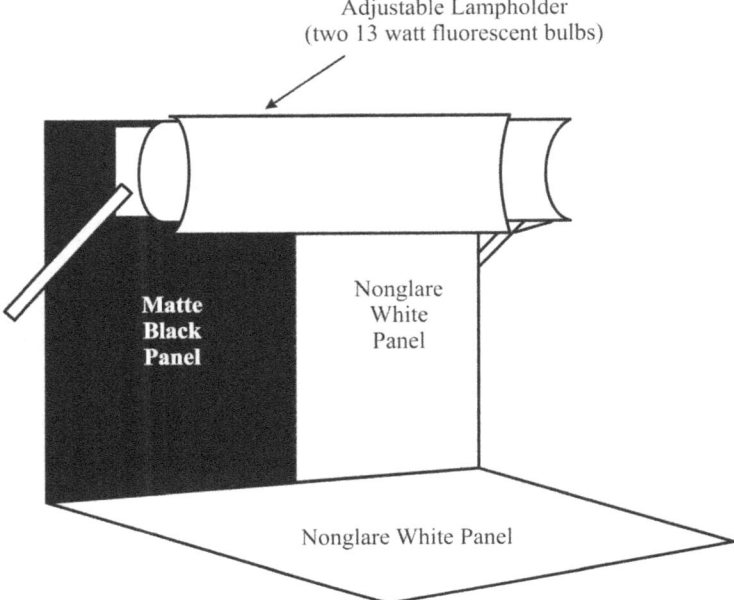

Fig. 10.9 Apparatus for visible particle inspection as presented in the European Pharmacopeia

For the assessment of particulate matter below visible size like in all large volume parenterals (LVP) for single use and small-volume parenterals (SVP), excluding IM and SC injections light obscuration and microscopic particle count test is done. Light obscuration is referred as Stage 1 and microscopic particle count is referred as stage 2. In light obscuration method equipment used to count and measure the size of particles by means of a shadow cast by the particle as it passes through a high-intensity light beam. In microscopic method sample is filtered through membrane filter (under ultra clean condition) and counting the particles on the surface of filter. If limit is exceeded for stage 1 the sample is subjected to stage 2.

Leakers Test

Ampoules sealed by fusion are subjected for leakers test. Negative pressure is built within an incompletely sealed ampoule (submerged entirely in deeply colored solution, i.e. methylene blue solution). All leakers are discarded

Note: Vials and bottles are not subjected to leakers test because the sealing material is not rigid.

Sterility and Sterility Test Regulations

Sterility is the most important and absolutely essential characteristic of a parenteral product. Sterility means the complete absence of all viable microorganisms. It is an absolute term; that is, a product is either sterile or not sterile. Building sterility into a product through meticulously validated cleaning, filtration, and sterilization procedures is more preferable than testing for sterility of a product subjected to marginal or inadequate production processes. The sterility test should never be employed as an evaluation of the sterilization process.

Sterility and quality cannot be tested into a product; they can only be components of controlled processes throughout the production sequence. The sterility test, however, should be employed as the last of several checkpoints in reaching a conclusion that the production process has removed or destroyed all living microorganisms in the product. The USP chapter 1 on injections states that preparations for injection meet the requirements under "Sterility Tests." After meeting these requirements—that is, all media vessels incubated with product sample reveal no evidence of microbial growth (turbidity)—the tested product may be judged to meet the requirements of the test. If evidence for microbial growth is found, the material tested has failed to meet the requirements of the test for sterility. Retesting is only allowed if there is unequivocal proof that the failed result was due to operator or accidental contamination. The FDA has stringent requirements for sterility retesting.

Evidence for microbial growth is determined by visual evaluation of a vessel containing the product sample in the proper volume and composition of nutrient solution. Provided that the growth conditions are optimal—proper nutrients, pH, temperature, atmosphere, sufficient incubation time, and so on—a single microbial cell will grow by geometric progression until the number of microbial cells and their metabolic products exceed the solubility capability of the culture medium. Manifestation of this "overgrowth" is visualized by the appearance of a cloudy or turbid solution of culture medium. A noxious odor may also accompany the turbid appearance of the contaminated medium. The sterility test is a failure when a product generates turbidity in a vessel of culture medium while the same lot of medium without the product sample shows no appearance of turbidity.

Sterility Test Methods

The USP and EP sterility tests specify two basic methods for performing sterility tests, the direct transfer (DT) or direct inoculation method and the MF method, with a statement that the latter, when feasible, is the method of choice. In fact, in some cases, membrane filtration may be the only possible choice. IP, USP and EP provide the detailed SOPs of these tests.

Direct Transfer Method

The DT method is the more traditional sterility test method. Basically, the DT method involves three steps:

1. Aseptically opening each sample container from a recently sterilized batch of product
2. Using a sterile syringe and needle to withdraw the required volume of sample for both media from the container
3. Injecting one-half of the required volume sample into a test tube containing the required volume of Fluid Thioglycollate medium (FTM) and the other half volume of sample into a second test tube containing the required volume of trypticase soy broth (TSB)

The sample volume must be a sufficient representation of the entire container volume and the volume, of medium must be sufficient to promote and expedite microbial growth, if present. Adequate mixing between the sample inoculum and the culture medium must take place to maximize interaction and facilitate microbial growth.

Membrane Filtration Method

The successful employment of this technique requires more skill and knowledge than that required for the DT method. Five basic steps are involved in the use of the MF sterility test method:

1. The filter unit must be properly assembled and sterilized prior to use.
2. The contents of the prescribed number of units are transferred to the filter assembly under strict aseptic conditions. The contents are filtered with the aid of a vacuum or pressure differential system.
4. The membrane is removed aseptically and cut in half.
5. One-half of the membrane is placed in a suitable volume (usually 100 ml) of FTM, and the other membrane half is placed in an equal volume of TSB.

A suitable membrane filter unit consists of an assembly that facilitates the aseptic handling of the test articles and allows the processed membrane to be removed aseptically for transfer to appropriate media or an assembly by which sterile media can be added to the sealed filter and the membrane incubated in situ. A membrane suitable for sterility testing has a rating of 0.45 µm and a diameter of approximately 47 mm.

Advantages

The MF method offers at least five advantages over the use of the DT method:

- Greater sensitivity.

- The antimicrobial agent and other antimicrobial solutes in the product sample can be eliminated by rinsing prior to transferring the filter into test tubes of media, thereby minimizing the incidence of false-negative test results.

- The entire contents of containers can be tested, providing a real advantage in the sterility testing of large-volume parenterals and increasing the ability to detect contamination of product lots containing very few contaminated units.

- Low-level contamination can be concentrated on the membrane by filtering large volumes of product. This results in faster reporting of test results since MF requires only 7 days incubation (for most terminally sterilized products).

- Organisms present in an oleaginous product can be separated from the product during filtration and cultured in a more desirable aqueous medium.

Disadvantages

- There exists a higher probability of inadvertent contamination in manual operations because of the need for greater operator skill and better environmental control in disassembling the filtration unit and removing, cutting, and transferring the membrane. (Newer systems such as the Steritest have eliminated this disadvantage.)

- The method is unable in differentiate the extent of contamination between units, if present, because all product contents are combined, filtered through a single filter, and cultured in single test tubes. Also, if accidental contamination has occurred, rather than this being detected in one or more vessels of the DT method, it manifests itself in the only container used per culture medium.

Interpretation of Results

If there is no visible evidence of microbial growth in a culture medium test tube, after subjecting the sample and medium to the correct procedures and conditions of the USP and EP sterility test, it may be interpreted that the sample representing the lot is without intrinsic contamination.

If microbial growth is found or if the sterility test is judged to be invalid (because of inadequate environmental conditions), the sterility test may be repeated.

Bibliography

- Akers MJ *Pharmaceutical Technology* 2001; July: 78-79.
- Akers MJ, Larrimore Daniel S, Guazzo DM. Parenteral Quality Control Sterility, Pyrogen, Particulate, and Package Integrity Testing, III Edn, 2003, Marcel Dekker, Inc. New York, Basel, US.
- Avis KE, In; Lachman L, Lieberman HA, Kanig JL. Eds. The Theory and Practices of Industrial Pharmacy. Varghese Publishing House, Bombay, pp. 430-78.
- Boylan JC, Nail SL, In; Banker GS, Rhodes CT (Eds). Modern Pharmaceutics. 2005 (Vol. 121) Marcel Dekker, Inc. New York, Basel, US, pp 381-414.
- Chapman DG, In: Winfield AJ, Richards RME (Eds). Pharmaceutical Practice, 3rd Edn, 2004, Churchill Livingstone, New York, pp. 247-63.
- Deluca PP, Boylan JC. In; Avis KE, Lieberman HA, Lachman L, (Eds.). Pharmaceutical Dosage Forms: Parenteral Medications vol. 1, 2nd Edn., 1992, Marcel Dekker, New York.
- Demorest LJ, Hamilton JG, In; Avis KE, Lieberman HA, Lachman L, Eds. Pharmaceutical Dosage Forms: Parenteral Medications, Vol 1, 2nd Edn, 1992. Marcel Dekker New York,
- Good manufacturing practices for pharmaceutical products. In: WHO Expert Committee on Specification for Pharmaceutical Preparations. Thirty-second Report. Geneva, World Health Organization, 1992, Annex 1 (WHO Technical Report Series, No. 823)
- Grandics P. *Pharmaceutical Technology April 2000.*

- Guide to Good Manufacturing Practice for Medical Products. Pharmaceutical Inspection Convention/ Pharmaceutical Inspection Co-operation Scheme, PE 009-2, 1 July 2004
- Indian Pharmacopoeia, Controller of Publications, Delhi, Vol. II, 1996.
- Remington: The Science and Practice of Pharmacy, Lippincott Williams & Wilkins, New York, Vol.–1, 21st. edn, 2006.
- Richards RME. In: Winfield AJ, Richards RME (Eds). Pharmaceutical Practice, 3rd Edn, 2004, Churchil Livingstone, New York, pp. 150-60.
- Sabra K, In: Winfield AJ, Richards RME (Eds). Pharmaceutical Practice, 3rd Edn, 2004, Churchil Livingstone, New York, pp. 298-312.
- The United States Pharmacopoeia (USP), 24th Ed., US Pharmacopoeial Convention, Rockville, MD, 2000.
- Williams KL. Endotoxin, pyrogens, LAL Testing and Depyrogenation, 2001, Marcel Dekker, Inc. New York.

CHAPTER 11

Sterile Processing: Quality Assurance and Validation

Introduction

In the era of Trade Related Intellectual Property Rights (TRIPS) quality has become the winning edge in each and every industry globally. To pace with the ever increasing competition of global pharmaceutical market Indian pharmaceutical industries can no longer rely on their traditional markets and have to take off for the global standards and challenges ahead.

In a global world where in the barriers to trade are coming down, the standards of quality have become more and more uniform or harmonized. Without achieving internationally acceptable quality, it will be impossible to make a mark in the global marketplace. According to the famous quality guru, Deming- Quality does not mean achieving perfection. It means the efficient production of the quality that the market expects. Quality is an achievable measurable, profitable entity that can be installed in any set up, if people are committed and prepared for hard work.

Juran, in his Quality Control Handbook, defines Quality Assurance (QA) as "the activity of providing evidence needed to establish confidence among all concerned that the quality function is being performed adequately." Quality assurance embodies the effort to assure that products have strength, purity, safety and efficacy as intended. The process of quality assurance includes in process, packaging, labeling, finished product testing, batch auditing, stability monitoring as well as raw material testing.

In a pharmaceutical manufacturing unit, sterile area is more sophisticated and can be more vulnerable to foreign particulate matter. Therefore it is essential to maintain stringent standards for particulate contamination which may be responsible for product failure in sterility and pyrogen test. Essentials of quality assurance are Quality system planning, Documentation, Quality system validation, Effective vendor control, Quality audits. Process validation is used to confirm that the resulting product from a specified process consistently conforms to product requirements, which is very critical and stringent in case of sterile products.

In this chapter we shall discuss the elements of quality system validation of sterile area in Pharmaceutical industry and highlight the important aspects of each element involved.

Essentials of Quality System Validation

Validation is an integral part of quality assurance. It involves the systematic study of systems, facilities and processes aimed at determining whether they perform their intended functions adequately and consistently as specified. A validated process is one which has been demonstrated to provide a high degree of assurance that uniform batches will be produced that meet the required specifications and has therefore been formally approved. Validation in itself does not improve processes but confirms that the processes have been properly developed and are under control. Validation provides an approach to prove quality, functionality and performance of a pharmaceutical/biotechnological manufacturing process. This approach can be applied to individual pieces of equipment as well as the manufacturing process as a whole. Guidelines for validation are set by the FDA, but the specifics of validation are determined by the pharmaceutical/biotech company.

Adequate validation is beneficial to the manufacturer in many ways:
- It deepens the understanding of processes; decreases the risk of preventing problems and thus assures the smooth running of the process.
- It decreases the risk of defect costs.
- It decreases the risk of regulatory noncompliance.
- A fully validated process may require less in-process controls and end product testing.

Table 11.1 shows some important definitions of the components of validation as per current good manufacturing practices (cGMP). Validation should thus be considered in the following situations:
- Totally new process;
- New equipment;
- Process and equipment which have been altered to suit changing priorities; and
- Process where the end-product test is poor and an unreliable indicator of product quality.

When any new manufacturing formula or method of preparation is adopted, steps should be taken to demonstrate its suitability for routine processing. The defined process should be shown to yield a product consistent with the required quality. In this phase, the extent to which deviations from chosen parameters can influence product quality should also be evaluated. When certain processes or products have been validated during the development stage, it is not always necessary to revalidate the whole process or product if similar equipment is used or similar products have been produced, provided that the final product conforms to the in-process controls and final product specification. There should be a clear distinction between in-process control and validation. In production, tests are performed each time on a batch to batch basis using specifications and methods devised during the development phase. The objective is to monitor the process continuously.

The Quality Assurance in manufacturing of sterile parenteral preparations involves the following elements.
- Validation of raw material
- Process validation
- Sterilization validation
- Validation of water system

- Cleaning validation
- Equipment validation
- Heating, ventilation and air conditioning (HVAC) system validations
- Machine validation
- Revalidation

Table 11.1 Definitions of validation and its components as per cGMP

Validation - Establishing documented evidence which provides a high degree of assurance that a specific process will consistently produce a product meeting its pre-determined specifications and quality attributes.

Process Validation - Documented evidence which provides a high degree of assurance that a specific process will consistently result in a product that meets its predetermined specifications and quality characteristics.

Qualification- Validation of facilities, equipment and services is called as qualification.

Design Qualification- Documented evidence that the premises, supporting systems, utilities, equipment and processes have been designed in accordance with the requirements of GMP.

Installation qualification - Establishing confidence that process, equipment and ancillary systems are capable of consistently operating within established limits and tolerances.

Operational qualification – Documented verification that the system or subsystem performs as intended over all anticipated operating ranges.

Process performance qualification - Establishing confidence that the process is effective and reproducible.

Product performance qualification - Establishing confidence through appropriate testing that the finished product produced by a specified process meets all release requirements for functionality and safety.

Prospective validation - Validation conducted prior to the distribution of either a new product, or product made under a revised manufacturing process, where the revisions may affect the product's characteristics.

Retrospective validation - Validation of a process for a product already in distribution based upon accumulated production, testing and control data.

Validation protocol - A written plan stating how validation will be conducted, including test parameters, product characteristics, production equipment, and decision points on what constitutes acceptable test results.

Validation for Raw Materials

Multicompendial grades for raw materials should be used and in house specifications should be put in place as early as possible in the development process. Raw material should be sourced from approved vendors or testing should be performed according to certificate of analysis until vendor qualification is complete. Protocol of validation of raw material should specify the following in detail:

1. Prepare the list of raw materials used in production batch i.e. active ingredient, excipient, vehicle, filter aids, solvent for extraction.
2. It is advisable to locate and validate at least two suppliers. It is better to deal with a manufacturer so that a direct line of communication with the organization is established to have better control rather than dealing with a third party.
3. If supplier is new. Visit the supplier's facility to evaluate his capacity to supply quantity and quality raw material required.
4. Obtain samples and supplier's certificates of analysis prior to approval of vendor.
5. Establish specification for each raw material and communicate to the vendor the requirement as to package to maintain sterility if aseptic manufacturing is to be done.
6. Establish test procedure for identity, purity and sterility.
7. Establish optimum package system and storage condition.
8. Establish shelf life.

Process Validation

Process validation is a requirement of the current good manufacturing practices. The FDA defines process validation as follows:

Process validation is establishing documented evidence which provides a high degree of assurance that a specific process will consistently produce a product meeting its predetermined specification and quality characteristics.

Elements of Process Validation

- **Prospective validation**

    In prospective validation, validation protocol is executed before the process is put into commercial use. This includes the following key factors.

1. *Equipment and process*:

   Equipment: Installation Qualification (IQ) and Design Qualification (DQ)

   Process: Operation Qualification (OQ)

   Product: Performance Qualification (PQ)

DQ is intended to ensure the proper equipment is purchased to meet the user requirements. IQ and OQ are intended to prove that the equipment is installed and operates per the manufacturer's specification. PQ is intended to prove that the equipment operates according to the user's requirements in its normal operating environment (Table 11.2).

Table 11.2 Elements of various types of qualifications

Type of Qualification	Elements
Design Qualification (DQ)	• Lists requirements of equipment / system. • Requirements are best created before "shopping" is undertaken. • Requirements are created by the needs of the system/process of which the equipment/ system will be a part.
Installation Qualification (IQ)	• Description of equipment/system including physical characteristics and function of key components. • List of manufacturer's specifications, drawings and operating manuals. • Verifying proper installation of utilities; water, steam, electrical, compressed air, ventilation, etc. • Calibration records for all instrumentation.
Operation Qualification (OQ)	• Verifies correct operation of critical components and operating ranges as defined by the specification and required performance. (Control System, Instruments, Mechanical Features) • Operational Tests (Empty Chamber Mapping, Component Operation)
Performance Qualification (PQ)	• Tests to demonstrate that the equipment/system performs in an actual as-used scenario. • Distribution Studies • Container Mapping • Heat Penetration Studies • Microbiological Challenge Studies

2. *System to assure timely revalidation*: In aseptic process the quality assurance producers should establish the circumstances under which revalidation is required. These may be based upon equipment, process and product performance observed during the initial validation challenge studies.

3. *Documentation*: Approval and release of the process for use in routine manufacturing should be based upon a review of all the validation documentation, including data from the equipment qualification process performance qualification, and product / package testing to ensure compatibility with the process.

(B) Retrospective Process Validation

All equipment, facilities and subsystems should be qualified and validated, which have been used for the production of batches of numerical data of in process and end product testing of which are included in retrospective validation.

Retrospective validation can also be useful to augment initial premarket prospective validation for new product or changed process, in such cases preliminary prospective validation should have been sufficient to warrant product marketing.

Following methods are used for retrospective validation:
- Collect numerical values of in process data and end product testing results.
- Organize these data in chronological order
- Include data for at least 20-30 batches for analysis
- Statistical analysis and evaluation of the data.

Sterilization Validation

The state of sterility of product is a sum total of control on raw material, sterile procession, and environmental monitoring. A batch of sterile preparations is released on the basis of end product sterility testing based on statistical sampling plan which incorporates a probability of non sterility of the object.

Sterilization is the process in which living microorganism are killed. Validation of the sterile process is very important when one deals with the parenteral products.

1. **Steam sterilization validation**

   Selection and calibration of thermocouple is very important in validation of steam sterilization because an error off 0.1 °C will produce a 2.3 % error in the calculated F value. The spore of *B. thermophillus* available in the form of strips or suspension is used as the biological indicator in steam sterilization. The efficiency of sterilization process is determined from design of F value and product heat transfer data.

2. **Validation of dry heat sterilization**

   Usually hot air oven is used for dry heat sterilization. The most difficult area to be heat up must be identified so that the thermocouple and biological indicators (BI) are placed at these spots to monitor. The most widely used BI for dry heat sterilization are the spores of *B. subtilis*. The number of survivors is determined by plate counting or fraction negative method.

3. **Ethylene oxide validation**

   Although the approaches for ethylene oxide validation differ from company to company the following are the general considerations:
   - Evaluate the product specification and package design.
   - Use the laboratory size ethylene oxide sterilizer during early phase of the validation.
   - Verify the calibration of all instrument involved in the monitoring the ethylene oxide cycle.
   - Temperature distribution study is performed using empty sterilizer.
   - Verify the accuracy and reliability of sterilizer control by repetitive run for each sterilization cycle.
   - Repetitive runs for heat penetration study.
   - Sterilization should on the final package product.

4. **Radiation sterilization validation**

   Radiation sterilization is used in heat sensitive materials. D value of the BI is used to monitor the process. *B. pumilus* can be used as a BI for the validation of the radiation sterilization process. Other factors must be considered in the sterilization by radiation, which are as followed:

- The physical appearance of container and contents.
- Stability of active ingredients and
- Safety of irradiated materials

5. Sterilizing filter validation

Filter integrity and filter efficiency test must be done daily prior to the filtration. A non destructive physical test (Bubble point test) is done to test the filter for its suitability for bacterial retention. In this test, the filter medium is wetted with a liquid and test gas pressure is slowly raised until a steady stream of bubble appear from a tube or hose attached to the blood stream pressure at which the bubble first appear is recorded as the bubble point.

Validation of water system for sterile products

Quality of water is important in the production of sterile products. Different qualities of water (which are used for different purposes) and their specifications should according to official standards. All water-treatment systems should be subject to planned maintenance, validation and monitoring.

In the validation of water system, water used in sterile product must be validated for engineering equipment, piping, valve filter, storage tank, carbon beds, deionizer and reverse osmosis (RO) units, ultraviolet lights, and heat sterilants, hoses and other attachment to the distribution piping.

The validation of the whole water system normally takes a year because of operation problems, equipment failure and engineering errors. Validation of water systems should consist of at least three phases:

Phase 1: investigational phase;

Phase 2: short-term control; and

Phase 3: long-term control.

During the period following phase 3 the objective should be to demonstrate that the system is under control over a long period of time. Sampling may be reduced from, e.g. daily to weekly.

The validation performed and revalidation requirements should be included in the "Water quality manual"

***Phase* 1:** A test period of 2-4 weeks should be spent monitoring the system intensively. During this period the system should operate continuously without failure or performance deviation. The following procedures should be included in the testing approach.
- Undertake chemical and microbiological testing in accordance with a defined plan.
- Sample the incoming feed-water to verify its quality.
- Sample after each step in the purification process daily.
- Sample at each point of use and at other defined sampling points daily.
- Develop appropriate operating ranges.
- Develop and finalize operating, cleaning, sanitizing and maintenance procedures.
- Demonstrate production and delivery of product water of the required quality and quantity.
- Use and refine the standard operating procedures (SOPs) for operation, maintenance, sanitization and troubleshooting.
- Verify provisional alert and action levels.
- Develop and refine the test-failure procedure.

***Phase* 2:** A further test period of 2-4 weeks should be spent carrying out further intensive monitoring while deploying all the refined SOPs after the satisfactory completion of phase 1. The sampling scheme should be generally the same as in phase 1. Water can be used for manufacturing purposes during this phase. The approach should also:
- demonstrate consistent operation within established ranges; and
- demonstrate consistent production and delivery of water of the required quantity and quality when the system is operated in accordance with the SOPs.

***Phase* 3:** Phase 3 typically runs for one year after the satisfactory completion of phase 2. Water can be used for manufacturing purposes during this phase which has the following objectives and features:
- Demonstrate extended reliable performance.
- Ensure that seasonal variations are evaluated.
- The sample locations, sampling frequencies and tests should be reduced to the normal routine pattern based on established procedures proven during phases 1 and 2.

Cleaning validation

Documented evidence to establish that cleaning procedures are removing residues to predetermined levels of acceptability, taking into consideration factors such as batch size, dosing, toxicology and equipment size.

- *(WHO Technical Report Series, No. 937, 2006)*

Cleaning validation plays the most important role in the validation of the sterile area. The objective of cleaning validation is to prove that the equipment is consistently cleaned of product, detergent and microbial residues to an acceptable level, to prevent possible contamination and cross-contamination. It is considered that the cleaning procedure consistently reduce the contaminant. The various sampling methods used for the evaluation are following:

(i) Direct surface sampling (direct method) or Swab sample collected after cleaning. It involves taking an inert material (e.g. cotton wool) on the end of a probe (referred to as a "swab") and rubbing it methodically across a surface. The type of sampling material used and its potential impact on the test data is important as the sampling material may interfere with the test.

(ii) Rinse sample (indirect method) for residual active ingredient is commonly used method to evaluate cleanliness. This method allows sampling of a large surface, of areas that are inaccessible or that cannot be routinely disassembled and provides an overall picture. Rinse samples may give sufficient evidence of adequate cleaning where accessibility of equipment parts can preclude direct surface sampling, and may be useful for checking for residues of cleaning agents, e.g. detergents.

Rinse samples should be used in combination with other sampling methods such as surface sampling.

(iii) Batch Placebo sample provide the best simulation of actual production of batch of product. This method relies on the manufacture of a placebo batch which is then checked for carry-over of the previous product. It is an expensive and laborious process. It is difficult to provide assurance that the contaminants will be dislodged from the equipment surface uniformly. Additionally, if the particles of the contaminant or residue are large enough, they may not be uniformly dispersed in the placebo batch.

The batch placebo method should be used in conjunction with rinse and/or surface sampling method(s). Samples should be taken throughout the process of manufacture.

Heating, ventilation and air conditioning (HVAC) system validations

Heating, ventilation and air conditioning (HVAC) systems are used for filtering air under positive pressure for maintaining desired environmental control in the manufacturing areas. HVAC system plays an important role in the protection of the product, the personnel and the environment.

For all HVAC installation components, subsystems or parameters, critical parameters and non-critical parameters should be determined. Some of the parameters of a typical HVAC system that should be qualified include:

- room temperature and humidity;
- supply air and return air quantities;
- room pressure, air change rate, flow patterns, particle count and cleanup rates
- unidirectional flow velocities and HEPA filter penetration tests(by D.O.P. (dioctyl phthalate) method; discussed in Chapter 10).

Machine validation: (filling, sealing, capping)

(i) The efficiency of any machine can be checked by the quality of the product. Whatever involved in it, like that in sterile area by the quality of the vial capping one can be predict, the machine functionality i.e. leakage test, system integrity test, closure displacement test,

(ii) The ampoule leaking can be calculated by the vacuum dry leak test, autoclave dye process, and electronic test.

Revalidation

Repeated validation of an approved process (or a part thereof) to ensure continued compliance with established requirements is termed as revalidation.

A revalidation of process validation must be done whenever there is a change in formulation equipment or process which could have impact on product effectiveness or product characteristics.

Bibliography

- Committee on Specifications for Pharmaceutical Preparations. Good Manufacturing Practices for Pharmaceutical Products. WHO Technical Report Series no. 82. Geneva: World Health Organization, 1992, pp 14-79.
- Cleaning Validation Guidelines. Ottawa, Canada: Health Products and Food Branch Inspectorate, Health Canada, May 2000, p 11.
- Chapman GM, Amer G, Boyce C, Brower G, Green C, Hall WE, Harpaz D, Mullendore B. Proposed Validation Standard VS1: Non-aseptic Pharmaceutical Processes. J Val Technol 2000; 6:502-20.
- Fetterolf DM. Developing a sound process validation strategy. Int. Biopharm. 207, 20,12, 38-46.
- Juran J.M. Section 2 Basic concept, In Quality control hand book, 3rd ed. Juran J.M., Gryna F.M.Jr, and Bingham, R.S. Jr (eds) McGraw-Hill, New York 1974.
- Guide to Inspections of Oral Solid Dosage Forms Pre/Post Approval Issued for Development and Validation. Washington DC: US Food and Drug Administration, 1994.
- Guide to Inspections Validation of Cleaning Processes. Washington DC: US Food and Drug Administration.
- Jatto E. and Okhamafe AO. *Trop J Pharm Res,* 2002, 1 (2) 115-122.
- Jenkins KM, Vanderwielen AJ. Pharm Technol 1994, 18(4), 60-74.
- WHO Expert Committee on Specifications for Pharmaceutical Preparations, WHO Technical Report Series, No. 937, 2006.
- *WHO good manufacturing practices: water for pharmaceutical use.* Geneva, World Health Organization 2005 (WHO Technical Report Series, No. 929)
- Silverman G.J.and Sinskey A.J. Sterilization by ionizing radiation. In Disinfection, Sterilization and Preservation,2nd ed. Block,S.S.(ed), Lea & Febiger, Philadelphia 1977, 552.
- Shenoy K.R.P. *Indian J Pharm Edu* 2000, 34 (3) 129-30.
- United States Pharmacopoeia and the National Formulary XXIII, 18th ed,. Rockville, MD: The United States Pharmacopoeia Convention Inc.,1995, pp 1982 – 1984.

CHAPTER 12

Stability Studies

Introduction

The aim of the development of a drug dosage form is to formulate a safe, effective and stable formulation (or a good quality product). The quality of a medicinal product is determined by its content of active substance(s), its purity (limitation or absence of decomposition products of the active substance(s)) and its organoleptic, physico-chemical and microbiological properties.

Purpose of Stability Tests

- To obtain information for estimation of the shelf-life of the medicinal product.
- To recommend storage conditions.
- To ascertain how the quality of a medicinal product varies as a function of time and under the influence of a variety of environmental factors.

- To ensure the safety to patients
- To fulfill the relevant legal requirements concerned with the identity, strength, purity and quality of the drug.
- To prevent the economic consequences of marketing an unstable product. (The sale of such a product is hardly the best advertisement for a manufacturer, and subsequent withdrawal and reformulation of the drug may lead to considerable financial loss.)

On the basis of the information thus obtained, storage conditions are recommended (the purpose of these studies is to produce recommendations) which will guarantee maintenance of the quality of the medicinal product, in relation to its safety, efficacy and acceptability, throughout the proposed shelf-life (i.e. during storage, distribution, dispensing and use). The design of the finished product stability studies for a medicinal product is based on the knowledge obtained from the studies on the active substance and from the Development Pharmaceutics studies.

Pharmaceutical products are degraded by various processes or methods (Chemical and physical degradation). The various modes of chemical degradation include hydrolysis, oxidation, isomerization, polymerization and decarboxylation. These chemical degradations are influenced by various physical factors like temperature, moisture, light and radiation.

Chemical Kinetics and Decomposition of Pharmaceutical Products

Chemical kinetics is defined as the study of the rate of chemical degradation or change and the factors affecting the rate of reactions such as concentration of reactants, temperature, composition of solvent system and the presence of catalysts.

Rates of Reaction

The rate of a reaction or process is defined as the velocity at which it proceeds and can be described as either *zero-order* or *first-order*.

Zero-order Reaction

If the loss of drug is independent of the concentration of the reactants and remains constant with respect to time, the rate is called Zero order.

$$\text{Rate} = K_0 C^0$$

Consider the rate of decomposition of drug 'A' changing into a product 'B', through a step in which it is get converted into liquid from the solid phase. If the amount of the drug Co, is decreasing at a constant rate, then the rate of elimination of A can be described as:

$$\frac{-dCo}{dt} = ko$$

where Ko = the zero-order rate constant.

The reaction proceeds at a constant rate and is independent of the concentration of A present in the body. The equation of zero order degradation reaction can be expressed as.

$$C_t = - K_o t + C_o$$

Where, C_t = remaining concentration.

C_0 = initial concentration.

t = time.

Unit of K_o = $(C_t - C_o)/t$

= conc. /time

= (mole/liter)/min

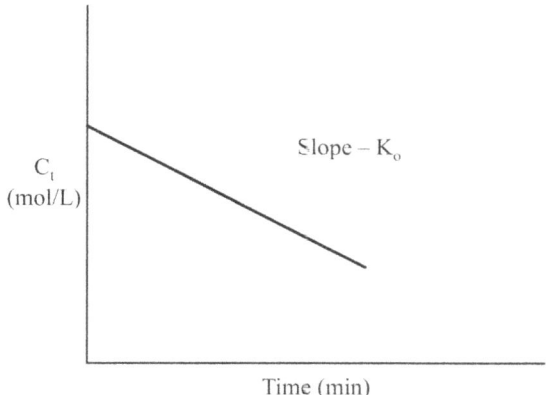

Fig. 12.1 Plot of zero order reaction rate.

Therefore, for a reaction following the zero order, the graph plotted between amount reacting and time (Fig. 12.1) should be linear with a positive slope (representing the rate of reaction (Ko)

Half life $t_{1/2}$ (t_{50})

It is the time required for decomposition of 50% of the initial concentration.

$$t_{1/2} = 0.5 C_o / K_o$$

Shelf life t_{90}

It is the time required to decompose 10% of the initial amount (i.e. drug potency = 90%).

$$t_{90\%} = 0.1 C_o / K_o$$

Example of Zero Order Reaction

Suspension is a case of zero order kinetics in which the concentration in solution depends on the drug solubility. As the drug decomposes in the solution more drug is released from the suspended particles so that the concentration remains constant. This concentration is of course, the drug equilibrium solubility in a particular solvent at a particular temperature. The important point is that the amount of drug in solution remains constant despite its decomposition with time, the reservoir of solid drug in suspension is responsible for this constancy.

Another example is the elimination of alcohol. Drugs that show this type of elimination will show accumulation of plasma levels of the drug and hence nonlinear pharmacokinetics.

First Order Reaction

A reaction is referred to be of first order, if the reaction rate depends on the first power of a single reactant.

If the amount of drug A is decreasing at a rate that is proportional to *A*, the amount of drug C_t remaining in the body, then the rate of degradation reaction of drug A can be described as:

$$\text{Rate} = K \cdot C_t$$

The drug is directly decomposed into one or more of the reacting substance in this type of reaction. Rate of concentration decrease may be expressed as:

$$\frac{-dc}{dt} = KCo$$

where K = the first-order rate constant.

The reaction proceeds at a rate that is dependent on the concentration of A present in the body. It is assumed that the processes of ADME follow first-order reactions and most drugs are eliminated in this manner.

The integration of above equation provides the equation of first order degradation reaction:

$$LogCt = \log Co - \frac{k.t}{2.303}$$

Therefore, for a reaction following the first order reaction, the graph plotted between log of percent remaining amount and time should be linear with a negative slope (Fig. 12.2).

The slope represents the rate of reaction K, which can be expressed as:

$$k = (2.303/t) \times \log \frac{a}{a-x}$$

Where   a = Co or the initial concentration time t = 0

x = Amount of drug reacting in time t

a – x = Amount remaining after time t

Unit of K = Sec^{-1} or hr^{-1} or min^{-1}

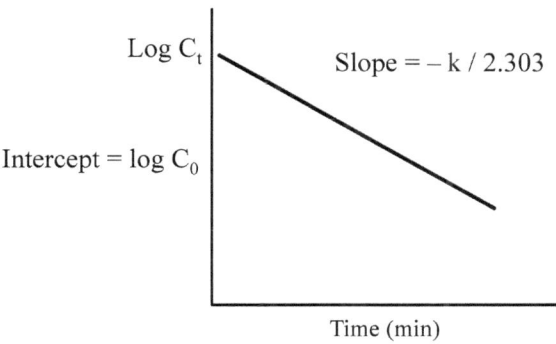

Fig. 12.2 Plot of first order reaction rate.

Half life

Half life of a drug is the time required for half of the drug to degrade. Half life can be expressed for drugs undergoing first order reaction, as followed:

$$t_{1/2} = (2.303/K) \times \log\frac{100}{50}$$

or $t_{1/2} = (2.303/K) \times \log 2$

or $t_{1/2} = 0.693/K$ (Independent of Co)

Shelf life

$$t_{90} = 0.105/K$$

Determination of the Reaction Order

1. **Substitution method**

    Substitute the values of Ct and the corresponding time t (at least 3 values) on the zero order equation Co = Ct – Kt
    - If you get a **constant value of K**, then the reaction is zero order.
    - If **not**, repeat the substitution for the **first order equation**:
      Log Ct = log Co – K t/2.303
    - If you get a **constant value of K**, the reaction is **1st order**,
    - If not repeat the using the **2nd order** equation and so on …

2. **Graphical method**

    Plot the remaining concentration Ct against time,
    - If you get a **straight-line** therefore the reaction is zero order.
    - If it gives a **curve** → plot log Ct against time.
    - If you get a straight line → the reaction is **1st order**.
    - If not try 2nd order plot and so on.

3. **t_{50} method**

    Carry out several experiments at least 3 and determine t_{50}
    - t_{50} increases by concentration → zero order
    - t_{50} decreases by concentration → 2nd order
    - t_{50} does not change by changing concentration → 1st order

Impact of Temperature on Process of Degradation

Process of degradation generally increases with the increase in temperature. As per a well experienced fact, the rate of a chemical reaction increases by a factor of between to three fold for every 10 °C rise in temperature. This may be understood by that fact that the reaction rates are proportional to the number of collisions per unit time. And the frequency of collisions increases with the increase of temperature.

Arrhenius studied the effect of temperature on the reaction rate constant (k) and expressed their relationship by the following equation (Arrhenius equation).

$$K = A\, e^{-Ea/RT}$$

Where A = a constant which is termed as the frequency factor

or $$\log K = \log A - \left(\frac{Ea}{2.303RT}\right)$$

Integrating the above equation between limits k_1 and k_2; and T_1 and T_2 the following equation is obtained.

$$\log \frac{K_2}{K_1} = -E_a / 2.303R \cdot \left(\frac{1}{T_2} - \frac{1}{T_1}\right)$$

or $$\log \frac{K_2}{K_1} = \frac{-E_a (T_2 - T_1)}{2.303R.T_1 T_2}$$

Where k_1 and k_2 are the reaction rate constant at temperature T_1 and T_2; Ea is the energy of activation (cal/mole): representing the minimum energy required by reacting molecule to undergo reaction; R is gas constant 1.987 (cal/mole. degree); T is absolute temperature (t °C + 273).

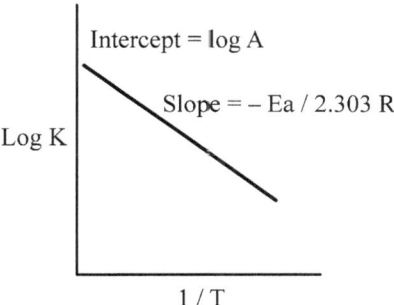

Fig. 12.3 Arrhenius plot.

Therefore, the common logarithms of the reaction rate constant at the various temperatures, plotted against the reciprocals of the absolute temperatures (1/T) will yield a straight line whose slope (negative) will be Ea/2.303R (Fig. 12.3).

Limitations of Arrhenius Equation
1. Arrhenius equation was based on the assumption that the reaction mechanism does not change as a function of temperature, i.e., Ea is independent of T, but this is not true practically for every case. Therefore, it may not be valid for some reactions, especially the complex reactions.
2. Higher temperature may evaporate solvents thus producing unequal moisture content at different temperatures.
3. At elevated temperatures, there is less relative humidity and oxygen solubility, which makes it difficult to predict the stability of drugs (which are sensitive to the presence of moisture and oxygen) at room temperature.
4. The viscosity of disperse systems is decreased at high temperatures, and thereby altering the physical characteristics.

Accelerated Stability Studies
These are the studies in which the performance or stability of the drug product is observed under accelerated conditions of degradation or high stress conditions (like elevated temperatures, high relative humidity etc.) and the reaction rates at elevated temperatures are extrapolated to that of normal room temperature's stability.

Stress testing of the drug substance can help identify the likely degradation products, which can in turn help establish the degradation pathways and the intrinsic stability of the molecule and validate the stability indicating power of the analytical procedures used. The nature of the stress testing will depend on the individual drug substance and the type of drug product involved. Arrhenius Equation forms the basis for the accelerated stability testing.

Stress testing is likely to be carried out on a single batch of the drug substance. It should include the effect of temperatures in 10°C increments (e.g., 50°C, 60°C, etc.) above that for accelerated testing), humidity (e.g., 75% RH or greater) where appropriate, oxidation, and photolysis on the drug substance. The testing should also evaluate the susceptibility of the drug substance to hydrolysis across a wide range of pH values when in solution or suspension. Photostability testing should be an integral part of stress testing. The standard conditions for photostability testing are described in ICH Q1B.

Objectives of Accelerated Stability Studies

The various kinds of accelerated stability studies are performed with the following objectives.

- **Establishing degradation pathways and developing and validating suitable analytical procedures.** However, it may not be necessary to examine specifically for certain degradation products if it has been demonstrated that they are not formed under accelerated or long term storage conditions.
- **Estimating/predicting the shelf life of the drug product:** Shelf life of a product may be predicted by accelerating the decomposition process and extrapolating to normal storage conditions. Shelf life may be predicted by various methods like direct use of Arrhenius equation, Q_{10} method, Free and Blyth method and Kennon method.
- **Rapid detection of deterioration in different formulations of same product:** This helps in selecting the best formulation of the same product.
- **Rapid means of QC:** This ensures that no unexpected change has occurred in stored product

Limitations of Accelerated Stability Studies

- It is not possible to predict the shelf life where product is to face fluctuating temperature in tropical regions.
- It is assumed that rate of reaction is not affected by increased temperatures but exceptions do exist e.g. suspension is a case of zero order kinetics but as the temperature increases solid turns into solution form and then first order degradation/reaction kinetics starts.
- Elevated temperatures may induce decomposition processes that are not otherwise present at normal storage conditions.
- For the products, which lose their physical integrity at higher temperatures, it holds no value or become meaningless e.g. breaking of emulsion, denaturation of proteins etc.
- Stability predictions at elevated temperatures are of little use when degradation is due to diffusion, microbial contamination, excessive agitation and photochemical reaction.

Shelf life Prediction

Accelerated stability testing is used to determine the shelf life at room temperature. Shelf life may be predicted by following methods.
- Application of Arrhenius equation
- Q_{10} method,
- Free and Blyth method
- Kennon method.

Application of Arrhenius equation

This method is based on accelerated stability testing for determining the shelf life at room temperature. The steps involved are as followed.

1. Determination of K value by plotting concentration versus time (according to the specified order) at different temperature.
2. The logarithms of the obtained rate constants are then plotted against the reciprocals of absolute temperature and the resulting line is extrapolated to room temperature (Fig. 12.4).
3. The obtained k value at 25 °C is a measure of the drug stability (t_{90} and t_{50}) under ordinary shelf conditions.

Drawing of Arrhenius plot

1. Draw in the upper 2/3 of the graph sheet, leaving the lower 1/3 empty.
2. X -axis is 1/ T × 1000 to enlarge the values.
3. Y -axis is Log K + I (integer) to make values positive.
4. Extrapolate the line, draw line from point of room temperature perpendicular to the line to get log K + I at room temperature.

Notes: Cut X -axis and never cut Y-axis.

If Log K + I = A , then Log K = A − I

K = anti log A-I.

Log A can not be computed from the graph since we cut X-axis (Log A = intercept at X = zero), only computed from the equation.

Slope = ΔY / ΔX /1000 (to return to original values)

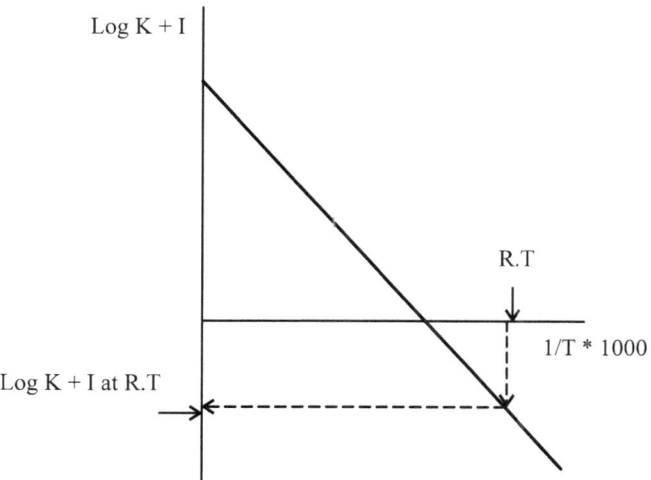

Fig. 12.4 Arrhenius plot in prediction of shelf life (from extrapolation of data obtained from accelerated studies).

Q_{10} method

The Q_{10} method is an approximate method based upon Ea (activation energy), which is independent of the order of reaction and is described as

$$Q_{10} = \exp[-Ea/R \{1/(T+10)-1/T\}]$$

Q_{10} is the ratio of different reaction rate constants and is the factor by which the rate constant increases with a 10 °C increase in temperature. Q_{10} may be defined as:

$$Q_{10} = K_{(T+10)} / K_T$$

Q values of 2, 3, 4 (with Ea values of 12.2, 19.4 and 24.5 Kcal/mol, respectively) are commonly used and related to Ea of reactions for temperatures ranging from 30-20 °C. Reasonable estimates can be made by Q value of 3 (Ea= 19.4 K cal/mol).

Steps involved in Q_{10} method

1. Calculate the Ea by studying variation in rate constant over a convenient temperature range. Determine the slope.

    Slope = Ea/2.303R

    or   Ea = Slope × 2.303R

2. If Ea is known, calculate Q_{10} value from the following equation

    $$Q_{10} = \exp[-Ea/R \{1/(T+10) - 1/T\}]$$

3. When Q_{10} value is known, shelf life (t_{90}) can be calculated by the following equation

$$t_{90}(T_2) = t_{90}(T_1) / Q_{10}^{\Delta T/10}$$

Where $t_{90}(T_2)$ = Shelf life at temperature T_2

$t_{90}(T_1)$ = Shelf life at temperature T_1

$\Delta T = T_2 - T_1$

Free and Blyth method

This method was coined on the names of scientist who developed it. The method includes the following steps.

- **Graph 1 (% residual drug Vs time in days)**: (A number of samples of similar drug in similar formulation is taken and each sample is subjected to high stress condition (generally of different elevated temperatures). At regular time intervals each sample is tested for drug content (amount of drug remaining/ present) accurately. Then a graph (Fig. 12.5) is plotted between % residual drug Vs time in days). Time for loss lines at several temperatures to reach 90 % of original potency is noted.

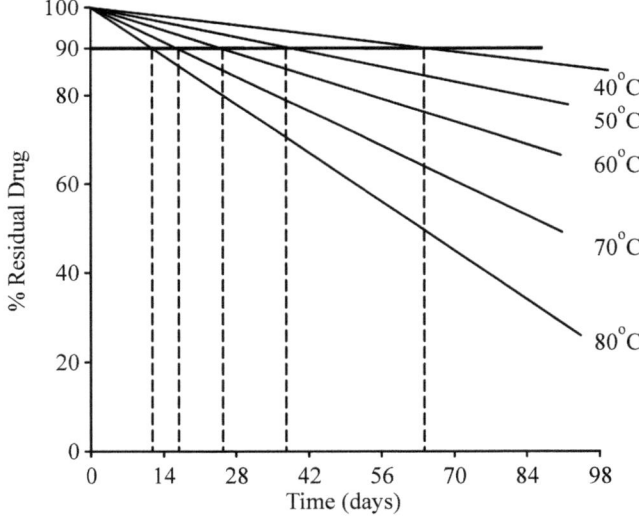

Fig. 12.5 Estimation of shelf life at elevated temperatures.
(For first order reaction)

- **Graph 2 (time V/S temperature):** Plot a graph (Fig. 12.6) between time values (log of days to 90 % potency) and temperature [reciprocal of absolute temperature (t °C + 273)]

- **Estimation of shelf life by extrapolation of Graph 2 to RT:** Extrapolate the time to room temperature (25 °C), time for 10 % loss of potency (shelf life) at room temperature can be obtained.

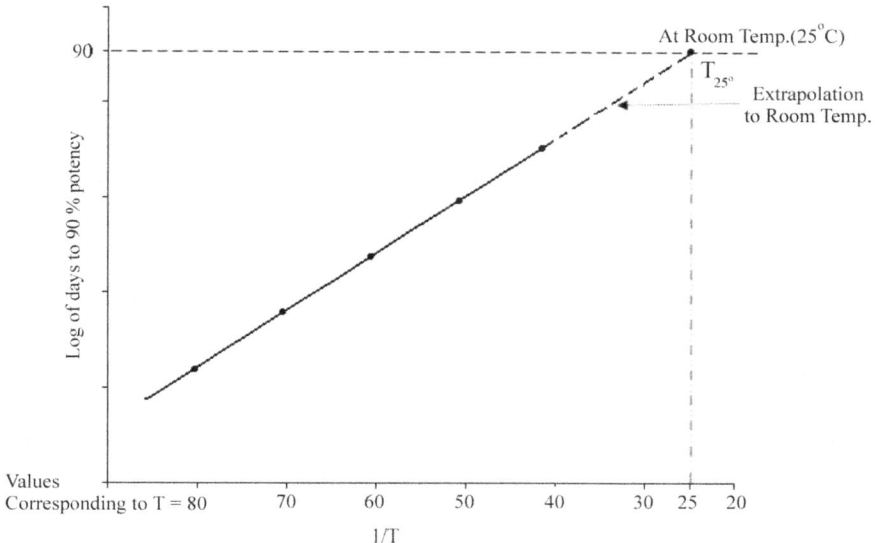

Fig. 12.6 Estimation of shelf life by extrapolation to Room Temperature (RT).

- **Graph 3 (% label claim Vs time in days) for Overage calculation :** If time ($t_{10\%}$) to reach 90 % potency at RT is too rapid to provide an adequate shelf life for the product, it is possible to determine the overages required for the product to maintain at least 90 % potency for prescribed time. This can be done by drawing loss line representative of 90 % potency value at RT (Fig. 12.7). Then a line (parallel to this) is drawn from desired shelf life to "Zero days". (It can be shown that by 10 % overages, shelf life of the product is almost doubled)

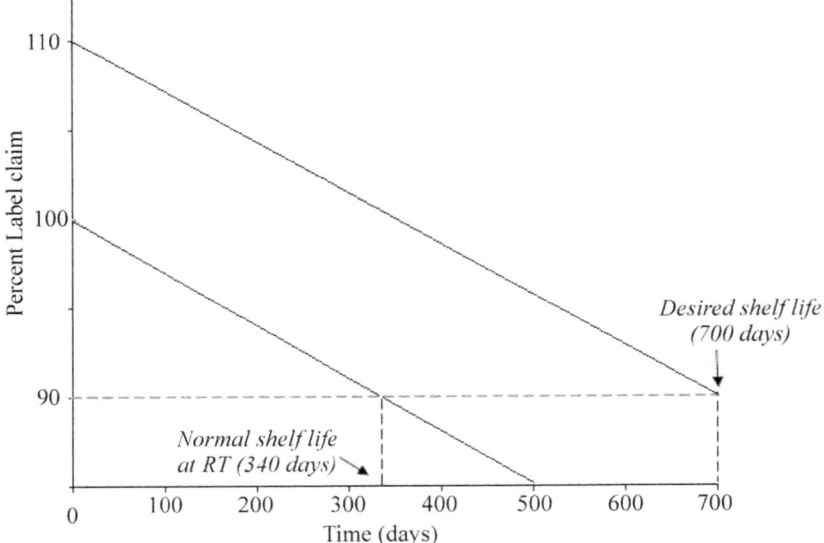

Fig. 12.7 Overage calculation.

Kennon method

Kennon studied the construction of certain kinetic path, which can be used for purposes of comparison during formulation development work.

Using standard kinetic equation Kennon calculated the path that reach or would be followed if 10 % loss in potency in 2 yrs at RT were permitted by chosing activation energy (Ea) of 10 and 20 Kcal/mol and by plotting time (months) to remain 90 % versus 1/T.

Table 12.1 Maximum and minimum time at which potency must be atleast 90 % of label claim at the temperature indicated in order to predict a shelf life of 2 yrs at RT.

Temperature (°C)	Maximum	Minimum
37	12 months	6.4 months
45	8.3 months	2.9 months
60	4.1 months	3 weeks
85	6 weeks	2.5 days

Steps involved are as followed

- Keep the formulations at specific temperatures for specific period of time as given in the table 12.1.
- If potency is above 90 % than there is a good assurance that formulation will meet requirement of 2 yrs' shelf life.
- If assay over 90 % at minimum time (Ea = 20 Kcal/mol) at respective temperature, it shows probability of having 90% potency after 2 yrs shelf life.
- If assay over 90 % at maximum time (Ea = 10 Kcal/mol) at respective temperature, it shows that product shall remain over 90% potency even after 2 yrs.

Accelerated Stability Studies with Physical Stress

The stability studies may also be done under physical stress conditions like e.g. cracking of emulsion, caking of suspension, crystal growth, change in crystal form, colour fading, colour development etc. As per the *Drug Stability Guidelines (2008) by USFDA,* the tests listed below, although not conclusive, should be considered as stability tests of the product (Table 12.2).

Table 12.2 Parameters of physical stability for finished pharmaceutical products

Dosage Forms	Specific Tests Indicated
Tablets	Hardness measurements
	Disintegration rate
	Dissolution rates, where appropriate
	Water content, microbial contamination
Capsules	Dissolution rates, where appropriate
	a. Soft-gelatin Inspection for leaks, pH, leakage, and pellicle formation.
	b. Hard-gelatin Visual Examination for brittleness
Suspensions	Viscosity, where appropriate
	Resuspendability
	Effects of freezing
	pH
Ointments, creams, gels and pastes	Homogeneity
	Viscosity, where appropriate
	Effects of freezing

Table 12.2 *contd...*

Dosage Forms	Specific Tests Indicated
Oral Powders	Completeness of solution/or dispersion
Powders for injections	Completeness of solution/or dispersion
Implants	Hardness Dissolution rate Friability
Injections	Sterility Syringeability, where appropriate Effects of freezing Multiple insertions/withdrawals pH Testing inverted container
Solutions	Sterility, where appropriate Effects of freezing pH
Emulsion	Globule size Cracking/ Phase separation, pH, viscosity
Aerosols	Delivered dose Particle size distribution Valve corrosion Spray pattern

Overages

Addition of an excess or overage of active ingredient for unstable drugs is required to cope with their declining potency. The International Pharmaceutical Federation (FIP) defined overages as *"the voluntary introduction of a specific excess during the manufacturer of pharmaceutical forms of medicaments that are unstable by nature and difficult to stabilize in order to maintain during their period of use, an active content within the limits compatible with therapeutic requirements."*

The overages are justified by FIP in following conditions:

- The liable active ingredient cannot possibly be standardized.
- The overages allow an even equilibrium of the constant active ingredient within the acceptable limits.

- The overages would not present a possibility of a therapeutic overdosage if the preparation were used during the early part of the products' shelf life.
- Clinically studies show that the overage is safe therapeutically.

FIP Guidelines on Overages

There are two types of overage recognized in EU guidelines: manufacturing overages (to allow for losses during manufacture) and stability overages (to allow for losses during the shelf life).

Manufacturing overages will not be reflected in the release or shelf life specifications - they should have been used during the manufacturing process, and the release specification should be nominal ± 5% unless otherwise justified.

Stability overages need to be justified by stability data. The amount of a stability overage will not be accepted if it represents a potential hazard from overdose of newly-made product or a toxic hazard (from the degradation products) at the end of shelf life. The release specification should be (nominal + overage) ± 5%.

The shelf life specification should be nominal ± 5% (or whatever variation can be justified by the stability data).

But overages should not be used to cover up imprecise or inaccurate analytical procedures or sub optimal manufacturing processes. The introduction of an overage of an active substance into a formulation should always be justified on the grounds of safety and efficacy of the product.

Bibliography

- Accelerated stability studies of widely used pharmaceutical substances under simulated tropical conditions. Geneva, World Health Organization, 1986 (WHO/PHARM/86.529).
- Guillaory JK, Poust RI, In; Banker GS, Rhodes CT (Eds). Modern Pharmaceutics. 2005 (Vol. 121) Marcel Dekker, Inc. New York, Basel, US, pp. 139-66.
- Lachman L, Hanna SA, Lin K, In; Lachman L, Lieberman HA, Kanig JL. Eds. The Theory and Practices of Industrial Pharmacy. 3rd Edn, 1986, Varghese Publishing House, Bombay, pp. 476-803.

- Rawlins EA, Bentley's Text book of pharmaceutics, Bailliere Tindall, London, pp. 140-70.
- Stability testing of active pharmaceutical ingredients and finished pharmaceutical products, WHO Technical Report Series, No. 953, 2009.
- Martin A. Physical Pharmacy, 4th Edn, 1993, BI Waverly, New Delhi, pp. 477-511.
- Pugh J. In: Aulton ME (Editor), Pharmaceutics: The science of dosage form design. 2nd Edn., 2002, Churchil Livingstone, New York, pp.101-12.
- USFDA, Guidance for Industry, Drug Stability Guidelines, 2008.
- WHO Expert Committee on Specifications for Pharmaceutical Preparations, WHO Technical Report Series, No. 937, 2006.

CHAPTER 13

ICH Guidelines on Stability

Introduction

In 1960s to 1970s, the pharma industry was opening up to global markets, but at that time also individual countries were only the registration authority for the registration of drugs. Each time when industry moves to market new products it has to repeat the time consuming process of evaluating the quality, safety and efficacy, and other detailed technical requirements as per different regulatory bodies of different countries. So, in order to reduce the cost of health, cost of R&D and the time delay in making safe and efficacious therapies, an urgent need to rationalize and harmonize regulation was felt.

When (in the 1980s) European Community or EC (now the European Union) moved towards the development of a single market for pharmaceuticals, the need of harmonization of regulatory requirements was felt among the various nations (US, EC, Japan China etc.).

In order to meet the objectives, at the WHO Conference of Drug Regulatory Authorities (ICDRA), in Paris, in 1989, the specific plans for action began to materialize. Soon afterwards, the authorities approached the International Federation of Pharmaceutical Manufacturers and

Associations (IFPMA) to discuss a joint regulatory-industry initiative on international harmonization, and ICH was conceived.

The birth of ICH took place at a meeting in April 1990, hosted by the EFPIA in Brussels. Representatives of the regulatory agencies and industry associations of Europe, Japan and the USA met, primarily, to plan an International Conference but the meeting also discussed the wider implications and terms of reference of ICH. The ICH Steering Committee which was established at that meeting has since met at least twice a year, with the location rotating between the three regions.

At the first Steering Committee (SC) meeting of ICH the *Terms of Reference* were agreed and it was decided that the Topics selected for harmonization would be divided into *Safety*, *Quality* and *Efficacy* to reflect the three criteria which are the basis for approving and authorising new medicinal products. It was also agreed that six-party Expert Working Groups (EWGs) should be set up to discuss scientific and technical aspects of each harmonization Topic. Eleven such Topics were selected for discussion at the First International Conference on Harmonization.

ICH

The complete name of ICH is the "International Conference on Harmonization of Technical Requirements for Registration of Pharmaceuticals for Human Use". ICH is a joint initiative involving both regulators and research-based industry representatives of the European Union, Japan and the USA in scientific and technical discussions of the testing procedures required to assess and ensure the safety, quality and efficacy of medicines.

ICH does not have "offices" as such because it is a voluntary cooperative effort of cosponsors from the three regions. The ICH Secretariat is based in Geneva. The biennial meetings and conferences of the ICH Steering Committee rotate between the EU, Japan, and the USA.

Purpose of ICH

The objective of ICH is to increase international harmonization of technical requirements to ensure that safe, effective, and high quality medicines are developed and registered in the most efficient and cost-effective manner. These activities have been undertaken to promote public health, prevent unnecessary duplication of clinical trials in humans, and minimize the use of animal testing without compromising safety and effectiveness

Goal of ICH

The goal of ICH is to promote international harmonization by bringing together representatives from the three ICH regions (EU, Japan and USA) to discuss and establish common guidelines.

Another goal of ICH is to make information available on ICH, ICH activities and ICH guidelines to any country or company that requests the information, and to promote a mutual understanding of regional initiatives in order to facilitate harmonization processes related to ICH guidelines regionally and globally, and to strengthen the capacity of drug regulatory authorities and industry to utilize them. The ICH Global Cooperation Group (GCG) was formed in 1999 and is charged with this task.

Members and Parties

ICH is comprised of representatives from six parties that represent the regulatory bodies and research-based industry in the European Union, Japan and the USA.

- In Japan, the members are the Ministry of Health, Labour and Welfare (MHLW), and the Japan Pharmaceutical Manufacturers Association (JPMA).
- In Europe, the members are the European Union (EU), and the European Federation of Pharmaceutical Industries and Associations (EFPIA).
- In the USA, the members are the Food and Drug Administration (FDA), and the Pharmaceutical Research and Manufacturers of America (PhRMA).
- Additional members include Observers from the World Health Organization (WHO), European Free Trade Association (EFTA), and Canada. The Observers represent non-ICH countries and regions.

The ICH Parties are the founding members of ICH and represent the regulatory bodies and research-based industry in the EU, US and Japan.

Products of ICH

ICH has developed over 50 harmonised guidelines aimed at eliminating duplication in the development and registration process, so that a single set of studies can be generated to demonstrate the quality, safety and efficacy of a new medicinal product. These guidelines also include the

Common Technical Document (CTD), which describes the common format for the preparation of a well-structured CTD for applications that will be submitted to regulatory authorities.

In addition, the ICH is working to facilitate international electronic communication through the provision of Electronic Standards for the Transfer of Regulatory Information (ESTRI) that will meet the requirements of the pharmaceutical companies and regulatory authorities. A product of this has been the Electronic Common Technical Document (eCTD), which allows for the electronic submission of the Common Technical Document (CTD) from applicant to regulator.

The Medical Dictionary for Regulatory Activities (MedDRA) Terminology has also been developed under the auspices of ICH.

Some important guidelines are as followed.

ICH Q1A(R2)	"Stability Testing of New Drug Substances and Products"
ICH Q1B:	"Photostability Testing of New Drug Substances and Products"
ICH Q1C:	"Stability Testing of New Dosage Forms"
ICH Q3A:	"Impurities in New Drug Substances"
ICH Q3B:	"Impurities in New Drug Products"
ICH Q5C:	"Stability Testing of Biotechnological/Biological Products"
ICH Q6A:	"Specifications: Test Procedures and Acceptance Criteria for New Drug Substances and New Drug Products: Chemical Substances"
ICH Q6B:	"Specifications: Test Procedures and Acceptance Criteria for New Drug Substances and New Drug Products: Biotechnological/Biological Products"

Applicability and Uses of ICH Guidelines

The ICH guidelines represent agreed-upon scientific guidance for meeting technical requirements for registration within the three ICH regions - EU, US and Japan. Each regulatory co-sponsor implements the guidelines according to its national/regional requirements. The ICH guidelines are not intended to be comprehensive guidance covering all aspects of product development and registration. They are intended to be used in combination with any regional requirements. An ICH guideline can be used by industry as a means of reducing testing duplication.

Industry and governments in ICH and non-ICH countries can use the ICH guidelines to address technical issues during the product development process. In addition to providing state-of-the-art guidance, the guidelines may well also serve as teaching tools. Harmonised ICH guidelines can reduce duplication in meeting technical requirements, thereby saving financial and material resources.

General Principles

The purpose of stability testing is to provide evidence on how the quality of a drug substance or drug product varies with time under the influence of a variety of environmental factors such as temperature, humidity, and light, and to establish a re-test period for the drug substance or a shelf life for the drug product and recommended storage conditions. The choice of test conditions defined in this guideline is based on an analysis of the effects of climatic conditions in the three regions of the EC, Japan and the United States. The mean kinetic temperature in any part of the world can be derived from climatic data, and the world can be divided into four climatic zones, I-IV.

Climatic Zone

The zones into which the world is divided based on the prevailing annual climatic conditions. Five climatic zones can be distinguished for the purpose of worldwide stability testing.

Table 13.1 Criteria of climatic zones

Climatic zone	Definition	Criteria Mean annual temperature measured in the open air/ mean annual partial water vapour pressure
Zone I	Temperate	≤ 15 °C / ≤ 11 hPa
Zone II	Sub-tropical with possible high humidity	> 15 to 22 °C / > 11 to 18 hPa
Zone III	Hot/dry	> 22 °C / ≤ 15 hPa
Zone IV a	Hot/humid	> 22 °C / > 15 to 27 hPa
Zone IV b	Hot/Very humid	> 22 °C / > 27 hPa

Stability Testing Conditions (Recent revision 2009 WHO)

The Secretariat reminded the Committee that the WHO guidelines had been revised in the light of harmonization efforts in collaboration with ICH. Subsequently focus had been placed within regional harmonization initiatives on the recommendations for hot and humid conditions (referred to as Zone IV). After extensive discussion the Committee reached consensus that the WHO stability guidelines be amended to reflect conditions for Zone IV as follows:

— Zone IVa (30 degrees Celsius and 65% relative humidity); and

— Zone IVb (30 degrees Celsius and 75% relative humidity).

It was agreed that each individual Member State within the former Zone IV would need to indicate whether its territory should be classified as Zone IVa or IVb.

Design of Stability Testing

The design of stability studies for the drug product should be based on the knowledge of properties and stability characteristics of drug substance(s). The design of the stability testing program needs to take into consideration the intended market and the climatic conditions of the area in which the drug products will be used.

A stability study is based on varying degrees of temperature, time, humidity, light intensity and partial vapour pressure, and their effects on the product in question. It should be pointed out that the effective or mean kinetic temperature reflects the actual situation more precisely than measured mean temperature, i.e. there is a difference between a product being kept for one month at 20 °C and one month at 40 °C, or two months at 30°C. Moreover, storage conditions often represent a higher temperature than the average meteorological data indicated for a country.

For some dosage forms, especially liquid and semi-solid dosage forms, the study design may also need to consider low temperatures, e.g. below zero – 10 °C to – 20 °C (freezer), freeze thaw cycles and temperatures between 2 °C to 8 °C (refrigerator). For certain preparations it is important to observe effects caused by their exposure to light.

Photostability testing (ICH Q1b) should be an essential part of the stability design. Photostability testing should be conducted on at least one primary batch of the drug product if appropriate.

Stability Testing Protocols

The protocol should contain an outline of the proposed plan to be used in generating stability data. The protocol should describe the type of product being tested, sampling process, duration and frequency of testing, number of samples and replicates per time interval, storage conditions (length of storage, type of storage, temperatures and packaging), methods of analysis (description or reference of published methods) with accompanying support data, if available, and other tests. The information listed in the ICH guidelines should be incorporated as appropriate in the development of a plan. These protocols are discussed as followed.

Selection of Batches

Data from formal stability studies should be provided on at least three primary batches of the drug substance. The batches should be manufactured to a minimum of pilot scale by the same synthetic route as production batches and using a method of manufacture and procedure that simulates the final process to be used for production batches. The overall quality of the batches of drug substance placed on formal stability studies should be representative of the quality of the material to be made on a production scale.

Container Closure System

The stability studies should be conducted on the drug substance packaged in a container closure system that is the same as or simulates the packaging proposed for storage and distribution.

Specifications

Specifications, which are a list of tests, references to analytical procedures, and proposed acceptance criteria, are addressed in ICH Guidance documents Q3A, Q6A and Q6B. Stability studies should include testing of those attributes of the drug substance that are susceptible to change during storage and are likely to influence quality, safety, and/or efficacy. The testing should cover, as appropriate, the physical, chemical, biological, and microbiological attributes. Validated stability-indicating analytical procedures should be applied. Whether and to what extent replication should be performed should depend on the results from validation studies.

Testing Frequency

Frequency of testing should be sufficient to establish the stability profile of the drug substance. The frequency of testing at the long-term storage condition should normally be every 3 months over the first year, every 6 months over the second year, and annually thereafter through the proposed retest period. At the accelerated storage condition for a 6-month study a minimum of three time points is recommended including the initial and final time points (e.g., 0, 3, and 6 months). Where an expectation (based on development experience) exists that the results from accelerated studies are likely to approach significant change criteria, increased testing should be conducted either by adding samples at the final time point or including a fourth time point in the study design.

Storage Conditions

In general, a drug substance should be evaluated under storage conditions (with appropriate tolerances) that test its thermal stability and, if applicable, its sensitivity to moisture. The storage conditions and the lengths of studies chosen should be sufficient to cover storage, shipment, and subsequent use (Table 13.2 to 13.6).

The long-term testing should cover a minimum of 12 months' duration on at least three primary batches at the time of submission and should be continued for a period of time sufficient to cover the proposed retest period. Additional data accumulated during the assessment period of the registration application should be submitted to the authorities if requested. Data from the accelerated storage condition can be used to evaluate the effect of short-term excursions outside the label storage conditions (such as might occur during shipping). Long-term and accelerated storage conditions for drug substances are detailed in the sections below. The general storage conditions should apply if the drug substance is not specifically covered by a subsequent section. Alternative storage conditions can be used if justified.

Table 13.2 General storage conditions

Study	Storage Condition	Minimum time period covered by data at submission
Long term*	25°C ± 2°C/60% RH ± 5% RH or 30°C ± 2°C/65% RH ± 5% RH	12 months
Intermediate**	30°C ± 2°C/65% RH ± 5% RH	6 months
Accelerated	40°C ± 2°C/75% RH ± 5% RH	6 months

*It is up to the applicant to decide whether long term stability studies are performed at 25 ± 2°C/60% RH ± 5% RH or 30°C ± 2°C/65% RH ± 5% RH.

**If 30°C ± 2°C/65% RH ± 5% RH is the long-term condition, there is no intermediate condition.

If long-term studies are conducted at 25°C ± 2°C/60% RH ± 5% RH and "significant change" occurs at any time during 6 months' testing at the accelerated storage condition, additional testing at the intermediate storage condition should be conducted and evaluated against significant change criteria (means failure to meet its specification). Testing at the intermediate storage condition should include all tests, unless otherwise justified. The initial application should include a minimum of 6 months' data from a 12-month study at the intermediate storage condition. WHO guideline (2009) recommends 30 °C /70% RH as confirmed long-term testing condition for India.

Table 13.3 Drug products packaged in semi-permeable containers

Study	Storage Condition	Minimum time period covered by data at submission
Long term*	25°C ± 2°C/40% RH ± 5% RH or 30°C ± 2°C/35% RH ± 5% RH	12 months
Intermediate**	30°C ± 2°C/65% RH ± 5% RH	6 months
Accelerated	40°C ± 2°C/not more than (NMT) 25% RH	6 months

*It is up to the applicant to decide whether long term stability studies are performed at 25 ± 2°C/40% RH ± 5% RH or 30°C ± 2°C/35% RH ± 5% RH.

**If 30°C ± 2°C/35% RH ± 5% RH is the long-term condition, there is no intermediate condition.

Table 13.4 Long-term testing conditions
(WHO Technical Report Series, No. 953, 2009)

Climatic zone	Temp. (^{0}C)	Relative Humidity (% RH)
Zone I	21	45
Zone II	25	60
Zone III	30	35
Zone IV a	30	65
Zone IV b	30	75

Table 13.5 Drug substances intended for storage in a refrigerator

Study	Storage condition	Minimum time period covered by data at submission
Long term	5°C ± 3°C	12 months
Accelerated	25°C ± 2°C/60% RH ± 5% RH	6 months

Data from refrigerated storage should be assessed according to the evaluation section of this guideline, except where explicitly noted below.

If significant change occurs between 3 and 6 months' testing at the accelerated storage condition, the proposed re-test period should be based on the real time data available at the long term storage condition.

If significant change occurs within the first 3 months' testing at the accelerated storage condition, a discussion should be provided to address the effect of short term excursions outside the label storage condition, e.g., during shipping or handling. This discussion can be supported, if appropriate, by further testing on a single batch of the drug substance for a period shorter than 3 months but with more frequent testing than usual. It is considered unnecessary to continue to test a drug substance through 6 months when a significant change has occurred within the first 3 months.

Table 13.6 Drug substances intended for storage in a freezer

Study	Storage condition	Minimum time period covered by data at submission
Long term	- 20°C ± 5°C	12 months

For drug substances intended for storage in a freezer, the re-test period should be based on the real time data obtained at the long term storage condition. In the absence of an accelerated storage condition for drug substances intended to be stored in a freezer, testing on a single batch at an elevated temperature (e.g., 5°C ± 3°C or 25°C ± 2°C) for an appropriate time period should be conducted to address the effect of short term excursions outside the proposed label storage condition, e.g., during shipping or handling.

Drug substances Intended for storage below – 20°C

Drug substances intended for storage below – 20°C should be treated on a case-by-case basis.

Evaluation

The purpose of the stability study is to establish, based on testing a minimum of three batches of the drug substance and evaluating the stability information (including, as appropriate, results of the physical, chemical, biological, and microbiological tests), a re-test period applicable to all future batches of the drug substance manufactured under similar circumstances. The degree of variability of individual batches affects the confidence that a future production batch will remain within specification throughout the assigned re-test period.

The data may show so little degradation and so little variability that it is apparent from looking at the data that the requested re-test period will be granted. Under these circumstances, it is normally unnecessary to go through the formal statistical analysis; providing a justification for the omission should be sufficient.

Statements/Labelling

A storage statement should be established for the labelling in accordance with relevant national/regional requirements. The statement should be based on the stability evaluation of the drug substance. Where applicable, specific instructions should be provided, particularly for drug substances that cannot tolerate freezing.

Recently in 2009, WHO recommended labelling statements for active pharmaceutical ingredients and for finished pharmaceutical products (FPPs) which are listed in Table 13.7.

Table 13.7 Recommended labelling statements for active pharmaceutical ingredients and finished pharmaceutical products *

Testing condition under which the stability of the API has been demonstrated	Recommended labelling statement
25 °C/60% RH (long-term) 40 °C/75% RH (accelerated)	"Do not store above 25 °C"
25 °C/60% RH (long-term) 30 °C/65% RH (intermediate, failure of accelerated)	"Do not store above 25 °C"
30 °C/65% RH (long-term) 40 °C/75% RH (accelerated)	"Do not store above 30 °C"
30 °C/75% RH (long-term) 40 °C/75% RH (accelerated)	"Do not store above 30 °C"
5 °C ± 3 °C	'Store in a refrigerator (2 °C to 8 °C)"
-20 °C ± 5 °C	"Store in freezer"

* Adapted from WHO Technical Report Series, No. 953, 2009

In principle, FPPs should be packed in containers that ensure stability and protect the FPP from deterioration. A storage statement should not be used to compensate for inadequate or inferior packaging. Additional labeling statements that could be used in cases where the result of the stability testing demonstrates limiting factors are listed in Table 13.8.

Table 13.8 Additional labelling statements for use where the result of the stability testing demonstrates limiting factors*

Limiting factors	Additional labelling statement, where relevant
FPPs that cannot tolerate refrigeration	"Do not refrigerate or freeze"
FPPs that cannot tolerate freezing	"Do not freeze"
Light-sensitive FPPs	"Protect from light"
FPPs that cannot tolerate excessive heat, e.g. suppositories	"Store and transport not above 30 °C"
Hygroscopic FPPs	"Store in dry condition"

* Adapted from WHO Technical Report Series, No. 953, 2009

Glossary

Some important definitions used in the guidelines are given as followed.

Accelerated testing

Studies designed to increase the rate of chemical degradation and/or physical change of a drug substance or drug product by using exaggerated storage conditions with the purpose of monitoring degradation reactions and predicting the shelf life under normal storage conditions. The design of accelerated studies may include elevated temperature, high or low humidity and intense light, low temperature and freezing/thaw cycling, as appropriate. Such test conditions are also applied to provide comparative evidence in short-term experiments of the equivalence of pharmaceutical products from various sources, such as those made by different manufacturers, processes, procedures, packaging, or where volumes and strengths of drug products are changed.

Data for these studies, in addition to long-term stability studies, can be used to assess longer-term chemical effects at non-accelerated conditions and to evaluate the effect of short-term excursions outside the label storage conditions such as that might occur during shipping. Results from accelerated testing studies are not always predictive of physical changes.

Climatic zones

The four zones in the world that are distinguished by their characteristic prevalent annual climatic conditions. This is based on the concept described by W. Grimm (*Drugs Made in Germany*, 28:196-202, 1985 and 29:39-47, 1986).

Dosage form

A pharmaceutical product type (e.g., tablet, capsule, solution, cream) that contains a drug substance generally, but not necessarily, in association with excipients.

Drug product

The dosage form in the final immediate packaging intended for marketing.

Drug Substance

The unformulated drug substance that may subsequently be formulated with excipients to produce the dosage form.

Expiration date

The date placed on the container label of a drug product designating the time prior to which a batch of the product is expected to remain within the approved shelf life specification if stored under defined conditions, and after which it must not be used.

Formal stability studies

Long term and accelerated (and intermediate) studies undertaken on primary and/or commitment batches according to a prescribed stability protocol to establish or confirm the re-test period of a drug substance or the shelf life of a drug product.

Intermediate testing

Studies conducted at 30°C/65% RH and designed to moderately increase the rate of chemical degradation or physical changes for a drug substance or drug product intended to be stored long term at 25°C.

Long term testing

Stability studies under the recommended storage condition for the re-test period or shelf life proposed (or approved) for labelling.

Mean kinetic temperature

A single derived temperature that, if maintained over a defined period of time, affords the same thermal challenge to a drug substance or drug product as would be experienced over a range of both higher and lower temperatures for an equivalent defined period. The mean kinetic temperature is higher than the arithmetic mean temperature and takes into account the Arrhenius equation. (When establishing the mean kinetic temperature for a defined period, the formula of J. D. Haynes (*J. Pharm. Sci.*, 60:927-929, 1971) can be used.)

Shelf life (also referred to as expiration dating period)

The time period during which a drug product is expected to remain within the approved shelf life specification, provided that it is stored under the conditions defined on the container label.

Stability Study Protocol

The detailed plan applied to generate and analyze acceptable stability data in support of the shelf life. It may also be used in developing similar data to support an extension to the shelf life.

Stability Tests

Stability tests are series of tests designed to obtain information on the stability of a drug substance or drug product in order to define its shelf life and utilization period for the drug product under specified packaging and storage conditions.

Stress testing (drug substance)

Studies undertaken to elucidate the intrinsic stability of the drug substance. Such testing is part of the development strategy and is normally carried out under more severe conditions than those used for accelerated testing.

Stress testing (drug product)

Studies undertaken to assess the effect of severe conditions on the drug product. Such studies include photostability testing (see ICH Q1B) and specific testing on certain products, (e.g., metered dose inhalers, creams, emulsions, refrigerated aqueous liquid products).

Bibliography

- Accelerated stability studies of widely used pharmaceutical substances under simulated tropical conditions. Geneva, World Health Organization, 1986 (WHO/PHARM/86.529).
- International Conference on Harmonisation. ICH Q1A (R2): Stability testing of new drug substances and products.
- International Conference on Harmonisation. ICH Q1B: Photostability testing of new drug substances and products.
- International Conference on Harmonisation. ICH Q1C: Stability testing of new dosage forms.
- International Conference on Harmonisation. ICH Q1D: Bracketing and matrixing designs for stability testing of new drug substances and products.
- International Conference on Harmonisation. ICH Q1E: Evaluation for stability data.
- International Conference on Harmonisation. ICH Q2R1): Validation of analytical procedures: text and methodology.
- International Conference on Harmonisation. ICH Q3A: Impurities in new drug substances.
- International Conference on Harmonisation. ICH Q3B: Impurities in new drug products.
- International Conference on Harmonisation. ICH Q5C: Stability testing of biotechnological /biological products.
- International Conference on Harmonisation. ICH Q6A: Specifications: Test procedures and acceptance criteria for new drug substances and new drug products: Chemical substances.
- International Conference on Harmonisation. ICH Q6B: Specifications: Test procedures and acceptance criteria for biotechnological/biological products.
- Stability testing of active pharmaceutical ingredients and finished pharmaceutical products, WHO Technical Report Series, No. 953, 2009.
- http://www.ich.org

APPENDIX

GLOSSARY

Antiadherent: The antiadherents stop the powder from sticking to the equipment as the tablet is being made. Example: Talc, Magnesium stearate, Starch derivatives.

Aromatic waters are clear, saturated aqueous solutions (unless otherwise specified) of volatile oils or other aromatic or volatile substances. Their odors and tastes are similar, respectively, to those of the drugs or volatile substances from which they are prepared, and they are free from empyreumatic and other foreign odors. Aromatic waters may be prepared by distillation or solution of the aromatic substance, with or without the use of a dispersing agent. (USP)

Pharmaceutical aerosols are products that are packaged under pressure and contain therapeutically active ingredients that are released upon activation of an appropriate valve system. They are intended for topical application to the skin as well as local application into the nose (nasal aerosols), mouth (lingual aerosols), or lungs (inhalation aerosols). These products may be fitted with valves enabling either continuous or metered-dose delivery; hence, the terms "Metered Topical Aerosols," "Metered Nasal Aerosols," etc. (USP)

Bioavailability is defined in § 320.1 of US FDA guidelines for industry as: the rate and extent to which the active ingredient or active moiety is absorbed from a drug product and becomes available at the site of action. For drug products that are not intended to be absorbed into the bloodstream, bioavailability may be assessed by measurements intended to reflect the rate and extent to which the active ingredient or active moiety becomes available at the site of action. (US FDA)

Biopharmaceutics is the study of the interrelationship of the physicochemical properties of the active pharmaceutical ingredient (API), and its pharmacokinetic and pharmacodynamic behavior.

Biopharmaceutical Classification System (BCS), is a drug development tool that allows estimation of the contribution of three fundamental factors including dissolution, solubility and intestinal permeability, which govern the rate and extent of drug absorption from solid oral dosage forms.

Bioequivalence is defined in as "the absence of a significant difference in the rate and extent to which the active ingredient or active moiety in pharmaceutical equivalents or pharmaceutical alternatives becomes available at the site of drug action when administered at the same molar dose under similar conditions in an appropriately designed study."
-21CFR 320.1 (US FDA)

Bioequivalence of a drug product is achieved if its extent and rate of absorption are not statistically significantly different from those of the reference product when administered at the same molar dose. (CDSCO, India)

Pharmaceutical Equivalence: it means drug products that contain identical amounts of the identical active drug ingredient, i.e., the salt or ester of the same therapeutic moiety, in identical dosage forms, but not necessarily containing the same inactive ingredients. (CDSCO, India)

Drug products are considered **pharmaceutical equivalents** if they contain the same active ingredient(s), are of the same dosage form, route of administration and are identical in strength or concentration (e.g., chlordiazepoxide hydrochloride, 5 mg capsules). Pharmaceutically equivalent drug products are formulated to contain the same amount of active ingredient in the same dosage form and to meet the same or compendial or other applicable standards (i.e., strength, quality, purity, and identity), but they may differ in characteristics such as shape, scoring configuration, release mechanisms, packaging, excipients (including colors, flavors, preservatives), expiration time, and, within certain limits, labeling. -CDER 2004 (US FDA)

Therapeutic Equivalence: the drug products that contain the same active substance or therapeutic moiety, and clinically show the same efficacy and safety. (CDSCO, India)

Drug products are considered to be **therapeutic equivalents** only if they are pharmaceutical equivalents and if they can be expected to have the same clinical effect and safety profile when administered to patients under the conditions specified in the labeling. -CDER 2004 (US FDA)

Pharmaceutical Alternatives: drug products that contain identical therapeutic moiety or its precursor but not necessarily, in the same amount or dosage form or as the same salt or ester. (CDSCO, India)

Drug products are considered **pharmaceutical alternatives** if they contain the same therapeutic moiety, but are different salts, esters, or complexes of that moiety, or are different dosage forms or strengths (e.g., tetracycline hydrochloride, 250 mg capsules vs. tetracycline phosphate complex, 250 mg capsules; quinidine sulfate, 200 mg tablets vs. quinidine sulfate, 200 mg capsules). Data are generally not available for FDA to make the determination of tablet to capsule bioequivalence. Different dosage forms and strengths within a product line by a single manufacturer are thus pharmaceutical alternatives, as are extended release products when compared with immediate- or standard-release formulations of the same active ingredient. -CDER 2004 (US FDA)

Difference factor (f1) calculates the percent (%) difference between the two curves at each time point and is a measurement of the relative error between the two curves.

Similarity factor (f2) is a logarithmic reciprocal square root transformation of the sum of squared error and is a measurement of the similarity in the percent (%) dissolution between the two curves.

Capsules are solid dosage forms in which the drug or a mixture of drugs is enclosed in Hard Gelatin Capsule Shells, in soft, soluble shells of gelatin, or in hard or soft shells of any other suitable material, of various shapes and capacities. They usually contain a single dose of active ingredient(s) and are intended for oral administration. (IP)

Capsules are solid dosage forms in which the drug is enclosed within either a hard or soft soluble container or "shell." The shells are usually formed from gelatin; however, they also may be made from starch or other suitable substances. (USP)

Extended-release capsules are formulated in such manner as to make the contained medicament available over an extended period of time following ingestion. Expressions such as "prolonged-action," "repeat-action," and "sustained-release" have also been used to describe such dosage forms. However, the term "extended-release" is used for Pharmacopeial purposes and requirements for Drug release typically are specified in the individual monographs. (USP)

Chemical Equivalence: it indicates that two or more drug products contain the same labeled drug substance as an active ingredient in the same amount.

Cold: any temperature not exceeding 8° (46°F) is "cold." A "refrigerator" is a cold place in which the temperature is maintained thermostatically between 2° and 8° (36° and 46°F). (USP)

Cool: any temperature between 8° and 15° (46° and 59°F) is "cool." An article for which storage in a cool place is directed may, alternatively, be stored and distributed in a refrigerator, unless otherwise specified by the individual monograph. (USP)

Conventional-release dosage forms are preparations showing a release of the active substance(s) which is not deliberately modified by a special formulation design and/or manufacturing method. In the case of a solid dosage form, the dissolution profile of the active substance depends essentially on its intrinsic properties. Equivalent term: immediate-release dosage form. BP

Creams are homogeneous, semi-solid or viscous preparations that possess a relatively fluid consistency and are intended for external application to the skin or certain mucous membranes for protective, therapeutic or prophylactic purposes especially where an occlusive effect is not necessary. (IP)

Creams are semisolid dosage forms containing one or more drug substances dissolved or dispersed in a suitable base. This term has traditionally been applied to semisolids that possess a relatively fluid consistency formulated as either water-in-oil (e.g., Cold Cream) or oil-in-water (e.g., Fluocinolone Acetonide Cream) emulsions. However, more recently the term has been restricted to products consisting of oil-in-water emulsions or aqueous microcrystalline dispersions of long-chain fatty acids or alcohols that are water washable and more cosmetically and aesthetically acceptable. (USP)

Delayed release dosage forms: It is defined as the dosage form that releases a discrete portion or portions of drug at a time (or times) other than promptly after administration. e.g. Enteric coated tablets. (USP)

Disintegrant: Disintegrants, such as starch help the tablet to break down into small fragments, when it is ingested. This helps the medicine to dissolve and be taken up by the body so that it can act more quickly.

Dissolution is defined as the process by which a known amount of drug substance goes into solution per unit of time under standardized conditions.

Excessive heat means any temperature above 40° (104°F). (USP)

Ear Drops are aqueous or oily solutions or suspensions of one or more medicaments intended for instillation into the outer ear. (IP)

Elixirs are clear, flavoured Oral Liquids containing one or more active ingredients dissolved in a vehicle that usually contains a high proportion of Sucrose or a suitable polyhydric alcohol or alcohols and may also contain Ethanol (95 per cent) or a dilute Ethanol. (IP)

Emulsions are Liquids containing one or more active ingredients and are stabilised oil-in-water or water-in-oil dispersions, either or both phases of which may contain dissolved solids. (IP)

Emulsions are two-phase systems in which one liquid is dispersed throughout another liquid in the form of small droplets. Where oil is the dispersed phase and an aqueous solution is the continuous phase, the system is designated as an oil-in-water emulsion. Conversely, where water or an aqueous solution is the dispersed phase and oil or oleaginous material is the continuous phase, the system is designated as a water-in-oil emulsion. Emulsions are stabilized by emulsifying agents that prevent coalescence, the merging of small droplets into larger droplets and, ultimately, into a single separated phase. (USP)

The **expiration date** identifies the time during which the article may be expected to meet the requirements of the compendial monograph, provided it is kept under the prescribed storage conditions. The expiration date limits the time during which the article may be dispensed or used. Where an expiration date is stated only in terms of the month and the year, it is a representation that the intended expiration date is the last day of the stated month. (USP)

Extended-release dosage forms: It is defined as the one that allows at least a twofold reduction in the dosing frequency as compared to that of conventional (immediate release) dosage form. For example: controlled release or sustained release tablets. (USP)

Eye Ointments are sterile, semi-solid preparations of homogenous appearance intended for application to the eye. They may contain one or more medicaments dissolved or dispersed in a suitable basis. (IP)

Ophthalmic ointments are ointments for application to the eye. Special precautions must be taken in the preparation of ophthalmic ointments. They are manufactured from sterilized ingredients under rigidly aseptic conditions and meet the requirements under Sterility Tests. (USP)

Freezer indicates a place in which the temperature is maintained thermostatically between -25° and -10° (-13° and 14°F). (USP)

Gels are homogeneous, semi-solid preparations usually consisting of solutions or dispersions of one or more medicaments in suitable hydrophilic or hydrophobic bases. (IP)

Gels (sometimes called Jellies) are semisolid systems consisting of either suspensions made up of small inorganic particles or large organic molecules interpenetrated by a liquid. Where the gel mass consists of a network of small discrete particles, the gel is classified as a two-phase system (e.g., Aluminum Hydroxide Gel). (USP)

Glidant: The glidants improve the flowability of the tablet granules or powder by reducing the friction between particles, preventing formation of lumps e.g. Talc, Corn starch, Colloids silicates.

The biological **half-life** or terminal half-life of a substance is the time it takes for a drug to lose half of its pharmacologic, physiologic, or radiologic activity.

HLB (Hydrophile-Lipophile Balance) is an empirical expression for the relationship of the hydrophilic ("water-loving") and hydrophobic ("water-hating") groups of a surfactant. The HLB system is particularly useful to identify surfactants for oil and water emulsification.

Implants are sterile solid preparations of size and shape suitable for implantation into body tissues so as to release the active ingredient over an extended period of time. They are normally presented individually in sterile containers. (IP)

Implants or pellets are small sterile solid masses consisting of a highly purified drug (with or without excipients) made by compression or molding. They are intended for implantation in the body (usually subcutaneously) for the purpose of providing continuous release of the drug over long periods of time. Implants are administered by means of a suitable special injector or surgical incision. This dosage form has been used to administer hormones such as testosterone or estradiol. They are packaged individually in sterile vials or foil strips. (USP)

Inhalation Preparations are liquid or solid dosage forms intended for administration as vapours or aerosols to the lung in order to obtain a local or systemic effect. They contain solutions or dispersions of one or more active ingredients which may be dissolved or dispersed in a suitable vehicle. (IP)

Inhalations are drugs or solutions or suspensions of one or more drug substances administered by the nasal or oral respiratory route for local or systemic effect. (USP)

The term **injectability** refers to the properties of the suspension during injection; it includes factors as pressure or force required for injection, evenness of flow, aspiration qualities, and freedom from clogging.

Injections are sterile solutions, emulsions or suspensions. They are prepared by dissolving, emulsifying or suspending the active ingredient(s) and any added substances in Water for Injection or in a suitable non-aqueous vehicle, or in a mixture of the two if they are miscible. (IP)

An **Injection** is a preparation intended for parenteral administration or for constituting or diluting a parenteral article prior to administration. (USP)

Infusions are sterile aqueous solutions or emulsions with water as the continuous phase. They are free from pyrogens or bacterial endotoxins, are usually made isotonic with blood and do not contain any added antimicrobial preservatives. (IP)

Insulin preparations are sterile preparations of human Insulin, bovine Insulin or porcine Insulin intended for subcutaneous injection into the human or animal body. They are either solutions or suspensions or they are prepared by combining solutions and suspensions. They contain not less than 90.0 per cent and not more than the equivalent of 110.0 per cent of the amount of insulin stated on the label. (IP)

In Vitro In Vivo Correlation (IVIVC): The establishment of a rational relationship between a biological property, or a parameter derived from a biological property produced by a dosage form, and a physicochemical property or characteristic of the same dosage form. (USP)

IVIVC is a predictive mathematical model describing the relationship between an in vitro property of a dosage form and a relevant in vivo response. Generally, the in vitro property is the rate or extent of drug dissolution or release while the in vivo response is the plasma drug concentration or amount of drug absorbed. (US FDA)

Linctuses are viscous Oral Liquids containing one or more active ingredients dissolved in a vehicle that usually contains a high proportion of sucrose, other sugars or a suitable polyhydric alcohol or alcohols. Linctuses are intended for use in the treatment or relief of cough, and are sipped and swallowed slowly without the addition of water. (IP)

Lozenges are solid preparations, that are intended to dissolve or disintegrate slowly in the mouth. They contain one or more medicaments, usually in a flavored, sweetened base. They can be prepared by molding (gelatin and/or fused sucrose or sorbitol base) or by compression of sugar-based tablets. (USP)

Lubricant: Lubricants ensure that the tablet has a smooth surface. They reduce the friction occurs between the walls of the tablets and the walls of the die cavity when the tablet is ejected e.g. Talc, Steric acid, magnesium stearate.

Mixtures are Oral Liquids containing one or more active ingredients dissolved, suspended or dispersed in a suitable vehicle. Suspended solids may separate slowly on keeping but are easily redispersed on shaking. (IP)

Modified release dosage forms is defined as "one for which the drug release characteristics of time course and/or location are chosen to accomplish therapeutic objectives not offered by the conventional dosage forms. (USP)

Molarity: The molar concentration, M, of the solution is the number of moles of the solute contained in one L of solution. (USP)

Molality: The molal concentration, m, is the number of moles of the solute contained in one kilogram of solvent. (USP)

A **mole** equals one gram atomic weight or gram molecular weight of a substance. (USP)

Nanosuspensions can be defined as colloidal dispersions of nano-sized drug particles that are produced by a suitable method and stabilized by a suitable stabilizer.

Nasal Preparations are liquid, semi-solid or solid preparations containing one or more medicaments and are intended for administration to the nostrils for local or systemic effects. (IP)

Nernst potential: for an ion passing across a membrane, the potential at which the diffusion force on the ion balances the electrical force acting on it. An electrical potential occurring in connection with the Nernst equation or the Nernst effect.

Normality: The normal concentration, N, of a solution expresses the number of milliequivalents (mEq) of solute contained in 1 mL of solution or the number of equivalents (Eq, gram-equivalent weight) of solute contained in 1 L of solution. (USP)

Ointments are homogeneous, semi-solid preparations intended for external application to the skin or certain mucous membranes for emollient, protective, therapeutic or prophylactic purposes where a degree of occlusion is desired. They usually consist of solutions or dispersions of one or more medicaments in suitable bases. (IP)

Ointments are semisolid preparations intended for external application to the skin or mucous membranes. (USP)

Ophthalmic solutions are sterile solutions, essentially free from foreign particles, suitably compounded and packaged for instillation into the eye. Preparation of an ophthalmic solution requires careful consideration of such factors as the inherent toxicity of the drug itself, isotonicity value, the need for buffering agents, the need for a preservative (and, if needed, its selection), sterilization, and proper packaging. Similar considerations are also made for nasal and otic products. (USP)

The **osmolality** of a real solution corresponds to the molality of an ideal solution containing nondissociating solutes and is expressed in osmoles or milliosmoles per kilogram of solvent (Osmol per kg or mOsmol per kg, respectively), a unit that is similar to the molality of the solution.

Thus, osmolality is a measure of the osmotic pressure exerted by a real solution across a sem(IP)ermeable membrane. (USP)

Osmolarity of a solution is a theoretical quantity expressed in osmoles per L (Osmol per L) of a solution and is widely used in clinical practice because it expresses osmoles as a function of volume. Osmolarity cannot be measured but is calculated theoretically from the experimentally measured value of osmolality. (USP)

Ostwald ripening is the process whereby larger droplets grow at the expense of smaller ones, because of the transport of dispersed phase molecules from smaller to larger droplets through the intervening continuous phase.

Overages: addition of an excess or overage of active ingredient for unstable drugs is required to cope with their declining potency. The International Pharmaceutical Federation (FIP) defined overages as *"the voluntary introduction of a specific excess during the manufacturer of pharmaceutical forms of medicaments that are unstable by nature and difficult to stabilize in order to maintain during their period of use, an active content within the limits compatible with therapeutic requirements."*

Parenteral Preparations are sterile products intended for administration by injection, infusion or implantation into the body. They may be preparations intended for direct parenteral administration or they may be parenteral products for constituting or diluting prior to administration. (IP)

Parenteral articles are preparations intended for injection through the skin or other external boundary tissue, rather than through the alimentary canal, so that the active substances they contain are administered using gravity or force, directly into a blood vessel, organ, tissue, or lesion. (USP)

Pastes are semisolid dosage forms that contain one or more drug substances intended for topical application. One class is made from a single-phase aqueous gel (e.g., Carboxymethylcellulose Sodium Paste). The other class, the fatty pastes (e.g., Zinc Oxide Paste), consists of thick, stiff ointments that do not ordinarily flow at body temperature, and therefore serve as protective coatings over the areas to which they are applied. (USP)

Pessaries are solid preparations containing one or more active ingredients and are suitable for vaginal insertion. They are normally intended for use as a single dose. (IP)

pH: quantitative measure of the acidity or basicity of aqueous or other liquid solutions. The term, widely used in chemistry, biology, and agronomy, translates the values of the concentration of the hydrogen ion—which ordinarily ranges between about 1 and 10^{-14} gram-equivalents per litre—into numbers between 0 and 14.

Polymorphism: many compounds are capable of crystallizing in more than one type of crystal lattice. At any particular temperature and pressure, only one crystalline form (polymorph) is thermodynamically stable. Since the rate of phase transformation of a metastable polymorph to the stable one can be quite slow, it is not uncommon to find several polymorphs of crystalline pharmaceutical compounds existing under normal handling conditions. (USP)

Powders are finely divided powders that contain one or more medicaments with or without auxilliary substances including, where specified, flavouring and colouring agents. (IP)

Powders are intimate mixtures of dry, finely divided drugs and/or chemicals that may be intended for internal (Oral Powders) or external (Topical Powders) use. Because of their greater specific surface area, powders disperse and dissolve more readily than compacted dosage forms. (USP)

Powders for injection are sterile, solid substances (including freeze-dried materials) which are distributed in their final containers and which, when shaken with the prescribed volume of the appropriate sterile liquid, rapidly form clear and practically particle-free solutions or uniform suspensions. (IP)

Propellants provide the driving force to expel product from its container. Propellants provide dispersion medium.

Pulsatile-release dosage forms are modified-release dosage forms showing a sequential release of the active substance(s). Sequential release is achieved by a special formulation design and/or manufacturing method. BP

Shelf life is the period of time after manufacturing in which the active pharmaceutical ingredient is assured to meet applicable standards of identity, strength, quality, and purity. (USP)

Spirits are alcoholic or hydroalcoholic solutions of volatile substances prepared usually by simple solution or by admixture of the ingredients. Some spirits serve as flavoring agents while others have medicinal value. Reduction of the high alcoholic content of spirits by admixture with aqueous preparations often causes turbidity. (USP)

Solutions are liquid preparations that contain one or more chemical substances dissolved, i.e., molecularly dispersed, in a suitable solvent or mixture of mutually miscible solvents. Since molecules in solutions are uniformly dispersed, the use of solutions as dosage forms generally provides for the assurance of uniform dosage upon administration, and good accuracy when diluting or otherwise mixing solutions. (USP)

Standard Operating Procedures (SOPs) for pharmaceutical compounding are documents that describe how to perform routine and expected tasks in the compounding environment, including formulation development, purchasing, compounding, testing, maintenance, training, materials handling and storage, quality assurance, labeling, beyond-use dating, cleaning, safety, and dispensing. SOPs are itemized instructions that describe how a task will be performed, who will do it, why it is done, any limits, and what to do if a deviation occurs. (USP)

Suppositories are solid bodies of various weights and shapes, adapted for introduction into the rectal, vaginal, or urethral orifice of the human body. They usually melt, soften, or dissolve at body temperature. A suppository may act as a protectant or palliative to the local tissues at the point of introduction or as a carrier of therapeutic agents for systemic or local action. (USP)

Suspensions are Liquids containing one or more active ingredients suspended in a suitable vehicle. Suspended solids may slowly separate on keeping but are easily redispersed. (IP)

Suspensions are liquid preparations that consist of solid particles dispersed throughout a liquid phase in which the particles are not soluble. Dosage forms officially categorized as "Suspensions" are designated as such if they are not included in other more specific categories of suspensions, such as Oral Suspensions, Topical Suspensions, etc. (see these other categories). (USP)

Syringeability refers to the handling characteristics of a suspension while drawing it into and manipulating it in syringe. It includes characteristics such as case of withdrawal from the container into the syringe, clogging and foaming tendencies, and accuracy of dose measurement.

Syrups are viscous Oral Liquids that may contain one or more active ingredients in solution. The vehicle usually contains large amounts of Sucrose or other sugars to which certain polyhydric alcohols may be added to inhibit crystallisation or to modify solubilisation, taste and other vehicle properties. (IP)

Oral Solutions containing high concentrations of sucrose or other sugars traditionally have been designated as **Syrups**. A near-saturated solution of sucrose in purified water, for example, is known as Syrup or "Simple Syrup." Through common usage the term, syrup, also has been used to include any other liquid dosage form prepared in a sweet and viscid vehicle, including oral suspensions. (USP)

Tablets are solid dosage forms each containing a unit dose of one or more medicaments. They are intended for oral administration. (IP)

Tablets are solid dosage forms containing medicinal substances with or without suitable diluents. They may be classed, according to the method of manufacture, as compressed tablets or molded tablets. (USP)

Dispersible tablets are uncoated or film-coated tablets that produce a uniform dispersion in water and may contain permitted flavouring and sweetening agents. (IP)

Chewable tablets are formulated and manufactured so that they may be chewed, producing a pleasant tasting residue in the oral cavity that is easily swallowed and does not leave a bitter or unpleasant aftertaste. (USP)

Effervescent tablets are uncoated tablets generally containing acidic substances and either carbonates or bicarbonates which react rapidly in the presence of water to release carbon dioxide. They are intended to be dissolved or dispersed in water before administration. (IP)

Modified-release tablets (Sustained-release tablets) are coated or uncoated tablets containing auxiliary substances or prepared by procedures that, separately or together, are designed to modify the rate or the place at which the active ingredient is released. (IP)

Delayed-release tablets: Where the drug may be destroyed or inactivated by the gastric juice or where it may irritate the gastric mucosa, the use of "enteric" coatings is indicated. Such coatings are intended to delay the release of the medication until the tablet has passed through the stomach. The term "delayed-release" is used for Pharmacopeial purposes, and the individual monographs include tests and specifications for Drug release. (USP)

Extended-release tablets are formulated in such manner as to make the contained medicament available over an extended period of time following ingestion. Expressions such as "prolonged-action," "repeat-action," and "sustained-release" have also been used to describe such dosage forms. However, the term "extended-release" is used for Pharmacopeial purposes, and requirements for Drug release typically are specified in the individual monographs. (USP)

Enteric-coated tablets (Gastro-resistant tablets) are delayed release tablets that are intended to resist the gastric fluid but to release their active ingredient(s) in the intestinal fluid. (IP)

Prolonged-release tablets, also known as **sustained-release tablets** or **extended-release tablets** are tablets formulated in such a manner as to make the contained active ingredient available over an extended period of time after ingestion. (IP)

Transdermal drug delivery systems are self-contained, discrete dosage forms that, when applied to intact skin, are designed to deliver the drug(s) through the skin to the systemic circulation. Systems typically comprise an outer covering (barrier), a drug reservoir, which may have a rate-controlling membrane, a contact adhesive applied to some or all parts of the system and the system/skin interface, and a protective liner that is removed before applying the system. The activity of these systems is defined in terms of the release rate of the drug(s) from the system. The total duration of drug release from the system and the system surface area may also be stated. (USP)

Tinctures are alcoholic or hydroalcoholic solutions prepared from vegetable materials or from chemical substances. (USP)

Warm: any temperature between 30° and 40° (86° and 104°F) is "warm."

Zeta (ζ) Potential: the potential difference across phase boundaries between solids and liquids. It's a measure of the electrical charge of particles are that are suspended in liquid. Since zeta potential is not equal to the electric surface potential in a double layer or to the Stern potential, it is often the only value that can be used to describe double-layer properties of a colloidal dispersion. Zeta potential, also known as electrokinetic potential, is measured in millivolts (mV).

Lightning Source UK Ltd.
Milton Keynes UK
UKHW022015091221
395336UK00004B/205